Prostate Cancer

FOR

DUMMIES®

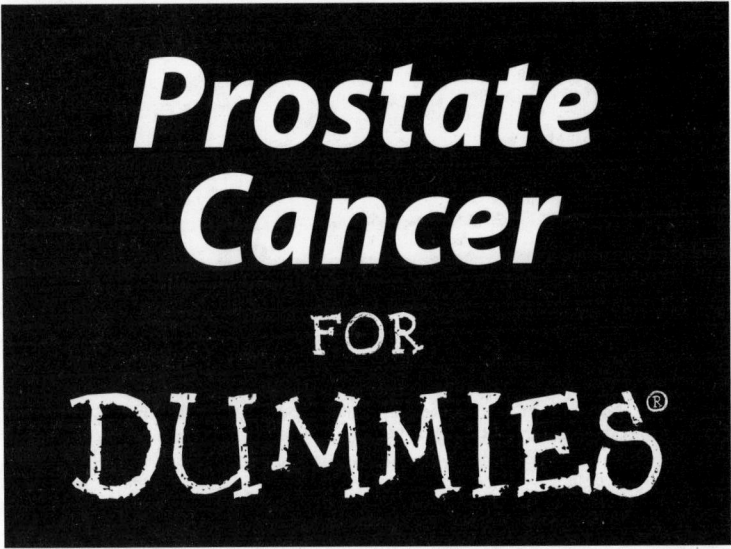

Prostate Cancer FOR DUMMIES®

by Paul H. Lange, MD,
with Christine Adamec

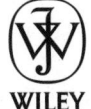

WILEY

Wiley Publishing, Inc.

616.99
LAN

Prostate Cancer For Dummies®

Published by
Wiley Publishing, Inc.
909 Third Avenue
New York, NY 10022
www.wiley.com

Copyright © 2003 by Wiley Publishing, Inc., Indianapolis, Indiana

Published by Wiley Publishing, Inc., Indianapolis, Indiana

Published simultaneously in Canada

For general information on our other products and services or to obtain technical support, please contact our Customer Care Department within the U.S. at 800-762-2974, outside the U.S. at 317-572-3993, or fax 317-572-4002.

Wiley also publishes its books in a variety of electronic formats. Some content that appears in print may not be available in electronic books.

Library of Congress Control Number: 2003101850

ISBN: 0-7645-1974-3

Manufactured in the United States of America

10 9 8 7 6 5 4 3 2

WILEY   is a trademark of Wiley Publishing, Inc.

About the Authors

Paul H. Lange, MD, a prostate cancer survivor himself, is an internationally renowned surgeon and a leader of cutting-edge research on urological malignancies, including prostate cancer. He is a medical school professor and chairman of the department of urology at the University of Washington in Seattle. Dr. Lange is also co-director of the Genitourinary Tumor Laboratory at the University of Washington.

Dr. Lange is the principal investigator of several large multi-disciplinary research grants on prostate cancer, including a prestigious SPORE (special programs in research excellence) grant from the National Institutes of Health. He is also the leader of an international clinical trial investigating whether radical prostatectomy or brachytherapy provides a better outcome for men with prostate cancer.

Dr. Lange has been on the editorial boards of many medical journals, including the *New England Journal of Medicine*, *Urology*, *Investigative Urology*, *Urologic Oncology*, and *Contemporary Urology*. He's a recipient of the Lattimer Medal from the American Urological Association for outstanding contributions to urology, and is a past president of the national Society of Urologic Oncology. Dr. Lange has authored or coauthored hundreds of articles in medical journals and several medical books on cancer, including prostate cancer.

Dr. Lange is a member of the American Urological Association, the American Association of Genitourinary Surgeons, the Society of Urologic Oncology, the American College of Surgeons, The American Society of Clinical Oncology, the American Association of Cancer Research, and the American Medical Association.

Christine Adamec is a freelance writer who has authored and coauthored 16 books, including *Fibromyalgia For Dummies* (Wiley Publishing) and *The Encyclopedia of Diabetes* (Facts On File, Inc.). Ms. Adamec is a member of the American Medical Writers Association, the American Society of Journalists & Authors, and the Authors Guild.

Dedication

Paul H. Lange, MD: This book is dedicated to my wife, Lucy Lange. Without her help and sacrifice, most of my career accomplishments would not have been possible.

Christine Adamec: This book is dedicated to my husband John Adamec, a prostate cancer survivor.

Authors' Acknowledgments

We want to acknowledge the assistance of Esther Gwinnell, MD, a psychiatrist in private practice in Portland, Oregon, and associate clinical professor of psychiatry at Oregon Health and Sciences University. In addition, we also thank Marie Mercer, reference librarian at the DeGroodt Public Library in Palm Bay, Florida, and Mary Jordan, interlibrary loan librarian at the Central Library Facility in Cocoa, Florida, for their research assistance. Thanks also to Alec Sohmer, Esq., an attorney from Brockton, Massachusetts, who assists people with Social Security disability claims.

Dr. Lange wishes to thank the following individuals for their expert advice on various sections in the book: William Ellis, MD, associate professor, department of urology, University of Washington in Seattle; Daniel Lin, MD, acting assistant professor, department of urology, University of Washington; R. Bruce Montgomery, MD, associate professor, department of medicine, division of oncology, University of Washington and VA Puget Sound HCS; Kenneth Russell, MD, professor, department of radiation oncology, Seattle Cancer Care Alliance; Paul Schellhammer, MD, professor of urology, Eastern Virginia Graduate School of Medicine, and and program director of the Virginia Prostate Center, Norfolk Virginia and Janet Stanford, PhD, research professor, department of epidemiology; Fred Hutchinson Cancer Research Center, Seattle, Washington.

We also want to thank Denise Chmela-Gerdon for her hard work during the days, evenings, and weekends that she devoted to helping manage this project, as well as for her continuous enthusiasm and support. Denise was integral to the successful completion of this book.

Publisher's Acknowledgments

We're proud of this book; please send us your comments through our Dummies online registration form located at www.dummies.com/register/.

Some of the people who helped bring this book to market include the following:

Acquisitions, Editorial, and Media Development

Senior Project Editor: Alissa D. Schwipps

Acquisitions Editor: Natasha Graf

Copy Editor: Greg Pearson

Acquisitions Coordinator: Holly Gastineau-Grimes

Technical Editor: J. Kellogg Parsons, MD

Editorial Manager: Jennifer Ehrlich

Editorial Assistant: Elizabeth Rea

Cover Photos: © Romilly Lockyer/ Getty Images/The Image Bank

Cartoons: Rich Tennant, www.the5thwave.com

Production

Project Coordinator: Maridee Ennis

Layout and Graphics: Amanda Carter, Jennifer Click, Seth Conley, Joyce Haughey, Stephanie Jumper, Michael Kruzil, LeAndra Johnson, Tiffany Muth, Shelley Norris, Barry Offringa, Janet Seib, Jeremey Unger

Special Art: Kathryn Born, medical illustrator

Proofreaders: John Tyler Connoley, John Greenough, Angel Perez, Carl William Pierce, Charles Spencer, TECHBOOKS Production Services

Indexer: TECHBOOKS Production Services

Publishing and Editorial for Consumer Dummies

Diane Graves Steele, Vice President and Publisher, Consumer Dummies

Joyce Pepple, Acquisitions Director, Consumer Dummies

Kristin A. Cocks, Product Development Director, Consumer Dummies

Michael Spring, Vice President and Publisher, Travel

Brice Gosnell, Publishing Director, Travel

Suzanne Jannetta, Editorial Director, Travel

Publishing for Technology Dummies

Andy Cummings, Vice President and Publisher, Dummies Technology/General User

Composition Services

Gerry Fahey, Vice President of Production Services

Debbie Stailey, Director of Composition Services

Contents at a Glance

Table of Contents

Introduction

• •

*H*earing that you have prostate cancer, or even that you *may* have it, is really very scary. I know this from both a professional and a personal point of view. I'm a medical professor and a clinical researcher, and I'm also a surgeon who specializes in treating prostate cancer. I see the fear in men's faces and hear it in their voices when they talk to me about their prostate cancer, and I've known for decades that this disease is very difficult for men to cope with.

And then it happened to me. A few years ago, I found out up close and personal how very hard it is to discover that you have prostate cancer. Even though I knew that I had an early stage of cancer that was curable and that I would be okay with few if any side effects, and even though I knew a great deal about the disease, it was still a major shock to me. I reacted in many of the ways that I've seen my patients react over the years: by continually worrying whether the treatment would work and if there was a better treatment option out there that I had somehow missed, and by wondering if I would be one of the rare ones who suffered significant complications from the treatment.

I had a prostatectomy. After I recovered, I resumed a demanding schedule of lecturing, performing surgery, doing clinical research, and writing books and medical journal articles. Now I want to share what I know about prostate cancer in the down-to-earth and understandable style of a *For Dummies* book.

You're no dummy, but you probably don't know a whole lot about prostate cancer. I can assure you that, in many cases, prostate cancer is a curable disease. But even if you have advanced cancer that's spread beyond the prostate, many treatments are available to help extend your life for years. You need good information to help you with the decisions that lie ahead, and my goal with this book is to provide you with this information. I believe that my perspective, as someone who treats prostate cancer and has personally experienced it himself, can help you.

About This Book

I have two primary goals with this book: first, to explain the key issues and problems that are associated with prostate cancer, and second, to assure you that, although the initial impact of being diagnosed with prostate cancer is devastating, you can take many actions to help extend your life. Read and then take the actions that best fit your particular situation so that you can live long and prosper.

You don't have to read this book from the first page straight on through to the end — although you can. You may want to read the first chapter to get a feel and flavor for the rest of the book. Then you can move to the chapters that affect you the most.

Conventions Used in This Book

To help you pick out information from a page, I use the following conventions throughout the text to make elements consistent and easy to understand:

- ✔ Any Web addresses appear in `mono font`.

- ✔ New terms appear in *italics* and are closely followed by an easy-to-understand definition.

- ✔ **Bold** highlights the action parts of numbered steps or keywords in bulleted lists.

- ✔ Sidebars, which look like text enclosed in a shaded gray box, consist of information that's interesting to know but not necessarily critical to your understanding of the chapter or section's topic.

Also, you may have noticed I use the singular pronoun *I* throughout the text, even though two names appear on the front cover. I do so because this book reflects my own views as a medical professional. However, Christine Adamec, an experienced medical writer, assisted me with the preparation and production of the book. Therefore, she's also credited on the cover.

Foolish Assumptions

In order to provide you with material to meet your unique personal needs, I make some basic assumptions. I assume that

- ✔ You have prostate cancer (or you think that you have it), or someone close to you has prostate cancer. Or you want to make sure that you or someone close to you doesn't have prostate cancer.

- ✔ You want information on treatments for prostate cancer as you form a treatment plan with your doctor. You may also be curious about alternative therapies.

- ✔ You want to know what actions you can take over the long-term to continue to fight your prostate cancer.

How This Book Is Organized

Prostate Cancer For Dummies is organized into seven major parts — the following sections explain what you find in each.

Part I: Prostate Cancer: What It Is and Is Not

In this part, I cover the realities of prostate cancer. You discover what the prostate gland is and does, and you find out about the few key symptoms of prostate cancer. I also include information on risk factors, who's most likely to have prostate cancer, and who's most likely to need annual screening and early screening — of course, you can still have prostate cancer even if you don't fit these categories. I also talk about other prostate diseases that often mimic prostate cancer by exhibiting symptoms similar but unrelated to prostate cancer, such as benign prostatic hyperplasia (BPH), prostatitis, and bladder infections.

Part II: Getting a Diagnosis

The chapters in this section walk you through the process of obtaining a diagnosis from your primary care physician and cover the key elements that should occur in your physical exam (such as the much-dreaded rectal exam, which is actually a very valuable test). I also cover the prostate specific antigen (PSA) test, a blood test used to screen for prostate cancer. The PSA test may also be used as a follow-up test for men who are diagnosed with prostate cancer.

You may also need to see specialists, such as urologists and oncologists (cancer doctors). I describe how to find the doctors who are right for your needs and let you know what questions you should ask them to make sure that they're the right doctors for you.

I also give you general information on key diagnostic tests, such as the bone scan, the ultrasound, and the cystoscopy. I devote an entire chapter to the *biopsy* (an analysis of extracted tissue), which is the definitive test for cancer. In addition, I explain how doctors stage and grade prostate cancer, and how the results help guide doctors in determining what therapies they need to recommend.

Part III: Getting to Wellness: Treating Prostate Cancer

In this part, I provide you with a general overview of various treatment options and discuss how you and your doctor can work together to come up with a plan to cope with your cancer. I include a chapter that discusses common fears associated with prostate cancer (including becoming impotent, developing incontinence, and losing your job) as well as the saving realities.

I also tell you what you can *do* about the cancer, whether it's *localized* (confined to the prostate gland) or more advanced. You're not helpless, and the situation is far from hopeless. I offer chapters on surgery, radiation therapy, hormone therapy, and other treatment options. I also include a chapter on such cutting-edge therapies as cryosurgery, microwave therapy, and genetic therapy.

Part IV: Changing Your Lifestyle to Combat Prostate Cancer

After you receive treatment for the cancer, you need to work on adopting a healthy lifestyle, which may decrease your risk of a recurrence of prostate cancer. . This part covers this topic in detail.

You don't have to dedicate your life to pumping iron, growing your own bean sprouts, or subsisting on berries. But you do need to take some practical steps toward a more healthy lifestyle, such as decreasing stress in your life (yes, even with prostate cancer looming over your head), eating right, and taking advantage of alternative preventive remedies that may help you. If you smoke or drink too much, I offer solutions for overcoming these habits and improving your odds for a healthy future.

Part V: Coping with the Aftermath Effects of Prostate Cancer

After your cancer is treated, you may experience serious side effects. The purpose of this part is to offer you practical coping suggestions. For example, sexual potency is extremely important to most men, and prostate surgery or radiation treatments may temporarily or even permanently curtail potency. A variety of effective options can help you cope with and overcome *erectile dysfunction* (problems getting and keeping erections).

Urinary problems (such as incontinence, blockage, or urinary irritability) are also possible side effects of treatment for prostate cancer. These urinary problems may be temporary or long-term. I cover the options available for dealing with these problems.

Many men who are treated for prostate cancer worry about the cancer coming back or moving to other parts of their body. I devote a chapter to this issue, including what to watch out for and what actions to take if you think you may have a recurrence of cancer.

Part VI: Handling Work and Family

You can't get away from it: Prostate cancer affects you at home and work. In this part, I discuss how to help others understand what you're going through, and how to tell them what you really need.

I discuss how to talk to your boss and co-workers about your condition. I also describe key federal and state laws that help protect you from being fired from your job when you're sick. In addition, I cover short-term and long-term work disabilities, and what you need to know if you must take a few weeks or more off from work while you recover. I also provide information on Social Security disability payments (if you aren't able to go back to work).

Family members may be terribly upset about your diagnosis, and it may be hard to help them with their fears and anxieties when you're feeling so distraught yourself. This section covers the basic emotional reactions your partner and family members may have, and tells what to say to them. I provide real-life examples of men who've been where you are, to help guide you through this tough time.

I also include a chapter for people who are very concerned about friends and relatives who have been diagnosed with prostate cancer. They love you and want to help, but maybe they just don't know what to do or say. I offer them some good suggestions to consider, so be sure to share this chapter with your loved ones.

Part VII: The Part of Tens

In this part, you can read about ten myths and realities of prostate cancer, ten must-do actions to take when you have prostate cancer, and ten ways to beat the blues.

At the back of the book, I provide two appendixes: a glossary of common terms that I use in the book and that you may hear from your doctor and an Internet resource guide of interesting Web sites that provide valuable resources and articles to read, as well as support groups that you can contact online. And, in case you're not a regular user of the Internet (or maybe you *never* use it), I include helpful organizations to contact by telephone or mail.

Icons Used in This Book

The icons in this book highlight things you need to pay special attention to when glancing through this book.

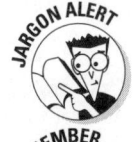

This icon marks paragraphs that define medical terms you're likely to hear around your doctor's office.

This icon points out essential information. Be sure that you not only read it but store it in your brain to recall later on.

When you see this icon, you can read about helpful hints for men with prostate cancer.

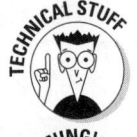

This icon marks information for those who want just a little bit more depth or detail on a particular subject. This information is interesting, but it's skippable if you want to stick to the basics.

This icon cautions you against things that can be potentially harmful.

Where to Go from Here

I know that it can be extremely hard to hear from your doctor that you or a loved one has prostate cancer. It was hard for me to hear my diagnosis, even though I'm a surgeon who has devoted much of my medical career to investigating and treating prostate cancer, and I knew that I was going to be cured. But after you recover from the initial shock of diagnosis, you need to educate yourself, and, with the help of your physician, make a plan for getting the best treatment possible. I hope *Prostate Cancer For Dummies* helps you achieve these goals and encourages you to maintain your commitment to managing your health.

Part I
Prostate Cancer: What It Is and Is Not

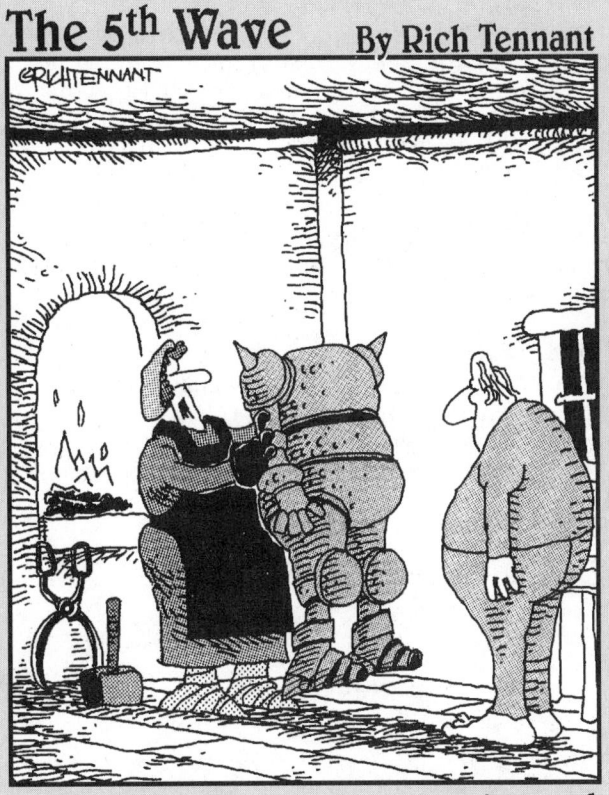

The 5th Wave   By Rich Tennant

"Okay, Sir Loungealot, I was able to pound out another inch in the waist, but you're gonna have to start taking care of yourself or buy a new suit of armor."

In this part . . .

Prostate cancer is no day at the beach, but it is treatable in most men when they talk to their physicians, educate themselves, consider the various forms of available treatment, decide what to do, and then do it.

If you're like most men, you rarely (or never) think about your prostate gland. Many men don't even know that they have a prostate. I provide basic information about the prostate and prostate cancer in Part I. In Chapter 1, I describe key aspects and symptoms of prostate cancer. (Most men with prostate cancer experience *no* symptoms.) In Chapter 2, I talk about the basic purpose and function of your prostate gland, including how it works when it's working right and how it can go wrong in you.

I tell you which men are most at risk for developing prostate cancer in Chapter 3. Keep in mind that even if you don't fit any of these risk categories, you can still develop prostate cancer. In Chapter 4, I talk about the symptoms of illnesses that sometimes may be confused with prostate cancer, such as bladder infections, benign prostatic hyperplasia (BPH), and prostatitis.

Chapter 1

Identifying Basic Realities of Prostate Cancer

*P*rostate cancer is a malignant tumor that starts in your prostate. Some prostate cancers are very slow-growing, causing you no trouble unless you live a very long time. On the other hand, quick-growing prostate cancers — and I think most of the ones picked up by doctors are this kind — can kill you if the cancer spreads beyond the prostate, if the cancer isn't diagnosed in time, or if you take no action after your diagnosis. However, you can often be cured of prostate cancer if the cancer is *localized* (or confined) to the prostate. I had surgery for my own localized prostate cancer in 1999. The surgery cured me, causing no side effects.

But even if a cure isn't possible, you can always be treated to at least temporarily shut down the cancer. Sure, you may experience side effects from treatment, just like you may end up with a scar from a wound your doctor sews up. But you're alive, and you likely have good prospects for many years ahead. So read this book, talk to your doctor, decide what to do about your cancer, and then do it.

In this chapter, I discuss what prostate cancer is, who's most at risk for developing the disease, what you can do about the disease, and how to handle the emotions you and your family may feel after a diagnosis of prostate cancer.

Understanding What Prostate Cancer Is and Who's at Risk

Any man can develop prostate cancer, but some men are at a greater risk for the disease. For example, if you haven't been diagnosed with prostate cancer, but your father, brother, or another male relative has (or has had) the disease, your risk for developing cancer increases, and you should have an annual screening for prostate cancer. Black men also have a higher risk for developing prostate cancer, although no one knows for sure why this is the case. Not to say that if you're not black, you don't have to worry about prostate cancer: All men are at risk for developing the disease. You can read more about the risks for developing prostate cancer in Chapter 3.

Prostate cancer isn't your fault. Experts really don't know what causes prostate cancer, so no one can blame you for making yourself sick. (And you shouldn't blame yourself, either.) At the same time, when you *know* that you have prostate cancer, you need to discover all you can about the disease and the treatment options. And then, with your doctor's help, you can select the best treatment for you.

Identifying Prostate Cancer Impostors

You may be experiencing some symptoms that may indicate prostate cancer, such as urinary frequency and urgency, or a poor urinary stream. Because men often don't experience any symptoms with prostate cancer, these same symptoms may indicate another illness altogether. The most common cancer impostors are

- **Benign prostatic hyperplasia (BPH):** The key word in BPH is *benign*. Benign is the opposite of cancer, and that has to be a good thing. However, BPH can be agonizingly painful for some men. BPH is a tissue overgrowth that can cause major pain and considerable trouble with urination. If you have symptoms of BPH, such as constantly having to urinate or having trouble urinating, you should see your doctor for treatment — which is often medication or sometimes surgery. Without treatment, BPH usually only gets worse, so don't try to ignore it.

- **Prostatitis:** This condition is characterized by inflammation and pain in the prostate. (When you find *-itis* at the end of a medical word, it usually refers to inflammation.) Prostatitis is sometimes caused by a bacterial infection that's treatable with antibiotics or other drugs. If you ignore the infection, it can spread to your bladder, kidneys, or other organs. See your doctor if you're having pain and trouble urinating.

- **Bladder infections:** As men age, they develop a greater risk for bladder infections. (This condition is also known as *cystitis,* another *-itis* word.) The symptoms of a bladder infection — difficulty with urination, for example — are similar to the symptoms that are characteristic of other *genitourinary* diseases (having to do with the kidney, bladder, prostate gland, penis, and testicles), including prostate cancer, BPH, and prostatitis.

If you have a bladder infection, you doctor usually prescribes antibiotics. Make sure that you take all the antibiotics your doctor orders. If you take your antibiotics for only two days when your doctor ordered medication for seven days, you only wipe out the weak germs. The stronger germs, which are still there, will continue to multiply. Bladder infections that are not treated properly can be dangerous, because the bacteria can spread to your kidneys.

Check out Chapter 4 for more detailed information on these medical problems, as well as on several others that may be confused with prostate cancer.

Working with Your Physicians

Working with physicians you trust is absolutely essential when you have prostate cancer. I say *physicians* plural because you usually deal with at least two different types: Your primary care physician, who usually performs your annual physical examinations, an important ritual that can help flag the early indicators of prostate cancer, and the specialist(s) who confirms and treats the cancer. You invariably need to see a *urologist* (an expert in treating diseases of the prostate, kidneys, bladder, and testes), but you may also need to work with urologic, radiation, or medical *oncologists* (physicians who specialize in treating cancer — some urologists subspecialize in treating cancers of the genitourinary system). See Chapter 6 for more about finding and working with specialists.

Discovering cancer

Your primary care physician may use several tests, including the rectal examination and the prostate specific antigen (PSA) blood test, to screen you for prostate cancer. (I describe the basics of the screening tests in Chapter 5.) If your primary care physician suspects you have prostate cancer, she recommends a biopsy. A pathologist analyzes the *biopsy* (excised tissue) of your prostate and determines, for sure, whether you have prostate cancer. Chapter 7 covers biopsies in great detail.

A self-test: Could you have prostate cancer?

Only a doctor can determine for sure whether you have prostate cancer. A self-test, such as the one I provide here, can give you *possible* indicators, at best. Keep in mind that in most cases, early prostate cancer has no symptoms whatsoever, which is why an annual physical examination and prostate specific antigen (PSA) blood test are so very important.

Get some scrap paper and jot down your answers to the following *yes* or *no* statements. Then read my analysis at the end of the list.

1. My father and/or brother has been diagnosed with prostate cancer.

2. I'm having trouble with urination. (You have trouble going or you have to go a lot. Or — Ouch! — you have both problems.)

3. I notice some blood in my urine.

4. I have constant, severe back pain.

5. I'm tired all the time.

6. I lose weight, even when I'm not trying to take off the pounds.

Now here's an analysis of your answers. If you answered yes to even one of these statements, you need to see your doctor.

✔ Question 1: If you answered yes to this question, you have an increased risk for developing prostate cancer. You should be diligent about having an annual physical exam, which includes a rectal exam (I know, I know, nobody likes this test, but it can save your life) and a PSA blood test, as well as a discussion with your doctor about your general health.

✔ Question 2: Trouble with urination may just be a sign of an infection or another

correctable problem. See your doctor so that he can zero in on the culprit. If you have prostate cancer, you need treatment. If you have a bladder infection, you also need treatment, because it may get worse.

✔ Question 3: If you see blood in your urine (doctors call it *hematuria*), don't panic, but do see your doctor right away. Having blood in your urine is *not* normal, and the cause needs to be investigated. It may be a sign of an infection, prostate cancer, or cancer of the urinary system. Your doctor can determine the source of the problem.

✔ Question 4: Back pain has numerous causes, ranging from infection to a pulled muscle to a disc problem (and on and on). Prostate cancer is another possible cause of back pain. Don't suffer in silence and wait for your severe back pain to magically disappear on its own. See your doctor and ask him to rule out prostate cancer, as well as other possible causes.

✔ Question 5: Being tired all the time is a possible sign of prostate cancer. Any cancer, especially if it spreads, can cause unexplained fatigue. Fatigue is also often caused by something other than cancer (such as depression from job stress), but you need to see your doctor to rule out any serious causes, including prostate cancer.

✔ Question 6: If you've lost weight (more than 10 or 15 pounds) without trying, and your weight continues to go down, this could be an indication of prostate cancer, or it could mean that you may have depression or another medical problem. See your doctor.

The next aspect of diagnosing prostate cancer, after its presence is confirmed, is determining how aggressively the cancer cells are growing and how much the cancer has spread. Doctors perform two types of cancer classifications when it comes to prostate cancer. First, they *grade* the cancer by checking your biopsy to see how different the cancer cells are from healthy cells and each other. Then they *stage* the cancer, mostly by using a system called *Tumor Node Metastasis (TNM)*. Doctors may also use special tests, such as CT scans, MRIs, or bone scans, to help stage the cancer. I cover grading and staging in much more detail in Chapter 8.

Planning your treatment

Deciding which treatment is best for you can be difficult. You must take several personal factors into account, including your general health (other than having prostate cancer), your life expectancy, and your race. With these and other factors in mind, you can work with your doctor to create both a short-term and long-term treatment plan. The short-term plan helps you cope with your cancer now (whether the cancer is localized or advanced), and the long-term plan allows for treatments down the road should the initial treatments not work and your cancer resurfaces. Chapter 9 helps you formulate a treatment plan, and Chapters 11 through 15 give you straight facts about your treatment options, including surgery, radiation, and hormone therapy.

Getting diagnosed with prostate cancer also can be unnerving because of the specific problems that are associated with the disease, such as impotence, incontinence, and the fear of death. Chapter 10 covers the major fears (as well as the realities) that men may experience when diagnosed with prostate cancer, including how to manage problems at home and work.

Opting for surgery

If your cancer is localized to the prostate, you're in reasonably good health (other than the cancer), and you have a health expectancy of at least ten years or more, a *radical prostatectomy* (or surgery that removes the entire prostate gland) may be the first line of treatment your doctor recommends. Surgery can be a pretty scary prospect, but it may cure you. If your cancer isn't localized, surgery may be able to at least delay the spread of cancer, if not stop it in its tracks altogether. Ask your doctor if he performs *nerve-sparing surgery,* where the nerve bundles that control erections are saved whenever possible. With nerve-sparing surgery, you have a 50 percent or better chance of regaining your sexual potency within a year of surgery (or sooner). Without nerve-sparing surgery, you run an almost certain risk of becoming impotent after the prostatectomy. (Chapter 11 covers the prostatectomy in much more detail.)

Considering radiation

Surgery isn't the one right answer for every man with localized prostate cancer. Some men do very well with radiation treatments. Two popular forms of radiation treatments are offered today:

- ✔ **Brachytherapy:** Radioactive seeds are implanted into the prostate gland in order to kill the cancer cells. (Don't worry — the radiation wears off after a few weeks.)

- ✔ **External beam radiation therapy (EBRT):** Given outside the body, this treatment focuses several beams of radiation on the cancerous prostate.

If you decide to have radiation therapy, your doctor will discuss whether brachytherapy or EBRT is the best treatment for you. (Some men receive both types of radiation treatment.) Read more about radiation therapy in Chapter 12.

Looking at hormone treatments

Your physician may recommend that you take hormones, which can slow the rate at which the cancer grows. Natural testosterone makes prostate cancer grow faster. Hormones put the brakes on your testosterone levels, slowing down the growth of the cancer. This approach often stops the cancer from spreading for many years. However, when hormone therapy is used as the only treatment, it doesn't cure the cancer.

Sometimes hormones are administered to decrease the size of the tumor before radiation treatments. If you have an advanced case of cancer when first diagnosed, hormones may be the only treatment option available to you. Hormones are also given to men whose initial treatments (usually surgery or radiation therapy) aren't effective at stemming the tide of the cancer.

The downside of taking hormones is that they can cause some nasty side effects, such as hot flashes, mood swings, and weight gain. You can rest assured that antidotes are available to help combat these side effects. I discuss everything you need to know about hormones and their side effects (of course, you need to talk to your own doctor, too) in Chapter 13.

Treating advanced cancer

Sometimes the cancer advances beyond the prostate gland, and surgery or radiation can't destroy it. Hormone therapy may also become ineffective after a certain period of time. Don't give up. You still have many good options to choose from, including using other forms of hormones, taking chemotherapy with cancer-killing drugs, and joining a clinical study. I cover these options in Chapter 15.

Discovering alternative therapies

Many people feel panicky after being diagnosed with prostate cancer. As a result, they may decide to turn to quick-fix remedies such as herbs, supplements, and special diets. Alternative therapies may help you feel better. For example, some herbs can help with the side effects of cancer treatments. Specifically, ginger may help with nausea caused by hormone therapy. And researchers are trying to determine more definitely whether supplements of vitamin E and selenium can help prevent prostate cancer, but already some studies indicate that they may be good for prevention.

But it's important to avoid relying on alternative therapies to treat prostate cancer because scientific evidence has not yet adequately proven their effectiveness. In Chapter 18, I discuss topics related to alternative therapy including what to watch out for when considering alternative remedies.

Making lifestyle changes

You can't cure cancer by dropping a few pounds or running around the block. But you can build up your overall stamina by making some lifestyle changes. In Chapter 17, I discuss the benefits of exercising and losing weight. I also talk about the effects of stress, and the actions you can take to reduce the stress in your life. (Yes, you can reduce stress even though you have one of the most stress-inducing problems on the planet — a diagnosis of prostate cancer.)

Coping with the side effects of treatments

You want to cure (or at least gain control over) your prostate cancer, so after discussing the best treatment options with your doctor, you go ahead and get treatment. Unfortunately, prostate cancer treatments sometimes cause side effects including frequent urination, diarrhea, hot flashes, fatigue, depression, weight gain, and muscle and bone loss.

Two of the biggest concerns for many men undergoing therapy for localized cancer, especially if they're considering having a prostatectomy, are impotence and incontinence, even though many men with prostate cancer never experience these problems, or they are only temporary problems for them. However, since they loom so large in most men's minds, I provide important details about these problems in Chapters 19 and 20. I'll give you the basics here.

- ✔ **Impotence:** If *impotence* (an inability to get or keep erections) becomes a problem for you after treatment, it may just be a short-term problem that time will resolve. But if the potency problem seems to be sticking around, don't worry: Solutions are available. You may want to try Viagra, the erection-inducing drug. Viagra isn't right for everyone, but it may do the job for you. You can also try vacuum devices (which can help you "pump up" an erection manually) or injectable drugs. If all else fails, and you're still unhappy, you may want to consider a penile implant. (Many men are very pleased with the results of the penile implant.)

✔ **Incontinence:** Many men worry about developing *incontinence* (loss of control over the release of urine) after undergoing treatment for prostate cancer. Sometimes surgery or radiation treatments may temporarily cause incontinence or other voiding problems, but most men recover within six months to a year.

If you face either (or both) of these problems after treatment, don't suffer in silence! Talk to your doctor. He can recommend the best road to success for you.

Dealing with the Effects of Your Cancer, at Work and at Home

A diagnosis of prostate cancer, even if you have no symptoms at all (and most men don't), can be a hard thing to cope with; it can weigh you down big-time. You may struggle to keep your anxiety from affecting you at work and at home.

I talk about how to deal with people at work and at home in Chapters 22 and 23. In Chapter 24, I offer a chapter for people who love someone who has prostate cancer. I specifically offer advice for wives and significant others who live with a men who may feel like they're imploding with emotions from being diagnosed with cancer and dealing with treatments. You may want to discreetly leave the book open to Chapter 24, where your loved ones will be likely to find it. Or you can just ask them outright to read it.

Chapter 2

Understanding the Prostate Gland and Recognizing Cancer Symptoms

I want to get one thing straight. It's your prosTATE gland, and *not* your prosTRATE gland. *Prostrate* means you're lying down, as in "he was prostrate with grief." You may feel pretty lousy when you think that you have prostate cancer — or *know* that you have it. And you may feel like lying down. But it's still your prostate, which (sort of) rhymes with *floss gate*. Studies have revealed that most men don't even know that they *have* a prostate gland in the first place (unless it gives them trouble), so the fact that thousands of people mispronounce "prostate" isn't that surprising.

Or, if they know that they have a prostate gland, many men think of it sort of as a superfluous organ, kind of like your appendix, which apparently just lies there doing nothing — unless it suddenly decides to get inflamed, making you rush to the hospital for an emergency appendectomy. However, in contrast to your appendix, your prostate gland *does* accomplish important functions. For example, your prostate is directly involved in your ability to father children, because it supplies essential nutrients to sperm fluid. However, when procreation is no longer in the picture, the prostate gland does nothing but cause trouble; it can interfere with urinating (blocking off urine flow), become infected and cause pain, or develop prostate cancer.

In this chapter, I cover the basics you need to know about the prostate gland and the symptoms that may indicate a variety of prostate diseases, including cancer. I cover the primary functions of your prostate when it's working well, as well as when you have symptoms indicating a problem. I talk about the basic anatomy of your prostate, inside and out, and I show you, with words and an illustration, where your prostate is in relation to other key parts of your body, such as your bladder, urethra, seminal vesicles, penis, and testicles.

Zeroing In on Your Prostate

Before you can understand the key problems that may develop with your prostate gland — especially the most serious problem of all, which is prostate cancer — you first need to understand exactly *where* your prostate gland is. You also need to know the basics of what the prostate does.

Understanding basic prostate anatomy

The healthy prostate gland is a walnut-sized organ that weighs in at about 15 grams, which is a little less than half an ounce, in young men (around age 20 or so) and 30 grams (about an ounce) or more in men who are age 50 or older. Unhealthy prostates can weigh as much as 100 grams or more, resembling the size of an orange or even a small grapefruit. Bigger is not better; in fact, it can be very bad.

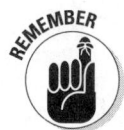

Keep in mind, however, that an enlarged prostate doesn't necessarily indicate prostate cancer. Instead, it may indicate a treatable common prostate disease, such as prostatitis or benign prostatic hyperplasia (BPH). (I describe these frequently occurring illnesses in Chapter 4.) The causes for these problems vary, but both diseases are usually treatable.

Location, location, location

Your prostate sits between your bladder and penis, just above your rectum. Your *urethra,* which is the tube that carries urine from your bladder through your penis and to the outside, runs through your prostate.

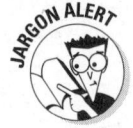

Two primary prostatic areas of concern are found inside the prostate gland itself: the peripheral zone and the transition zone.

- ✔ The *transition zone* is located more toward the middle of your prostate gland.
- ✔ The *peripheral zone* encompasses most of the outer part of your prostate, especially on the side facing the rectum.

The peripheral zone is the area where problems with prostate cancer are likely to be located and identified. If the doctor feels a suspicious bump or lump on your prostate when he performs a rectal examination, it will likely lie within the peripheral area. (Read more about the all-important rectal exam in Chapter 5.)

The Energizer Bunny of growth

For reasons that no one really understands — although it may have something (or a lot) to do with male hormones — the prostate gland has a fascinating propensity to continue to grow and grow. In fact, the prostate is the only organ within your body that keeps growing larger as you get older. Other glands max out during or after puberty, remaining about the same size for your entire life (unless they become inflamed or cancerous, or you develop another serious medical problem). Of course, the prostate gland grows at a much slower rate than your other organs; otherwise, everyone would die at a young age from exploding prostate glands. (Prostates don't really explode, but they can sometimes hurt a lot and feel like they're ready to explode.)

Medical experts know that testosterone is required for the continued growth of the prostate, but so far no one has discovered the details of why the prostate keeps on growing and growing. This growth isn't necessarily a good thing; it can lead to diseases of the prostate. An enlarged prostate is more likely to get into trouble. An enlarged prostate may also be an indicator of prostate cancer. However, a large prostate isn't always a sign of prostate cancer. You can have a small prostate gland and have cancer, and you can also have a very large prostate and *not* have cancer.

The main thing to keep in mind is that the rectal examinations performed during routine physical exams will almost always detect a very enlarged prostate. If your prostate is enlarged, your doctor will figure out the cause and recommend what you should do next.

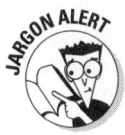

The entire prostate gland is surrounded by what's called the *capsule,* a thin, tough membrane that is stronger than the cells found within the interior of the prostate. Prostate cancer cells can sometimes penetrate through and grow outside the capsule. This penetration can occasionally be detected through tests, but usually it can only be detected after surgery, when the whole prostate is removed during surgery and then examined by the pathologist. When penetration occurs, doctors consider the cancer to be *not localized* (or no longer limited to the prostate itself), meaning that the cancer has spread. The spread may be minimal (such as just outside the capsule), it may be in lymph nodes near the prostate, or it may be in other distant parts of your body. When the cancer spreads to the lymph nodes or other regions, doctors call it advanced cancer, or cancer that has *metastasized.*

A routine physical examination or prostate biopsy rarely can tell your doctor if your cancer has spread. Your doctor may need to order some tests, such as a CT scan (to examine the lymph nodes) or a bone scan, to determine whether the cancer has invaded your bones. (Read more about bone scans and other tests in Chapter 6.) If the cancer has advanced, many good anti-cancer treatments are available to work against the cancer invaders. (I describe them all in Chapters 14, 15, and 21.)

Considering the surrounding organs

The prostate gland affects and is affected by the surrounding organs, such as the urinary bladder, the seminal vesicles, and the testicles. (See Figure 2-1 for the location of these organs.)

- **Urinary bladder:** A prostate that functions normally doesn't affect the bladder. Consider them neighbors who wave as they pass but don't visit each other's houses. But when the prostate starts having some problems, the neighboring bladder also begins to feel the effects. And the bigger the prostate problem becomes, the greater the impact on the bladder. For example, prostate problems can cause an intense urge to urinate frequently when the prostate is blocking the flow of urine. When the flow of urine is blocked, the bladder has to work harder, causing it to become hyperactive when filling with urine.

- **Seminal vesicles:** The seminal vesicles supply nutritious fluid to sperm. When the prostate becomes enlarged or infected, it can cause the seminal vesicles to swell up and impede the delivery of seminal fluid. Blocked seminal vesicles can cause pain.

- **Testicles:** The testicles are sex organs that produce sperm and *testosterone,* a male hormone. The testosterone is sent to the prostate and throughout the bloodstream to the other organs. Testosterone causes male sexual characteristics, such as a deep voice, body hair, greater muscle tissue than that found in women, and so on.

  Prostate cancer thrives and grows when testosterone is around. With advanced prostate cancer, doctors often do things to eliminate testosterone (see Chapter 13). These testosterone-cutting steps can lead to hot flashes, a loss of muscle mass, mood swings, and other symptoms that are also common to women who are in the throes of menopause.

Functions affected by the prostate

In general, the prostate affects two primary functions: reproduction and urination. When you have a problem with your prostate, you may also have a problem with fertility or normal urination. (Remember, though, you can still have prostate cancer and not have any problems with urinating, which I can't emphasize enough.)

Sexually speaking

Because most people are far more interested in having sex (or at least in thinking or reading about it) than they are in urinating (unless they start having some serious trouble with the basic function of emptying their bladder), I start with the topic of sex.

The prostate is a major player in the production and release of *seminal fluid,* which is the white stuff that's ejaculated, or expelled, when a man has an orgasm. Most of the volume that comprises the seminal fluid comes out of the seminal vesicles and from the prostate. A smaller volume comes from the testicles and contains the sperm. You have two seminal vesicles (shown in Figure 2-1 behind the bladder on either side.)

During orgasm, the fluid from the seminal vesicles and testicles arrives at the prostate and mixes with substances produced by the prostate. One of these substances is *prostate specific antigen (PSA).* PSA thins out the ejaculate and makes it easier for sperm to travel up a woman's uterus after intercourse in order to reach, penetrate, and fertilize the egg that is released (at that special time of the month) into the upper uterine tube. (See Chapter 5 for more information about PSA.)

Your prostate isn't directly involved in your ability to get an erection. However, the nerves that control erections run right next to the prostate, and these nerves can become damaged if the prostate is injured in an accident or if you're treated for prostate cancer with x-rays or surgery.

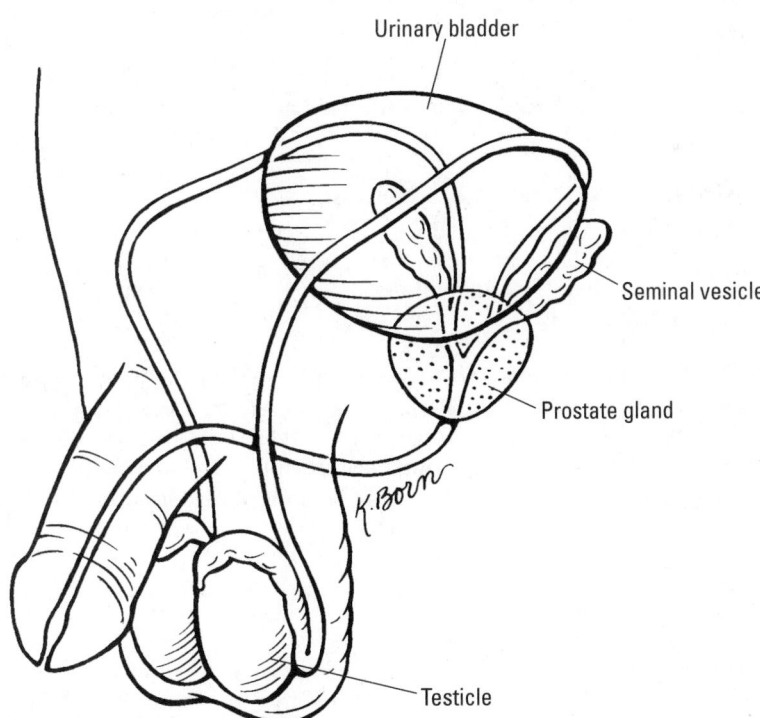

Figure 2-1:
The prostate gland and other key reproductive organs.

Urinary bladder

Seminal vesicle

Prostate gland

K. Born

Testicle

Comparing bird and turtle cancers

When I think about prostate cancer, I compare it to birds and turtles growing in a box. To me, birds are like cancers that grow very fast, leave their box (the prostate) quickly, and move on to attack the man's lymph nodes and the bones. In contrast, turtles are like slow-growing cancers that stay within the prostate for years, hanging around and not doing much of anything until they get very large. Turtle cancers may cause some minor urinary symptoms and be somewhat aggravating, but they're generally not life-threatening.

Telling the difference between the two types of cancer is the major challenge for doctors. They have to determine whether the cancer is a bird or a turtle. (Another problem they may face is that, in contrast to the animal kingdom, sometimes the turtle cancers somehow transform with the passing of time into bird cancers.)

Researchers are working hard to try to determine more precisely what kind of cancers are the bird type and what kind are the turtle type. When this code is broken, the diagnosis and treatment of patients with prostate cancer will improve. Because researchers know that cancer is caused mostly by defective genes, and because they also know a lot about how to work with genes, I believe that the code will be broken (at least partially) very soon.

For now, doctors pretty much have to depend on broad risk factors to figure out whether your prostate cancer needs to be treated quickly. These factors include your prostate specific antigen (PSA) blood test scores (for example, are they going up and, if so, how fast), the apparent size of your prostate cancer, and other factors that I discuss in more detail in Chapter 5. Remember, even if you have serious prostate cancer, you can still have no symptoms.

Urinating matters

The prostate doesn't actually assist the bladder with urination in any way. Instead, it usually just allows it to happen by not interfering with the flow of urine. But a swollen and malfunctioning prostate can impair your urination considerably.

If you flip back to Figure 2-1, you'll notice that the bladder is right on top of the prostate gland. Narrow tubes called *ureters* carry the urine from your kidneys to your bladder. The urethra travels right through the prostate gland, like a pipeline that cuts through a state. If prostate tissue grows inward and toward your urethra, urinating can become very difficult. If the clog or blockage becomes too severe, you may not be able to urinate at all.

If you can't urinate at all, you're facing a medical emergency, and you must get to your doctor or the emergency room immediately. This emergency situation requires the insertion of a *catheter,* which is a tube that the doctor or nurse manually inserts through your penis and into your bladder. The catheter moves the urine out and alleviates the pain and suffering. The catheter only represents a temporary solution. You still have to resolve the problem that's causing the blockage, or you'll find yourself in this situation again and again.

This type of serious urination problem is usually caused by a prostate disease, such as prostatitis or BPH. In some cases, however, the true culprit may be a urinary tract infection that you're harboring in your bladder. These diseases are described in much more detail in Chapter 4, because their symptoms can mimic those of prostate cancer.

Urination problems (such as frequency and urgency) can also be caused by prostate cancer. If you have problems urinating, see your doctor. He can determine the cause of your symptoms and tell what you can do about them.

When Good Prostates Go Bad: Symptoms That May Occur

Some men who've been diagnosed with prostate cancer have symptoms, but in many cases, men have no symptoms or warnings at all: The lack of symptoms is especially common for men who are in the early stages of prostate cancer that's localized to the gland, with no spread beyond it.

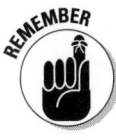

If you're 50 years old or older, insist on having an annual PSA blood test, as well as an annual rectal exam, to screen for prostate cancer. If you're at a higher risk for prostate cancer because you're black or if you have a brother or father who's had prostate cancer, you should receive annual prostate testing after age 40.

The following symptoms may be an indication of prostate cancer:

- Problems with urination, including frequent urination (especially at night), painful urination, blood in the urine, a weak urine stream, and a urine stream that stops and starts

  If *hematuria* (blood in the urine) is visible to your naked eye, report it to your doctor right away. The blood can indicate a minor or a major problem, so let your doctor determine what is causing it.

- Bone pain (may be a symptom of advanced prostate cancer)

- Constant fatigue

- An unintended weight loss of ten or fifteen pounds or more

- Chronic and severe lower back pain

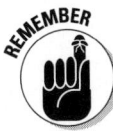

If you suffer from one or more of the symptoms in this list, you don't necessarily have prostate cancer. But you do need to see your doctor to find out what's actually going on with your body.

Chapter 3

Investigating Who's at Risk for Prostate Cancer

*M*en who are diagnosed with prostate cancer often wonder to themselves *why* this awful problem has been laid at their doorstep. Many of them also think, "Was it something that I did — or maybe something that I failed to do — that caused this problem to happen to me?" The fact is most men have no control over the known risk factors for prostate cancer. (A *risk factor* refers to an increased probability that a health problem may occur because of one or more specific traits.) It's not their fault. Even so, it still helps to know about the risk factors for prostate cancer, in case you or other family members have one or more of them. They're mostly factors that you can't control, like your age, your race, or the family that you were born into. But if you have even one risk factor for developing prostate cancer, I hope that you'll be more vigilant about the factors that you *can* control, such as getting regular checkups, eating right, minimizing stress, and so forth.

It's important to keep in mind that you're not doomed to develop prostate cancer merely because you check "yes" in one or more boxes asking you about risk factors. Even if you're black, older than age 50, and have both a brother and a father with prostate cancer, your risk of getting the disease is still low. But your risk is higher than it is for people who don't have all these risk factors, so it's important for you to be diligent in obtaining annual screenings and receive prompt treatment if your doctor does find prostate cancer.

In this chapter, I cover the known risk factors as well as the possible risk factors for prostate cancer. I also discuss research that shows that there are risk factors you actually *can* change, either before cancer occurs (preventive action) or after your diagnosis and treatment have already happened (when you're working on avoiding a recurrence of the disease). Finally, I discuss a group of people that the federal government has determined may be at an increased risk for prostate cancer — military veterans who served in the Vietnam War.

Aging Matters

Men can develop prostate cancer at virtually any age. However, it's extremely unusual for doctors to find prostate cancer in men younger than 40 years old (although it can happen). In general, men older than age 50 have a greater risk of developing prostate cancer than younger men, and prostate cancer is very common among men age 65 and older. The risk continues to increase with age.

Table 3-1 illustrates the *incidence* (the number of people in one year who are diagnosed with a disease while they're alive divided by the number of men in the same population) of prostate cancer in the United States. (In this case, by age and race per 100,000 men.) The statistics in Table 3-1 provide scientific proof that the risk of being diagnosed with prostate cancer increases with age.

Table 3-1	Incidence of Prostate Cancer in the United States by Age and Race: The Rate per 100,000 Men		
Age at Diagnosis	*All Races*	*White Males*	*Black Males*
40 – 44	5.4	4.6	13.2
45 – 49	32.0	28.3	79.2
50 – 54	127.5	120.9	254.3
55 – 59	310.2	299.9	573.4
60 – 64	570.5	552.4	1,018.1
65 – 69	859.2	842.3	1,274.7
70 – 74	1,070.6	1,041.9	1,645.3

Source: SEER (Surveillance, Epidemiology, and End Results) Cancer Statistics Review 1973 – 1999, National Cancer Institute

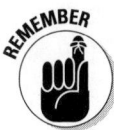

Because few men younger than age 40 develop prostate cancer, screening for the disease (including a PSA test and a rectal exam discussed in Chapter 5) is rarely performed before age 50. However, if you have risk factors for the disease, such as being a black man and/or having a family history of prostate cancer, you need to lower the age for starting annual testing to about 40 or 45. The more risk factors you have, the greater your need for annual screenings beginning at age 40.

Should older men (age 70 and older) be screened for prostate cancer? I really don't like age cutoffs when it comes to screening, so I vote yes, on a case-by-case basis. I primarily consider the man's life expectancy, and whether a man is likely to live for ten or more years from now. Some men who are 70 years old have the physical health and stamina of a man who's 60 or younger. Other men are age 70, and they're severely ill with heart disease, diabetes, and other serious medical problems, and they're unlikely to live for 10 more years, whether or not they have prostate cancer.

If you're *under* age 50, you're in one or more of the high-risk groups discussed in this chapter, and your doctor or insurance company doesn't recognize your need for an annual screening for prostate cancer, seriously consider paying for it yourself. (The PSA test usually costs about $35.)

Regarding Racial Risks

Men of all races can develop prostate cancer, but the risk is markedly increased for black men. The risk of death from prostate cancer is also greater for black men, followed by the death rates for white men, and then Hispanics, American Indians, and Asians. (See the sidebar, "Looking at racial death rates for prostate cancer" in this chapter for further information.)

According to the 2002 report on prostate cancer risk factors from the American Council on Science and Health, black men from the United States have a 69 percent higher risk of developing prostate cancer than white men. The National Cancer Institute in Washington, a federal government cancer agency, reports that black men from the United States have the highest rates of prostate cancer in the world. According to the Centers for Disease Control and Prevention (CDC), black men develop prostate cancer at a younger age than white men, and they also have a greater risk of dying from prostate cancer.

If you're a black man, you need to be screened for prostate cancer early (around age 40 or 45). You also need to act aggressively if cancer is detected, because there's some evidence that the cancer can be especially aggressive in black men, although it's not known why this is true.

Researchers are seeking to identify the causes for the higher risk of prostate cancer in black men so that they can create solutions for saving black men from disability and death by prostate cancer.

Identifying Your Genetic Risks: Tracing Your Family (Cancer) Tree

Your own genetics can affect whether or not you develop prostate cancer. Researchers believe that this genetic risk may be caused by a genetic mutation that is passed on, so they are trying to find the location of the defective gene.

How powerful are genes in causing prostate cancer? This is a topic that's likely to be debated for years to come. In fact, many research groups, including my colleagues in Seattle, are working hard to determine the exact hereditary genes that come into play in some prostate cancers. However, studies in various populations (such as twins in Sweden) have shown that genetic factors are definitely at work in some families.

Reviewing the medical histories of the men in your family

Researchers have determined that if your father and/or brother has had prostate cancer, your risk for developing the disease is approximately double to five times that of other men whose fathers and brothers didn't have the disease. Your risk is higher if your father and/or brother had an early onset of prostate cancer before the age of 55.

It's a good idea to contact men in your family to figure out your potential risks for developing prostate cancer. Your physician will appreciate this additional family tree information; it will help him determine how aggressive your screening should be. For example, if you have one or more relatives with prostate cancer, and your PSA level is slightly high, your doctor may decide to do a *biopsy* (tissue removal to check for cancer). (You can read more about PSA levels and their significance in Chapter 5, and more about biopsies in Chapter 7.)

If you're not sure whether any of your male family members died of cancer, ask other family members. If no one in the family really knows for sure, you can

Looking at racial death rates for prostate cancer

According to the Centers for Disease Control and Prevention (CDC), the racial rates for death from prostate cancer per 100,000 men of the same race living in the United States look like this:

- ✔ Blacks 48.7
- ✔ Whites 19.6
- ✔ Hispanics 14.5
- ✔ American Indians 11.3
- ✔ Asian/Pacific Islanders 8.0

Source: "At A Glance: Prostate Cancer: The Public Health Perspective 2001," Centers for Disease Control and Prevention, 2001

request a copy of the death certificate, which will include the cause of death, from the state in which the male family member died. You can also check obituaries, but the cause of death is often not listed in newspaper reports.

People may confuse one type of cancer for another. For example, when prostate cancer spreads, it spreads first and mostly to bone. It is this spreading of the cancer that actually kills. In such a case, the man would die from prostate cancer and not bone cancer, because the cancer started in the prostate gland. However, some people may assume that the man died of bone cancer. So, if someone says a relative of yours died of bone cancer, ask if he had prostate cancer before he died. If so, the man may have died from prostate cancer that spread into his bones. (Cancer that starts in the bones is very rare.)

Looking at the medical histories of the women in your family

The medical histories of the women in your family can also signal a risk for prostate cancer. According to research, men whose mothers or sisters had either breast cancer or ovarian cancer have a greater risk for developing prostate cancer than men whose mothers and sisters have been cancer-free. Pretty lousy deal for both you and your mom or sister, but there it is. It's better to know about such risks so that you can schedule annual screenings to help allay your own fears as well as the fears of the people who love you.

Considering Other Factors That May Put You at Risk

The known and accepted risk factors for developing prostate cancer are age, family history, and race. However, you should also consider other health habits that may be risk factors, such as drinking alcoholic beverages and smoking tobacco. (Surprise! They're both bad for your health, and some experts believe that these habits may further increase your risks for developing prostate cancer. Or they may aggravate the disease after it develops.) It's best to adopt healthy habits as a good preventive strategy.

Other potential risk factors include:

✔ **Physically inactive lifestyles:** If you're physically inactive, you're more likely to be overweight or obese. Together, these factors may contribute to your risk of developing prostate cancer (although research has not definitively proven this connection). Doctors do know that obesity can impair treatment when cancer is diagnosed. For example, obese men may be ordered by their surgeons to lose weight, simply because it's dangerous to cut through a lot of fat tissue during surgery.

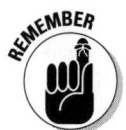

It's best to get off the couch as soon as possible and create a healthier lifestyle for yourself, even if you've already been diagnosed with prostate cancer. A strong body can fight off illnesses, including cancer, more effectively.

✔ **Heavy consumption of red meat and fatty foods:** According to clinical studies in the United States and other countries, chowing down on too many overly generous portions of steak and roast beef, and skimping on your intake of vegetables and fruits may lead to prostate cancer. Some studies suggest that a diet high in fat content may lead to prostate cancer. Don't worry, you don't have to subsist entirely on a diet of just tofu and bean sprouts to avoid prostate cancer or prevent a reoccurrence, if you've already had cancer. But if you're addicted to milk shakes and burgers, you may want to seriously rethink your diet — or at least make some changes to it.

✔ **High stress levels:** Studies indicate that very high levels of stress can raise your levels of prostate specific antigen (PSA). It's not known if this may cause prostate cancer to occur (or recur), but to be on the safe side, try to minimize your stress levels as much as possible. Check out Chapter 16 for some ideas on how to do that.

✔ **Excessive smoking and drinking:** Some studies indicate that smoking and heavy drinking may contribute to the development of prostate cancer, although it is not known by what mechanism this occurs. You can improve your health and lower your chances for developing prostate cancer by ending these problem health habits as soon as possible.

Adopting a healthier lifestyle is easier said than done, I know. That's why I include advice in Chapter 17, which I hope helps you achieve this goal.

Possibly Linking Prostate Cancer to Vietnam War Veterans

The Vietnam War was a difficult time for many people, especially for the U.S. military personnel who served in Southeast Asia. The National Academy of Sciences has determined that American servicemen who served inside the country of Vietnam during the Vietnam War may have been exposed to prostate-cancer–causing conditions. The U.S. Congress subsequently created a benefits program for some Vietnam veterans who have developed prostate cancer since that time.

Note: I'm *not* saying that I personally believe that prostate cancer was caused by Agent Orange or any other substance that was used in Vietnam during the Vietnam War. As a clinical researcher, I'd have to study and analyze the data myself before I could say it was valid, and I haven't done so. Instead, I'm providing the information in this section *solely* as a service to readers who are Vietnam veterans, so that they can take advantage of existing government programs that they may be eligible for.

Being exposed to Agent Orange

Many servicemen were exposed to Agent Orange and other herbicides. These herbicides were sprayed in Vietnam to eliminate the heavy foliage that made it difficult or impossible to see. Some researchers think that exposure to these herbicides may have caused many of the health problems (such as prostate cancer, diabetes, and other illnesses) that were later experienced by Vietnam veterans. It's unclear if or how the spraying of Agent Orange actually led to the ultimate development of prostate cancer and other diseases in people who served in Vietnam. Nor is it clear how many Vietnam veterans would've developed prostate cancer anyway, had they never served in Vietnam. But the U.S. government has accepted the presumption that Agent Orange and other herbicides have caused prostate cancer and other diseases among the men who were stationed in Vietnam.

Combating the stress

The actual stress of the war itself is one other possibility that may have contributed to the development of prostate cancer among Vietnam veterans. Some studies have shown that extremely high stress can be linked with abnormally high PSA levels. Because prostate cancer can take years to develop, it's not a stretch to imagine that combat stress may be a contributing factor to the later development of prostate cancer.

Receiving support

If you served in Vietnam during the Vietnam War, and you've developed prostate cancer since then, you're eligible to apply for the Agent Orange program.

In 2001, Congress passed the Veterans Education and Benefits Expansion Act. This law established a presumption that veterans who served in Vietnam were exposed to herbicides. If you're a Vietnam veteran who served in Vietnam between the years of 1962 and 1971, you may qualify for medical coverage (and in some cases, monthly compensation) under this law. You don't have to prove that you were ever exposed to Agent Orange, nor do you have to prove that this presumed exposure caused you to get prostate cancer years later.

The Agent Orange program is described in detail in the Department of Veterans Affairs (VA) pamphlet "Agent Orange: Information for Veterans Who Served in Vietnam," which is available from your local VA office (or you can call the national toll-free help line at 1-800-749-8387). You can download the pamphlet from the VA Web site at www.va.gov/agentorange.

You can also contact veterans service organizations to request further information and help. You may want to try contacting the American Legion at 800-433-3318, the Veterans of Foreign Wars of the United States (VFW) at 800-VFW-1899, the Disabled American Veterans (DAV) at 877-426-2838, or the Vietnam Veterans of America at 800-882-1316. These organizations have chapters throughout the United States.

Chapter 4

Identifying Diseases That May Mimic Prostate Cancer

Tom didn't see his doctor because he feared that his symptoms, which included frequently having to go to the restroom, pain with urination, and lower back discomfort, probably meant that he had prostate cancer. He didn't really want to think about the problem at all. Hoping that the symptoms would eventually just go away, Tom chose to ignore them.

Tom's symptoms got worse and worse. Finally, after hearing several co-workers laughing and joking about "Tommy Toilet" and "Thomas Tinkle," who was always rushing to the bathroom, Tom decided that it was past time to see his doctor. After the doctor examined Tom, asked him some questions, and ran a few tests, he discovered that it wasn't cancer at all. Instead, the symptoms were caused by a bacterial infection in Tom's prostate, a condition that can be treated with antibiotics. Tom had suffered needlessly for months.

Sometimes men have prostate problems that are aggravating but have nothing to do with prostate cancer. The symptoms of these problems (urinary urgency, frequency, and so on) are sometimes similar to those found in prostate cancer. You need to be aware of the diseases that mimic prostate cancer so that your doctor can determine whether you have cancer or something else. No matter what health problem you have, you need to get it identified and treated.

In this chapter, I talk about benign prostatic hyperplasia (BPH), prostatitis, and bladder infections — medical problems that mimic prostate cancer. I discuss what these medical problems are, what causes them (what is known thus far), their key symptoms, and how they're usually treated. I also cover other medical problems that may cause urinary symptoms, such as diabetes, sexually transmitted diseases, interstitial cystitis, and bladder cancer.

Dealing with Benign Prostatic Hyperplasia

Benign prostatic hyperplasia (BPH), which is also known as benign prostatic hypertrophy, is present to some extent in all men as they age. BPH is an overgrowth of noncancerous cells that causes an enlargement of the prostate gland. In some men, this overgrowth of cells may impede the flow of urine. Although annoying and sometimes very painful, this blockage is rarely fatal. You will, however, usually need to receive medical treatment to resolve the problem eventually.

BPH is increasingly common in men older than the age of 50, although many men experience no symptoms for years. One-third of all men older than age 60 have BPH that causes problems. So if you have symptomatic BPH (I describe the symptoms in the next section of this chapter), you're a member of a large group — even though you never asked to join this club, and you would have declined if invited!

The increased risk of BPH with age is due in part because the prostate gland is the only gland that continues to grow in size as you age, aided by the output of a form of testosterone called *dihydrotestosterone.* Consequently, your prostate may be twice as big (or more) at age 50 (when your prostate gland may weigh 30 or more grams) than at age 20. In this case, however, bigger is not better. An enlarged prostate doesn't inevitably mean that you have symptomatic BPH or other medical problems, but BPH is more likely to occur in a larger prostate.

Detecting symptoms of BPH

If you have BPH, you likely have at least a few symptoms. The most common symptoms are

- Frequent urination.
- A slow weak stream of urine (dribbling or difficulty getting any urine out at all). This may result in a need for more time to urinate. Because your stream is slow, and you may have a lot of stopping and starting,

it basically takes a long time to get all the urine out, which can be really embarrassing when you're holding up a long line of fans at the men's room during a football game!

It's a natural reaction to try even harder to urinate when you can't get much (or anything) out with the usual effort. Yet such straining can worsen your BPH symptoms, so don't split a gut trying to urinate. See your doctor if your straining gets that bad.

✔ A feeling of urgency when you feel like voiding.

Beware of the following serious symptoms often associated with BPH, and get immediate medical attention if you suffer from either:

✔ Blood in your urine is a definite sign that you need medical attention. It may indicate may indicate a more serious condition than BPH, such as bladder or kidney cancer, especially if your urinary bleeding is painless.

✔ If you can barely urinate, or if your bladder feels totally full for one hour or more, and you feel like you're going to burst, but your bladder is still continuing to fill up, this constitutes a medical emergency. That urine needs to come out, and the longer that it stays in your bladder, the more likely you're going to suffer from extreme pain, possible infection, a backing up of urine, and other serious medical consequences. Call your doctor, and if he's not available, insist that this emergency information be relayed to him immediately. If your doctor doesn't get back to you within a few hours, go to the emergency room of the nearest hospital or to a walk-in clinic so that you can be treated.

Testing for BPH

In addition to a rectal exam (see Chapter 5), your doctor will ask you a series of questions to get an idea of the type and severity of your prostate symptoms. He may also want to order one or more of the following tests:

✔ **A urinalysis:** This urine test is used to rule out a bladder infection. You're given a sterile wet cleaner for wiping off the end of your penis. The doctor is interested in whether there's any bacteria *inside* your bladder, not on your penis, so be sure not to skip the cleaning part. Then you merely urinate in a cup. You don't have to fill up the whole cup. Even just a little bit of urine is usually enough. Sadly, you can have both BPH and a bladder infection.

✔ **An ultrasound examination of your prostate:** This test involves a probe being inserted into your rectum. Ultrasound uses sound waves, which don't hurt you — you can't even feel them. The ultrasound makes images (sort of like shadows) on a screen. The doctor then reads these images and determines how big the prostate is. The ultrasound occasionally can detect if the prostate might contain cancer, in which case a biopsy might be performed at that time or later. (Read about the biopsy in Chapter 7.).

✔ **A urodynamic examination:** This test uses a small *catheter* (a tube inserted through the penis and into the bladder) to measure the pressures on your bladder. Measuring bladder pressures can help your doctor determine whether a bladder problem is due to either a hyperactive bladder or blockage.

The urodynamic examination is not painful, and the only slight discomfort comes from the insertion of the catheter. The doctor fills your bladder with fluid so that he can see what it looks like on an x-ray when it's full. Then you're told to urinate. The doctor looks at whether your bladder is contracting *before* it should. If your bladder does contract before it should, you have a hyperactive bladder. The doctor also measures the pressures in your bladder as you urinate. If the pressures are high, your bladder is overworking — it may also be a sign of BPH. These high pressures may also signal an underlying problem of prostate cancer (but this situation is rare).

How BPH differs from prostate cancer

BPH is a treatable illness, and although it can be painful, it's rarely fatal. In most cases, it can be treated with a course of medication. Surgery is only necessary in severe cases. In contrast, many cases of prostate cancer are curable, but it's a fatal disease for about 30,000 men per year in the United States alone. Treatment is much more aggressive for prostate cancer. Prostate cancer is treated with surgery, radiation therapy, hormone therapy, and/or chemotherapy — all of which are more difficult to deal with than the treatments for BPH.

Men with BPH are not more prone to developing prostate cancer than men who never had BPH.

Treating BPH

If you have a minor case of BPH, your doctor will probably recommend that you limit your consumption of alcohol and caffeine, because these substances can aggravate your problem. Your doctor may also advise you to cut back on fluids before you go to bed, so that you don't wake up repeatedly, having to urinate right away. Other than that, your doctor will tell you to come back if your symptoms get worse. If the problem becomes chronic or troublesome, further treatment is generally required. I describe the various treatments for BPH, including surgery, in the following sections.

Finding relief with saw palmetto

Some doctors (although I'm not one of them) recommend saw palmetto, an herbal remedy that has been shown in some studies to reduce the size of the prostate gland in some patients with minor cases of BPH and relieve inflammation in patients with prostatitis. Saw palmetto is not effective in severe cases, however. You can find saw palmetto in health food stores, as well as in many pharmacies and supermarkets.

The key drawback to saw palmetto, as with other herbal remedies and supplements, is that it's not nearly as closely regulated by the Food and Drug Administration (FDA) as prescribed drugs or over-the-counter drugs (such as Tylenol, heartburn remedies, and so on). The FDA can't pull an herbal remedy or supplement off the market unless it's been proven dangerous (rather than being merely ineffective). As a result, you can find a great variation among the different preparations of saw palmetto that are sold. You shouldn't expect any uniformity between brands.

If you try saw palmetto, after first discussing it with your doctor, be sure to purchase saw palmetto that's packaged and sold in the United States, to be on the safe side. Also, if you find that the drug does help you (and it *is* a drug, don't imagine it isn't), stay with the same brand. If another brand is having a big sale, ignore it; go for what works for you (even if it costs a little more).

Medications usually work

Today, early cases of symptomatic BPH are treated with a category of medications known as *alpha blockers* (which block special nerves to the prostate that normally make the prostate opening contract, and thus, they relax the prostate somewhat and make urinating easier), such as Flomax (generic name: tamsulosin), Minipress (generic name: prazosin), Hytrin (generic name: terazosin), or Cardura (generic name: doxazosin). Doctors may also prescribe Proscar (generic name: finasteride), a hormonal drug that works to shrink the size of your prostate gland by reducing your production of dihydrotestosterone, the male hormone mentioned earlier in this chapter. These alpha blocker drugs can cause some side effects, such as drowsiness, dizziness, insomnia, and headaches, but these side effects are rare. Proscar can also cause breast enlargement and tenderness, diarrhea, diminished libido, decreased ejaculate volume, and impotence, but these side effects are rare and they go away when the drug is discontinued.

BPH drugs usually help relieve the frequency of urination and the feeling of urgency, allowing you to get through your business meetings, your long commute home, or your golf game without having to dart back and forth to the bathroom constantly. These drugs can help you lead your normal life.

Heating up and destroying the problem

If you have mildly symptomatic BPH, your doctor may decide to resolve the problem by superheating the prostate using microwave, laser, or electrical energy. I believe these lesser procedures sometimes help, but often they only work for a little while, and then you'll need a more definitive formal surgical procedure.

- **Microwave treatment:** This procedure was approved by the Food and Drug Administration (FDA) in 1996. Nobody's going to ask you to stick your penis in a microwave oven. Rather, a special catheter is placed through your urethra into your bladder and microwave energy from a special device in the catheter is precisely focused into your prostate, superheating the prostate tissue so that it's destroyed. Over the next several weeks to months, the prostate shrinks and, theoretically, urinating becomes easier.

- **Transurethral needle procedure:** During this procedure, an instrument is passed through your urethra and special needles are inserted directly into the prostate in several areas. These needles can transmit either a certain type of laser heat energy or electrical energy. In both cases, the energy heats up the prostate tissue, destroys it, and eventually shrinks the prostate.

Generally, both procedures are safe and can be done in the office (or a surgical outpatient facility), and do not require hospitalization. Generally, the recovery time is much faster than with formal surgery (discussed in the next section). Be sure to work with a doctor who has experience performing these procedures because the more experienced the doctor is, the more adeptly he'll perform the procedure.

If surgery is needed

If medications and/or heat treatments aren't effective, or if your doctor feels that your case is too severe for these treatments, you may require more formal surgery. Three basic procedures can get you back to urinating better. If your prostate is very large, the surgeon will make an incision in your lower abdomen, open up the prostate capsule, shell out the BPH part of the prostate, and then close the capsule. This process is much like scooping out the inside of a melon and leaving the outer skin intact. This is called an *open simple prostatectomy*, and shouldn't be confused with the radical prostatectomy (which is done for cancer and not BPH), where the whole prostate is removed.

More commonly, surgery for BPH includes one of the following two procedures in which the doctor goes through the urethra and cuts the prostate from the inside. In both cases, electrical energy or special laser cutting energy is used:

✔ **Transurethral incision of the prostate (TUIP):** This is the less common procedure for treating serious cases of BPH. The surgery only requires one or two incisions, which are made to relieve bladder pressure, and no tissue is removed. Usually TUIP is done for small prostates.

✔ **Transurethral resection of the prostate (TURP):** This procedure removes the prostate tissue that's blocking the flow of urine. Urologists liken this procedure to an apple corer, because the surgeon actually cores out your prostate from the inside. A small percentage (less than 2 percent) of men have some trouble controlling their urine after this procedure.

The Inflamed Prostate: Prostatitis

Prostatitis refers to an inflammation of the prostate gland that may occur for a variety of reasons, such as from an infection of the prostate gland, and can cause the prostate to swell up as large as a lemon. (***Note:*** In some cases, prostatits isn't caused by an infection, but rather by undeterminable factors. In fact, many experts now use the more general term "pelvic pain syndrome" instead of prostatitis to describe this condition.) Researchers believe that this condition affects several hundred thousand men a year in the United States alone. Aggravatingly, you can have no bacteria at all present in your prostate but still experience the inflammation and pain anyway. Studies show that other possible causes of prostatitis include:

✔ **Trauma:** Some aggressive activities, such as frequent bumpy truck rides, may aggravate the prostate.

✔ **Diets heavy on alcohol, caffeine, and spicy foods:** Your diet may cause, or at least worsen, prostatitis.

According to researchers who study the *epidemiology* of prostatitis (who's most likely to suffer from it), prostatitis is more common among younger and middle-aged men. Men between the ages of 36 and 50 have the highest risk for developing prostatitis, while men older than 66 have the lowest risk. Black men and white men have the highest risks for developing prostatitis. Studies also indicate that men living in the southern and western regions of the United States have a higher risk than men elsewhere in the country. The reason for the higher risk in these areas is unknown.

Detecting symptoms of prostatitis

In addition to the obvious symptom of inflammation, prostatitis may also bring other symptoms, including

✔ Pain in your testicles and/or back and/or pelvis and/or the area between the scrotum and the anus

✔ Difficulty urinating

✔ Pain with urination

✔ Pain with ejaculation

✔ A difficult-to-describe sick feeling within your pelvic area

✔ Fever and/or chills

Testing for prostatitis

Your doctor will determine whether you have prostatitis based on your symptoms, your lab work, and your physical examination. You can also expect to have a rectal examination. (Rectal exams don't usually hurt, but if you have prostatitis, they can be painful.) The doctor will massage your prostate gland to elicit prostatic fluid. He cultures this fluid to find out if you have an infection and, if so, what kind of infection you have. The culture also helps him determine the best antibiotic for treating your infection.

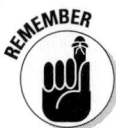

Don't try to figure out the source of your prostate problem on your own, and don't rely on a "diagnosis" from your friends or family. Regardless of what your Uncle Frank says you should do, or what your cousin Susie tells you that her boyfriend did when *he* had a problem that was just like yours, the reality is that you're a unique individual. You need to see your doctor so that you can get diagnosed and treated.

How prostatitis differs from prostate cancer

Prostatitis is an inflammation, not a cancerous condition. Although prostatitis can be very painful, it's usually managed with a course of medications. Sometimes prostatitis can go away without treatment (although it usually comes back). In contrast, prostate cancer usually requires more extreme measures, such as surgery or radiation treatments, and never goes away on its own without treatment. Prostatitis, unlike prostate cancer, is never fatal. Prostatitis is also very painful, unlike prostate cancer, which is usually not painful unless the condition is advanced.

Treating prostatitis

After you've been diagnosed with prostatitis, your doctor can treat it effectively. If an infection is causing the condition, antibiotics should work. Your doctor will prescribe the best antibiotic for you and determine how long you should take it. (***Remember:*** Be sure to follow your doctor's instructions very carefully. Many people fail to take their medicine for more than a few days, which generally isn't long enough to kill the bacteria.)

Usually the problem clears up when treated with antibiotics, although some men may develop a nasty chronic case of prostatitis. Often this condition isn't easy to treat, especially if the prostatitis isn't caused by infection at all. See your doctor, and if that doesn't work, ask the physician for a consultation with a urologist who is an expert in this condition.

In addition to or instead of consulting a doctor, some patients try to treat prostatitis with over-the-counter (OTC) medications, such as anti-inflammatory drugs, or herbal remedies, such as saw palmetto. (Check out the "Finding relief with saw palmetto" sidebar in this chapter.) If your medical problem stems from an inflammation that isn't an infection, these remedies *may* make you feel a little better, but they won't eradicate the germs. If you *do* have an infection, however, without receiving medical treatment and antibiotics, your infection will only worsen.

Some men (and some doctors) find that prostatitis symptoms improve with taking over-the-counter or prescribed nonsteroidal anti-inflammatory medications such as Motrin or Advil (generic name: ibuprofen) or Vioxx (generic name: rofecoxib). Others may feel better by taking muscle relaxants such as Flexeril (generic name: cyclobenzaprine hydrochloride).

Be sure to consult with your physician before treating your problem with any drugs, including OTC medications or saw palmetto.

Some symptoms, such as low back pain, difficulty with urination, and a hesitant, slow stream of urine, can occur with infections as well as with prostate cancer. If you have such symptoms, don't assume that they're nothing to worry about, and that you can just take care of them later. Even if your problem *is* just a minor infection, you still need to see your doctor. Untreated infections can get worse, and you can end up a very sick puppy. You also need to rule out prostate cancer when such symptoms occur. Don't wait. Be safe now, not sorry later.

Looking at Bladder Infections

Women are much more prone to developing bladder infections than men, because women have much shorter *urethras* (the tube that carries your urine from your bladder to the outside). But men can develop bladder infections, too. Bladder infections are no day at the beach. They can drive you wild.

Here's the thing: Your urethra travels right through your prostate, sort of like an interstate highway cutting through a state. If you get a bladder infection, your urethra and bladder will be sore, and the problem may mimic the symptoms of prostatitis or other prostate ailments, such as BPH. The condition may even mimic the symptoms of prostate cancer. The true culprits, however, are those nasty bacteria that are proliferating inside your bladder. The prostate gland itself is fine.

Detecting symptoms of a bladder infection

A bladder infection, also known as *cystitis,* can be a very annoying problem. When infected, your bladder becomes unhappy and inflamed. The most common symptoms of bladder infections in men are

- ✔ **Pain with urination:** You may feel a straining or pressure pain. You may also feel temporarily better after you urinate — until the next time, which comes all too soon.

- ✔ **Difficulty urinating:** A lot of effort and straining produces precious little urine.

- ✔ **Frequent and urgent urination:** You may feel like you have to keep rushing to the bathroom, even though you produce very little when you do go. The feeling is similar to how you feel after you drink six soft drinks very fast.

- ✔ **Blood in your urine:** It may not be noticeable to the naked eye, but it's detectable by a laboratory or the doctor.

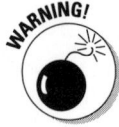

   If you see blood in your urine, even just a little bit, or if you notice that your urine is a pinkish color, contact your physician immediately, even when you don't have any pain or other symptoms. It may be a minor infection, or it may mean something more serious, such as bladder or kidney cancer. Don't panic, and don't ignore this indicator of a problem.

- ✔ **Back pain.** You may experience a feeling of pressure or strain, especially in your lower back.

- ✔ **A low or moderate fever.** The fever is often accompanied by a very cranky and tired feeling.

Testing for a bladder infection

Doctors usually diagnose a bladder infection in one of two ways:

✔ A simple urinalysis, which involves checking the urine for red or white blood cells or bacteria. Normal urine is sterile and has neither red nor white blood cells nor bacteria in it. Often a dipstick is used to perform the test.

✔ A urine culture, which involves sending the urine to a laboratory, where the technicians attempt to grow bacteria over a 48-hour period. Sometimes infection that doesn't show up in a simple urinalysis will be revealed in a urine culture, making a urine culture more reliable than a simple urinalysis.

The down side of a urine culture is that the results won't come back for at least a few days, while a simple urinalysis can be performed while you wait.

How bladder infections differ from prostate cancer

Bladder infections are caused by bacteria, unlike prostate cancer. As with prostatitis and BPH, bladder infections are usually readily treatable with a course of medications, while prostate cancer requires more invasive types of therapy, such as surgery or radiation. If you have recurrent cases of bladder infection, the doctor may put you on a low "maintenance" dose of antibiotics, so that the few remaining germs never get a chance to multiply. These medications generally have few side effects. However, in contrast, the side effects of anti-cancer medications, such as incontinence, impotence, or hot flashes, can be much tougher to deal with.

Treating your bladder infection

The best way to manage a bladder infection is to take the medicine your doctor orders (almost always an antibiotic), drink copious quantities of water (about a liter a day), and realize that you'll usually recover from this problem after about a week or ten days and then feel fine again.

Most bladder infections are treatable with antibiotics such as Cipro (generic name: ciprofloxican), Floxin (generic name: ofloxacin), and Bactrim (generic name: trimethoprim and sulfamethoxazole). (Doctors aren't limited to these antibiotics; they have a lot to choose from.) The antibiotics that are commonly used for bladder infections don't have that many side effects, but they do have a few. Some of these medications may cause headaches and nausea in some people, while others, such as Floxin, may cause a strange metallic taste in your mouth. The taste goes away when you finish taking the drug.

Unlike in women, whose bladder infections are caused by germs that enter from outside the body, bladder infections in men are often caused by more serious conditions, such as congenital urinary tract defects. So, when your bladder infection is over, your doctor may order other tests to make sure that nothing else is wrong.

If you're having pain and irritation with urination, and your doctor says that no infection is present, try eliminating caffeine from your diet to see whether it helps relieve the problem. The underlying problem may be those eight cups of coffee or all those colas you drink each day. Another possible cause: Over-the-counter cold medicine with decongestants, which can cause bladder irritation in some men. Stop taking the cold medicine and see whether you notice a difference.

Regarding Other Possibilities

If you don't have BPH, prostatitis, or a bladder infection, and you're experiencing aggravating symptoms that seem to be emanating from the prostate or bladder, you may be suffering from another condition. The key candidates are as follows:

- ✔ Type 2 diabetes
- ✔ Sexually transmitted diseases
- ✔ Interstitial cystitis
- ✔ Bladder cancer

Dealing with Type 2 diabetes

Type 2 diabetes, formerly called *adult onset diabetes,* is the most common form of diabetes. It represents about 90 percent of all cases of diabetes. Type 2 diabetes, like prostate cancer, is a serious chronic disease that can be fatal, although treatment with medication and dietary control enables many people to live a normal life.

If your doctor suspects that you have Type 2 diabetes, he may order a blood test to confirm the problem. In fact, if the first blood test says "yes" loud and clear, most doctors will still order a second test to make sure that the first one wasn't just lab error. Your doctor may suspect that you have diabetes because people with untreated diabetes are constantly urinating. (Constant urination may be a sign of one of the other diseases I describe in this chapter, including prostate cancer.)

You may also fit other risk factors for diabetes, such as being overweight, being older than age 50, and having other medical problems, such as high blood pressure, that are common among people with diabetes.

Type 2 diabetes is a disease that is primarily characterized by high blood sugar. This condition usually doesn't require self-injections, although some people with Type 2 diabetes need insulin injections after many years. (People with Type 1 diabetes must have insulin to stay alive.) If you are diagnosed with Type 2 diabetes, you can take daily oral medications to treat the illness. You also need to test your blood frequently and watch your diet. (It's *not* true that you must give up all your favorite foods forever when you have diabetes. But you do need to be more careful with your diet than you probably were in the past.)

Considering STDs

A sexually transmitted disease (STD), such as gonorrhea or syphilis, can cause back pain, difficulty with urination, and a need to constantly urinate. These symptoms may also occur with prostate cancer. If you have an STD, you may also notice a discharge from your penis that you haven't seen before, which isn't a symptom of prostate cancer.

If you've had sex with a new partner, consider the possibility that you may have contracted an STD; even if you haven't had sex with a new partner lately, it's possible that your current partner may have passed the infection to you. Sexually transmitted diseases aren't pleasant, but fortunately most STDs, with the exception of herpes or the human immunodeficiency virus (HIV), are easily eradicated with common antibiotics.

Pondering your painful bladder: Interstitial cystitis

Interstitial cystitis (IC) is a painful bladder condition that causes frequent urination and pain — symptoms you may also experience with prostate cancer — usually without an infection. Interstitial cystitis is primarily found in women, as men only make up about 10 percent of those suffering from IC. This condition may occur when there's a breakdown of the normal mucosal layer (a thin layer of tissue that protects the bladder) in the bladder. (What initiates this destructive process is unknown.)

IC can be very painful yet difficult to diagnose because so few men have IC, and it may easily be confused with prostatitis or BPH. But rest assured, IC isn't a fatal disease. It usually can be treated with medication and dietary changes, although the treatment often just controls rather than cures the condition.

Most doctors recommend that you avoid spicy foods and caffeine. Medications such as Elmiron (generic name: pentosan polysulfate) or Detrol (generic name: tolterodine tartrate) may be effective. A low dose of an anti-depressant such as Elavil (generic name: amitriptyline) may help, as well. The dose is usually lower than the amount used to treat depression, and you *don't* need to see a psychiatrist to receive a prescription for it.

Checking for bladder cancer

Another medical problem that can cause frequency of urination, difficulty urinating, a feeling of irritation in the bladder, and blood in the urine is bladder cancer. Bladder cancer kills about 12,400 men in the United States each year, a much smaller number than the statistics for prostate cancer. But this form of cancer can share some of the symptoms of (especially advanced) prostate cancer (such as pain in the pelvic area or bloody urine).

If your doctor suspects bladder cancer, he may perform a *cystoscopy,* where he looks at your bladder by inserting a special thin instrument into your bladder. (Read more about the cystoscopy in Chapter 6.) A urologist usually performs this test. The doctor may also remove sample tissue during the cystoscopy so that he can perform a *biopsy,* a test to determine whether cancer is present. (To discover more about biopsies, read Chapter 7.) However, don't assume that your doctor is convinced that you must have bladder cancer if he does a cystoscopy. This procedure is sometimes used to diagnose the cause of many different diseases, including recurrent infections, BPH, and other medical problems common to the bladder.

Bladder cancer is often treated with surgery. It may also be treated with chemotherapy and/or radiation treatment. Your urologist and oncologist, can help you determine the best treatment to resolve the problem.

Part II
Getting a Diagnosis

The 5th Wave   By Rich Tennant

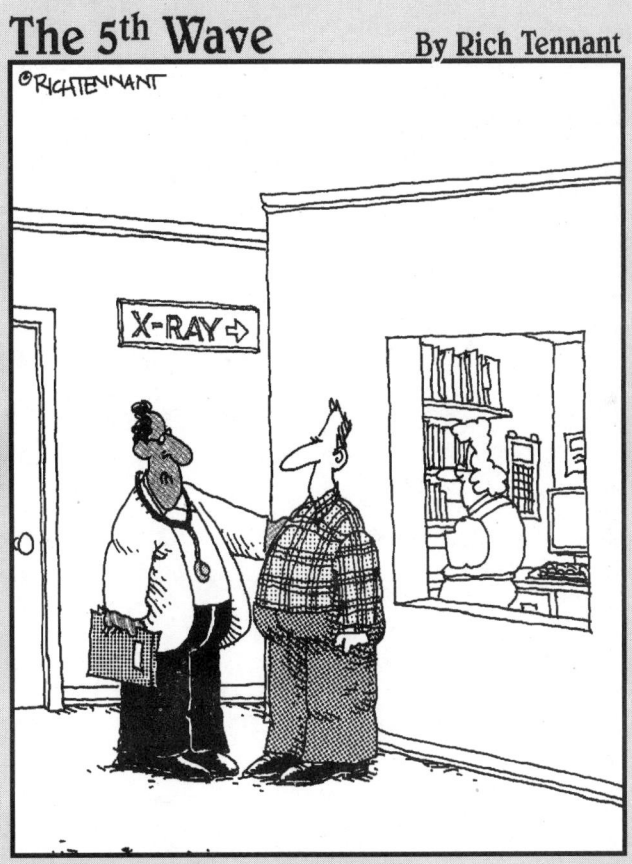

"I'd like you to see a specialist. A gentleman I take a self-defense class with is an oncologist. He'll ask you for your family's medical history, your present treatment, and for you to sneak up behind him and try to put him in a choke hold."

In this part . . .

This part is all about getting diagnosed with prostate cancer. When you have prostate cancer, you need good doctors on your side. In Chapter 5, I talk about the role of your primary care physician, who may be the one who flags prostate cancer in the first place. I also describe how prostate cancer is detected. The prostate specific antigen (PSA) blood test is one tool that doctors can use to help diagnose prostate cancer and monitor your progress after treatment. I discuss the PSA and how doctors use it in Chapter 5. I also talk about the rectal examination. This test is universally hated, but it's very important in diagnosing prostate cancer.

If you're diagnosed with prostate cancer, you'll need to consult with specialists, such as urologists, radiation oncologists, and medical oncologists. In Chapter 6, I describe what these doctors do. I also talk about the tests they may order. In Chapter 7, I tell you about the biopsy, a special test used to verify that cancer is present. In Chapter 8, I explain how doctors use the biopsy to classify how aggressive your cancer is. I also talk about a special grading system for prostate cancer — the Gleason grade — and cover other classification systems used to evaluate how bad the cancer is.

Chapter 5

Working with Your Doctor to Detect Prostate Cancer

* *

In This Chapter

▶ Relaying important medical information to your doctor

▶ Getting through the digital rectal exam

▶ Understanding the meaning and importance of the PSA test

▶ Keeping in contact with your primary care physician

* *

$\mathcal{B}$ecause prostate cancer frequently causes few symptoms — or no symptoms at all — it's often first detected by primary care physicians (PCP) during routine testing. Your doctor may discover a possible problem during your rectal examination or note red flags raised by the results of your prostate specific antigen (PSA) blood test. Because your primary care physician often plays such an important role in diagnosing your cancer, I focus this chapter on working with your physician and understanding the basic tests that primary care doctors perform to help diagnose prostate cancer.

Your primary care physician may be an *internist* (a physician who specializes in medical illnesses of the internal organs), a *family practitioner* (a generalist who treats routine medical problems that are found both inside and outside your body), or a *specialist* (a doctor who specializes in treating certain areas of the body; for example, a *urologist,* who focuses on treating diseases of the bladder, kidneys, testis, and prostate,, or an *oncologist,* who specializes in treating cancer — I discuss both specialties in Chapter 6). Some doctors (like me) specialize in *both* urology and oncology. No matter what type of doctor you see, be sure to get a routine rectal exam and a prostate specific antigen (PSA) blood test. If you're 50 years old or older, you need to have these tests once every year. (Some men who are younger than 50 also need to have annual PSA tests. See the section "Pondering the PSA," later in this chapter.)

Reporting Your Medical History to Your Doctor

To check your health and diagnose any medical problems that you may have, your doctor needs a basic understanding of you, including both the you of the past and the you of the present, to help ensure the healthy you of the future. (Getting a feel for your overall health is important whether you're seeing your usual primary care physician, whom you've known for years, or a specialist you're meeting for the first time.) Your doctor will ask many questions about past illnesses, your current physical status, and what medications, if any, you're currently taking. Your doctor also will ask some questions that you may consider very personal, such as "Do you consume alcohol, and if so, how much do you drink on an average day?" When you answer these questions, you provide your doctor with the information she needs to evaluate your general health as well as the results of your laboratory tests.

To receive the best medical analysis, answer your doctor's questions honestly. (The doctor is sworn to protect your confidentiality, sort of like your priest or rabbi.) If you hold back information, you'll be shortchanging yourself and others who care about you and want you to live as long as possible.

Asking about your past illnesses

With every physical examination, your doctor (or sometimes the nurse) should go over your medical history with you, in part by reviewing your past illnesses. A review of your general health and medical history is important, because medical problems that you experienced in the past can have a direct effect on the medical problems you're having right now.

Your body is made up of a series of systems (digestive, nervous, skin, urinary tract, and so on), as well as of many different organs within the systems, and all of these individual organs and systems come together to make up one person: you. And when one system or organ has a problem, it often has an effect on other parts of your body. Because your doctor understands the relationship between the different systems of your body, she may ask you questions about past illnesses to determine the causes for your current illness.

If anyone in your family has had prostate cancer, you should report this fact to your doctor when she reviews your medical history. Cancer isn't contagious, but it may be hereditary. If your father and brother had prostate cancer — and now you're age 50 and you're having urinary problems — you definitely need to be screened for prostate cancer.

Natural drugs are still drugs

Many people are under the false assumption that if drugs are natural, they're always automatically safe. Taking an herbal remedy is often essentially the same as taking a drug that your doctor prescribes. (Many medications prescribed by doctors are derived from plants and thus are essentially natural, as well.) Too many people assume that herbs, minerals, and other supplements are risk-free.

Ironically, sometimes people expect major results from herbs and supplements without the risk of any side effects. It doesn't work that way.

When you assume that supplements are inherently safe, and you purchase any vitamins or supplements whose labels purport to cure what ails you (whether you're having some difficulty urinating, or you want to lose weight, or you want to resolve a host of other common medical problems), you may be unwittingly jeopardizing your health.

I'm not saying that alternative remedies are inherently bad or that you should never use them. Alternative medicines may play a valuable preventive role in prostate cancer. I devote an entire chapter (Chapter 18) to discussing important alternative therapies for men diagnosed with prostate cancer. I also cover saw palmetto, an herb used to treat some prostate ailments (but not prostate cancer!), in Chapter 4. I just don't want you to automatically assume that herbs and supplements are always safe or effective. Be a skeptical consumer.

Inquiring how you're doing right now

How you're feeling right now is relevant, even if you're feeling just fine. But don't assume that you can't possibly have any medical problems just because you don't have any symptoms. Prostate cancer usually doesn't come with early symptoms, just as some other diseases are symptomless (such as kidney disease, which may not cause problems in the early stages but can often be detected by testing the creatinine level in your blood or urine). It sounds weird, but you can feel just fine as prostate cancer cells insidiously multiply inside your prostate gland.

Even if you're experiencing a problem that seems pretty minor, report it to your doctor and let her decide if it's significant. For example, if you have any problems with urination, be sure to tell your doctor, whether the problem is frequent urination, a slow stream, trouble with stopping and starting, pain with urination, or all of the above. Make sure that you report even minor urinary problems that continue, because they may be indicators of a developing serious medical problem. Your doctor can treat medical problems in the initial stages of development easier than she can treat them in the full-blown stages.

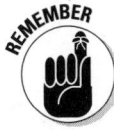

Of course, your urine stream won't be as powerful at age 55 as it was when you were a young man of 20. If you're nearing middle age, you probably can't write your name in the snow like you could when you were younger. In fact, you may even have trouble hitting the top of your shoes! (It may sound gross, but nearly every man has done something like this at some point.) You shouldn't worry if your stream is less powerful than it was when you were a teenager. You don't need to feel like you're a very sick man who must have cancer! Instead, your weak stream may be the result of normal aging or, if it's a medical problem, something else altogether (such as benign prostatic hyperplasia, which is described in more detail in Chapter 4). But a weak urine stream is important information that your doctor needs to know about. So make sure that you tell her about it.

Discussing medications you take

In order to get the best advantage of that medical brain your doctor has, you need to report any drugs you're currently taking. Be sure to leave nothing out! If you're taking any of the following types of medications, tell your doctor:

- **Prescribed medications:** The prescription medications you take can interact with medications that the doctor may wish to prescribe for you in the event that you have a bladder infection, *prostatitis* (an inflammation of the prostate, described in detail in Chapter 4), or another medical problem. In fact, sometimes the medications you're currently taking are not the best ones for you anymore. Your primary care physician should reevaluate your medications at least once a year. If she doesn't do this, remind her to do so. If you see any other doctors, they will also need to know what drugs you take.

- **Over-the-counter drugs:** If you're like most people, you may think that the over-the-counter drugs you take don't actually count as medicine. So when you report to your doctor the drugs you're taking, you may forget about the acetaminophen or ibuprofen (over-the-counter pain relievers) you take frequently, the heartburn medicine you take almost everyday, or the laxative you take periodically. Yet these are important omissions; for example, constantly taking acetaminophen can hurt your liver. And if you're taking heartburn drugs everyday, you may have a digestive disorder that your doctor should treat before it gets worse and causes serious damage.

- **Alternative or natural remedies:** Natural remedies can boost or diminish the effect of other drugs you're taking. For example, if you're taking the blood thinner Coumadin (generic name: warfarin), you should never take gingko biloba, a natural blood thinner. Some people have nearly bled to death because they didn't tell their surgeons that they were taking herbal remedies such as gingko biloba. Also, some natural remedies may be harmful to you, depending on the diseases and medical conditions you may currently have. Finally, you should report all natural drugs you're taking, because you may be taking herbs or supplements in an attempt to treat a condition that you really should see your doctor about.

Always tell any new doctor about any drug allergies you may have, such as an allergy to penicillin, sulfa, or any other drug. Allergies can affect what medication your doctor will consider prescribing for you. It can't hurt to remind your regular doctor about any drug allergies, as well, especially when he's preparing to write you a prescription for a medication you haven't taken before.

When you see a doctor for the first time, bring a printed list of all your medications, along with the dosages. If you don't have time to make such a list, put all your medicines in a bag and bring them with you.

Volunteering important info when the doctor doesn't ask

Be sure to volunteer important information even if, for some reason, your doctor doesn't ask you for it. Jot down some notes ahead of time, and refer to these notes when you see your doctor. Don't bring a scroll of complaints to discuss. Narrow your list down to three or four key issues or problems, if at all possible.

Here are some examples of information to volunteer during a physical examination:

- ✔ Symptoms pertaining to the urinary tract (pain, difficulty, frequency, or any other trouble with urination)

- ✔ Significant changes in your weight (such as a weight loss or gain of more than ten pounds when you haven't been trying to gain or lose weight)

- ✔ Changes in your overall sleep habits or energy levels (The problem may be that you're overworking, but it's also possible that a medical problem may be impairing your sleep or draining your strength.)

- ✔ Instances of cancer in your family (especially your parents and siblings)

- ✔ Any pain you have, especially significant pain that's getting worse (When prostate cancer spreads, it mostly goes to the bone. In rare cases, the first sign of prostate cancer can be bone pain.)

The Digital Rectal Exam: You Can Get Through It

After you discuss your medical history and current medical status, your doctor may want to perform a digital rectal exam. In general, rectal examinations are performed annually. (Most men should have rectal exams once a year after age 50.)

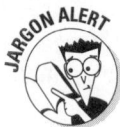

The *digital rectal examination* (DRE) is just one aspect of a complete physical examination; it takes a maximum of 15 seconds to perform. The DRE is a physical examination of your rectal area and prostate gland. When your doctor performs this test, he looks for any deviations from the way your prostate should normally feel, which is fairly smooth and pliant. Of course, just because your prostate feels strange to your doctor, it *doesn't* automatically mean that you must have prostate cancer. What it does mean is that you'll need some further testing and evaluation.

Some men actually avoid having routine physical examinations specifically because they hate the digital rectal examination. Other men try to talk their doctors into skipping that part of the exam altogether. Don't make this mistake. The rectal exam is sometimes the first step in diagnosing prostate cancer. If you have prostate cancer, the exam can help you obtain the treatment you need to combat the problem effectively. Yes, a rectal exam can be embarrassing, annoying, and slightly uncomfortable, but it can also save your life.

Understanding how the DRE is performed

Doctors perform digital rectal examinations in a variety of ways. Some doctors have you stand up, spread your legs, bend over, and lean against the examining table. Others have you lie on your side on the examination table. Still others have you get up on the table on your elbows and knees. Your doctor will ask you to assume a position that he finds works best for the exam — try to work with him on this one.

The doctor uses a lubricated gloved finger to probe the area for possible problems. (Check out Figure 5-1 to see how the rectal exam is performed.) When he performs the exam, you may feel brief, slightly cold pressure in the area of your prostate. The doctor feels for bumps and lumps that shouldn't be there. Suspicious bumps and lumps can tell him if you have a problem that should be evaluated further.

For the best and fastest results with a rectal examination, make sure that you don't tense up your body. Of course, it isn't easy to relax when your doctor is probing a private part of your body. But the more your body tenses up, and the more you think about how awful and aggravating the procedure is going to be (or about whether the exam is ever going to end), the harder you make it on yourself, and the longer the exam will last. If you can relax and concentrate on other things for the short period of time necessary to perform the rectal exam, you'll feel better, and you'll make it easier for the doc to do his thing and get it over with.

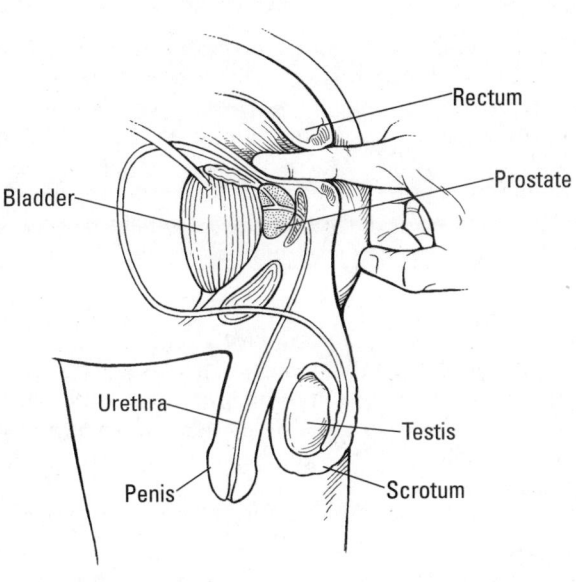

Figure 5-1:
The digital rectal examination. This drawing shows the relationship of the prostate to other nearby organs, as well as how the doctor's gloved finger can probe the prostate through the rectum.

Rectum

Prostate

Bladder

Urethra

Testis

Penis

Scrotum

Usually, the more rectal exams a doctor has performed, the better he is at doing them fast and efficiently with little discomfort. Of course, if you have a problem in Prostate Land (especially a raging infection), the exam may hurt some, even if you have the most talented doctor on the planet. (This does *not* mean that if the rectal exam hurts you, you must invariably have a major problem. Sometimes it hurts a little, and you're still just fine. The problem may be that you unconsciously tightened up your muscles, even though you tried to relax them.)

If your doctor thinks that your prostate may be infected, he'll press on it during the rectal exam, which can hurt a bit. The doctor may press long enough to generate some prostatic fluid, which will come out of the tip of your penis. This fluid is checked for infection, either under the microscope or in a culture.

Prostatic fluid is a substance produced by the prostate to nourish sperm; it also helps sperm move along faster. (Sperm are sluggish critters without prostatic fluid.) The prostatic fluid and the sperm mix together just before orgasm and ejaculation. (You can read more about the anatomy of the prostate in Chapter 2.)

Interpreting the results of your DRE

Your doctor may suspect the presence of prostate cancer based on the findings from your digital rectal examination. When cancer is present, the prostate gland may feel different than normal. It may feel uneven, lumpy, or bumpy, rather than its normal smooth self. If your doctor has performed rectal exams on you before, he has a general feel for what your prostate usually feels like and can tell if something is potentially wrong. If your doctor detects any deviations, he may refer you to a specialist (usually a urologist) for further evaluation. (I discuss working with a specialist in Chapter 6.)

If your doctor feels some lumps or bumps on your prostate, it doesn't necessarily mean that you have cancer. Your doctor won't know if it's cancer for sure until a biopsy test confirms that cancer is present. (I discuss biopsies in Chapter 7.) The lumps may be a result of prostatitis or some other problem, so don't panic if your primary care doctor sends you to a urologist for a further check of your prostate gland. Be glad, instead, that your doctor is looking out for your best health interests.

Pondering the PSA

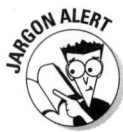

All men who are 50 years old and older, as well as all men who are 40 (or older) and at risk for cancer (such as black men or men who have a family history of cancer), should have an annual PSA test, along with a rectal exam, as part of their routine physical exam. The PSA test (a relatively painless blood test) helps your doctor identify the possible presence of prostate cancer by checking for *prostate specific antigen* (a protein substance produced by the prostate gland), which is present in high levels in many people who have prostate cancer. I consider the PSA test to be as important a screening device for detecting prostate cancer among men as the mammogram is for detecting breast cancer among women.

The only thing you may need to do to prepare for the PSA test is to avoid engaging in sexual activities 24 hours before the test. Intercourse or other sexual acts as well as bicycling may artificially raise your levels of PSA, giving you a flawed test result. Because this effect is so rare, I don't offer this precaution during the first test. Instead, I discuss it with patients before a second test if the results of the first test are elevated.

Deciphering the results

PSA levels can be anywhere from zero to a thousand or more. But generally, in men who still have their prostate gland, a normal value is considered to be 4 nanograms per milliliter or lower.

PSA: How it became a screening tool

Prostate specific antigen (PSA) was first discovered in the 1970s by several researchers in Japan and the United States. It wasn't actually named until 1979, when Dr. Ming Wang described PSA in an article in *Investigative Urology*. In 1980, Dr. Wang and his colleague, Lawrence Papsidero, created a blood test for PSA. The Food and Drug Administration (FDA) began approving PSA blood tests in 1985.

The test was initially approved for (and was most useful for) determining whether anti-cancer therapies were working in men who already were being treated for prostate cancer. My colleagues and I were fortunate enough to be very involved in some of these early studies. In 1990 and 1991, several groups, including mine, discovered and published that PSA was also effective at screening and diagnosis. The most comprehensive and well-documented paper on the topic, "Measurement of Prostate-Specific Antigen in Serum as a Screening Test for Prostate Cancer," was published by Dr. William Catalona and his colleagues in the April 25, 1991, issue of the *New England Journal of Medicine*. Today, PSA is the definitive test for detecting early prostate cancer in the United States and other countries.

Your PSA levels may affect whether the doctor chooses to order a biopsy. Even if your prostate feels okay to your doctor during your rectal exam, he may still order a biopsy if he considers your PSA level to be high. Because some men with PSA levels under 4 have prostate cancer, some doctors argue that the normal level of PSA (and the point at which doctors should consider doing biopsies of the prostate) should be *lowered* to 2.5 or 3 so that even more cases of cancer can be caught before they advance further.

Your doctor may also take into account your *PSA velocity,* which is how fast your PSA levels go up. If your PSA level was 1 last year, and now it's 2.4, your doctor has cause for concern, and more frequent testing (and even a biopsy) may be advised. To determine the frequency of the screening needed to diagnose prostate cancer, your doctor may consider the size of your prostate gland compared to your PSA level. This comparison is called *PSA density.* Generally, a high PSA level in a man with a small prostate is more disturbing than the same PSA level in a man with a large prostate.

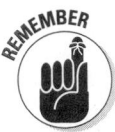

An above-normal PSA test result may indicate cancer. It may also indicate prostatitis or benign prostatic hyperplasia. (I describe both of these prostate illnesses in Chapter 4.) Frequently, above-normal PSA tests indicate "none of the above." Men can be healthy and well despite an elevated PSA.

Reviewing reliability issues

The PSA test isn't foolproof. Men with high scores (4 nanograms per milliliter or higher) don't necessarily have cancer. On the other hand, men whose scores are below the cutoff level of 4, and who would generally be screened as normal by their doctors, may actually have prostate cancer. Despite these drawbacks, the PSA is an extremely effective test that can help save lives.

Virtually any laboratory can perform a PSA test, but some labs are more efficient and careful than others. If you have a blood test, and your blood is then split up and placed into three separate vials and sent to three different laboratories, it's possible that you may receive three slightly different PSA measurements. For this reason, your doctor will order a recheck of your blood, particularly if you have an elevated PSA level, to rule out any possible lab errors. If you or your doctor is very concerned about lab error, you may wish to have your PSA level evaluated at a different laboratory than you normally use or even at the hospital, where the equipment is usually checked more carefully than at a standard lab. Also, for the second test, I recommend that you abstain from sexual activity and bike riding 24 hours before the test, because these activities may occasionally raise your level of PSA.

A note about testing frequency

The American Cancer Society and the American Urological Society agree with my recommendation for annual PSA tests. However, some organizations, such as the American Academy of Family Physicians, question whether annual screenings are a good idea and worry that too many unnecessary biopsies may be performed if all men ages 50 and older are screened with PSAs. The basis for this concern is that the test isn't foolproof. In fact, if your PSA is mildly elevated (between 4 and 10), chances are that you don't have prostate cancer (about 70 percent of the time). In addition, long-term studies showing whether PSA screening saves lives have not yet been completed. Thus, some experts worry that PSA testing is a waste of money. However, I strongly believe that the price of the extra biopsies is well worth it. PSA tests can help identify men with prostate cancer and save lives. One qualifier: Testing and aggressive treatment may not be a good idea if a man has less than a ten-year life expectancy because he's very elderly or he's in poor medical shape. Prostate cancer often grows slowly, so a less aggressive approach is probably okay in this circumstance.

Looking at Other Lab Work

Your primary care doctor may also request general laboratory tests to go along with the rectal exam and PSA test. For example, he may want to request

Excluding a few good men from PSA testing

Some researchers believe that some men can be excluded from annual PSA testing (getting tested less frequently), especially if they have very low PSA levels. A study released by the National Cancer Institute in 2002 (the Prostate, Lung, Colorectal and Ovarian [PLCO] trial) followed the PSAs of about 30,000 men, noting changes in their PSA levels. Of the men who still had their prostates and whose PSA was at a very low level (between 0 to 1 nanograms per milliliter or ng/ml), 98.7 percent continued to have PSA levels at or below 4 for the next four years.

However, with the men whose initial PSAs were higher than 1 ng/ml, the risk of their PSA levels rising over time was higher than among those whose PSAs were 1 or less. This was especially true for men with PSAs of 3 to 4 ng/ml; 24 percent of them showed higher readings a year later, and 83 percent showed elevated readings within the next four years. (How many of these men had prostate cancer, prostatitis, or another prostate ailment is unknown.)

These results confirm that you should be monitored every year if your PSA level is 3 or above, and that you should probably also be monitored annually if your PSA level is 2 or above. However, because a large number of men have PSA levels that are less than 2, doctors may want to consider doing the test less often in these men.

a *complete blood count (CBC),* a determination of the number of white and red blood cells in your blood, or a *blood urea nitrogen (BUN)* test, a blood test that may be abnormal in the presence of prostate cancer blocking the urine flow. The doctor may also order a urinalysis or urine culture to check your urine for possible infection. These tests aren't markers for cancer, but they're important because they can provide your doctor with information on your overall health.

Some doctors may also order a blood test of your prostatic acid phosphatase (PAP), which is a tumor marker, because elevated levels of PAP are sometimes found in men with prostate cancer. However, the PSA is a far more effective and targeted test for prostate cancer.

Keeping in Touch with Your PCP

Although you need to consult with one or more medical specialists to discover whether you have prostate cancer (and to receive treatment if cancer is discovered), you still need to keep in touch with your primary care physician. Here are several key reasons why your primary care physician needs to stay active on your healthcare team:

> ✔ Your primary care physician tracks all your health problems and acts as a sort of program manager of your health. Other specialists concentrate on specific problems, such as prostate cancer, kidney disease, and so

on. (You don't get a free pass that exempts you from other health problems if you have cancer, even though it seems like you should.)

✔ You may need authorization from your primary care physician to obtain services from specialists. (Your HMO may require advance permission from your primary doctor before authorizing payment for you to see another doctor or have a specific treatment.)

✔ Your primary care physician usually manages your medications, ensuring that you won't experience any interactions from drugs that don't go well together.

If Cancer Isn't Found

If your prostate gland feels completely normal during a rectal examination, and your other tests, such as the PSA, are within the normal range, you may proceed to thank the fates or your god that you're still okay. But remember, get tested again a year from now! Things can change, and some cancers, especially if they're small, can be missed. You want to catch any problems in the early stages, when it's far easier for your doctor to treat the problem.

Free PSA will cost you

The *free PSA* test is another tumor marker. It's newer than the regular PSA test. Free PSA is a special version of PSA; specifically, it's the inactive form of the antigen. Doctors still rely on the regular PSA test to screen patients for prostate cancer, but free PSA can provide extra help to doctors, especially if they have any question about whether another biopsy should be performed. The free PSA test costs around $65 or more (depending on the lab) — about twice the cost of a regular PSA. (The term *free* obviously doesn't refer to the test itself!)

With regular PSA tests, low scores are good. A score below 4 is desirable, and a score below 2 is even better. However, when it comes to free PSA, the value is expressed as the free PSA divided by the total PSA, and a low percentage score is bad. Generally, scores of 20 percent and above are considered good, while scores of 15 percent and below mean the chances of cancer are higher.

Chapter 6

Diagnosing and Treating Prostate Cancer with the Help of Specialists

. . . .

In This Chapter

▶ Considering the different types of cancer specialists

▶ Finding the right specialist for you

▶ Asking smart questions

▶ Understanding the tests your specialist may order

. . . .

Maybe you've never needed a medical specialist, because your family doctor was able to treat everything that ailed you. But when your primary care physician suspects that you have prostate cancer, you need to see specialists who are skilled at treating the problem.

In this chapter, I talk about how to find a good specialist and, after you've found him or her, what questions to ask. I also cover important tests that specialists may order, such as the bone scan, the ultrasound, and the cystoscopy. I also briefly cover the biopsy, which I describe in more detail in Chapter 7.

Getting the Gist of Urologists and Oncologists

Because your primary care physician usually can't diagnose and treat prostate cancer, you need to see other medical specialists, including a urologist, and maybe an oncologist, too. (Sometimes urologists can provide all the treatment you may need, as a "one-stop shop," and sometimes they can't.)

Urologists

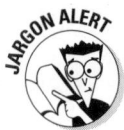

If your primary care physician suspects that you have prostate cancer, his first course of action is to refer you to a urologist for a definite diagnosis. *Urologists* are medical doctors that specialize in treating problems associated with the *genitourinary tract,* which includes the kidney, bladder, prostate gland, penis, and testicles. Most urologists are generalists who treat many different diseases of the genitourinary tract, while some urologists subspecialize in a variety of areas, such as urologic oncology, where almost all of their practice is treating genitourinary cancers, including prostate, bladder, kidney and testis cancer. Urologists are also surgeons, and they can perform such operations as the *radical prostatectomy* (surgical removal of the prostate gland; see Chapter 11).

If your urologist thinks that your prostate feels somewhat (or a lot) abnormal, or if your prostate specific antigen (PSA) test shows that the levels of PSA in your blood are higher than normal, he may decide to perform a *biopsy,* which is a removal of tissue to check for the presence of cancer. If the biopsy comes back positive for cancer, the urologist then will tell you how serious the cancer is, based on the staging and grading of the cancer (which I discuss in Chapter 8). The urologist will also discuss treatment options with you. If you decide upon surgery or hormone therapy, the urologist you're seeing will likely treat you (unless you decide that you want to see another urologist). If you decide on radiation therapy, the urologist will refer you to a radiation therapist. If you need chemotherapy, the urologist will recommend a medical oncologist.

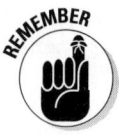

All urologists are not created equal. Some urologists are very talented doctors who are up on the latest medical knowledge and surgical techniques, while others may not keep up with the latest info. It's important to find a urologist who meets your needs. I discuss how to find the best one for you later in this chapter.

Oncologists

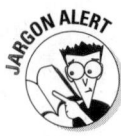

An *oncologist* is a doctor who specializes in treating patients who have cancer. *Radiation oncologists* treat cancer with radiation therapy, and *medical oncologists* treat cancer with chemotherapy. *Urologic oncologists* are urologists who subspecialize in treating cancer, but many urologists are generalists who treat all diseases of the genitourinary system, including cancer. If you're diagnosed with prostate cancer, you'll be treated by a urologist and possibly by one or more oncologists.

Oncology can be divided into further subdivisions.

✔ Urologic oncologists are urologists who, with extra training and experience, subspecialize in treating urologic cancers, such as prostate cancer, bladder cancer, kidney cancer, and testicular cancer. These subspecialists usually work in academic medical centers and perform research. Genitourinary cancer is a very important part of the education and qualification requirements for all urologists, including generalists.

✔ Radiation oncologists are concerned with taking care of *localized cancer* (cancer that hasn't spread from the prostate gland) if surgery isn't the plan. They use radiation to destroy cancer (a pleasing thought to anyone with cancer), when it's first diagnosed. They know exactly how much radiation is required to kill the cancer, and where and when to apply it for the best effect. Radiation oncologists also treat cancer that's spread to the bone, helping stop pain. (See Chapter 12 for more information about radiation therapy.)

✔ Medical oncologists are doctors who treat cancer with medicine. As do urologists, sometimes medical oncologists treat patients when *hormone treatment* is needed (a treatment that is often used to fool your body into making less testosterone; testosterone can make cancer grow faster). If hormone treatment is tried and fails, a medical oncologist may treat your cancer with cancer cell-killing drugs, a form of treatment that's referred to as *chemotherapy* (discussed in Chapter 15). Medical oncologists are specially trained to administer chemotherapy, and urologists usually don't give chemotherapy to patients.

Sometimes medical oncologists talk to patients when they're first diagnosed (to help them decide what treatment to select), because medical oncologists usually aren't involved in the primary treatment (radiation or surgery), and, consequently, they may be less biased toward one therapy or another.

Finding a Good Specialist

If you ever need a truly excellent doctor, it's now, when you are in the process of being diagnosed with prostate cancer. You need the best specialists you can find to advise you on possible treatments as well as to provide those treatments. Your regular primary care physican may refer you to a specialist, or you may locate a specialist on your own by networking with friends and family or researching specialists online.

Keeping a few things in mind

As you prepare to undergo the process to determine whether you have prostate cancer, hold the following thoughts in the forefront of your brain:

✔ Don't choose a specialist in the heat of a panic, fearing that your days are numbered because you have (or fear that you have) prostate cancer. Take at least several weeks to make sure you're selecting a really good doctor.

✔ Work with a specialist you feel comfortable with. If your specialist makes you feel uncomfortable, because he seems indifferent to you, won't answer your questions, or just somehow feels wrong to you, find another doctor. The doctor shouldn't have to be your new best friend, but he should be someone you feel that you can trust.

✔ Try to work with specialists who are in your health insurance company's network. When doctors are in the network, they're on the insurance company's approved list of doctors, and most of the bill will be taken care of by your health insurance. Another added bonus of choosing an in-network specialist is that most insurance companies check out the doctors that they cover and hold them to strict standards. Insurance companies have access to information about physicians that you would have a hard time obtaining on your own, such as information about malpractice lawsuits.

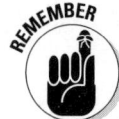

However, not being on some list doesn't necessarily mean a doctor is bad. Sometimes it's worth it to go out of network, especially if you want special expertise, such as a surgeon who reliably performs nerve-sparing prostate surgery that may preserve your sexual potency. (Read more about this procedure in Chapter 11.)

✔ When you're considering two different doctors, make appointments to see both of them. That way, if Dr. Admirable, the first doctor you see, is great, and you decide you really want him to treat you, you can always cancel your appointment with Dr. Braveheart.

✔ You may want to travel to see what people consider one of the best urologists in the business. If you have the means and feel you'd get the best from Dr. Faraway, then go with him. But realize that you usually see Dr. Faraway for a consultation before surgery and when you have the surgery, but you need to see a local urologist for follow-up care after surgery or other treatments.

Don't assume that all the best doctors are out of state — you may have excellent physicians in your very own backyard. It's also wise to pick your doctor not only on the basis of the doctor's reputation but also on how comfortable you feel with him. Just because a urologist is famous doesn't make him the right one for you.

✔ If you choose a surgeon because he's performed hundreds of prostatectomies, and you're seeking his experience, make sure he *knows* that you expect *him* to perform your surgery. Some men have automatically assumed that the urologist they consulted with in an appointment is the same one who's going to perform the surgery. To their later dismay, they found out that the first doctor handed the job off to another doctor, and, in some cases, the original doctor wasn't even present during the surgery.

✔ If you're diagnosed with prostate cancer, consider taking a day or two off from work to concentrate on gathering information on the illness and available specialists. (Ask your partner to help, too, but don't expect your loved one to do all your research.) Write down information you gather — it's easy to forget who said what, when, and where.

Receiving a referral from your doctor

Your primary care physician may be able to refer you to the best specialists in your area for diagnosing and treating prostate cancer. Nearly all urologists are very good at performing biopsies of the prostate. You don't need to shop around for a doc to do your biopsy. When it comes to choosing the doctor who performs the treatment, however, you need to decide whether to go with the urologist who performed your biopsy or to find a more experienced and well-known specialist. Your primary care doctor may be able to make a recommendation. In addition, the urologist who did your biopsy may be very well-versed in doing nerve-sparing surgery, and if not, may be able to recommend another urological specialist in the area who does nerve-sparing surgery well.

Networking

Your primary care doctor usually knows the names of reputable urologists or oncologists in your local area. If he doesn't, or if you want to go beyond your local area to find a specialist, or you want your specialist to be located in a bigger hospital, you may need to find your own urologist or oncologist. You can network by asking your friends, family members, and acquaintances if they know of any good doctors for treating prostate cancer.

When you network to find a specialist, friends and family give you their open opinions (the key advantage of networking). On the other hand, everyone has their own biases (the key disadvantage of networking). Some patients may blame a negative outcome on the doctor rather than the disease — for example, the patient's cancer may have been advanced, and no doctor could have prevented incontinence. Keep your skeptical ears open as you ask for recommendations.

Also, don't be afraid to ask all the doctors you've ever consulted for any reason (and ask your partner to ask her doctors) what urologist or oncologist they'd see if they or someone in their family had prostate cancer. (You can even contact health professionals, such as dentists and optometrists, and ask for recommendations.) If you need a radiation oncologist, ask for a recommendation from any radiologists or x-ray technicians you may know.

TIP

Faxing and e-mailing for referrals

It can be hard to reach busy doctors, but when you need a recommendation for a specialist to treat cancer, you can't wait months and months. You probably don't want to make an appointment to see various doctors merely to ask them for the names of urologists or oncologists. You can call, but you may be worried that if you call a doctor's office, the doc will never get the message (a valid fear).

What can you do? Consider faxing your doctor a note requesting a recommendation for a specialist. Most doctor's offices will give you the doctor's fax number. Or you can take a twenty-first century approach and e-mail doctors you already know, asking them to reply with specialist recommendations. (You can often find e-mail addresses through a doctor's Web site — if she has one — or you can call the office and ask the receptionist for the doctor's business e-mail address.)

Keep your note brief (a few paragraphs), and include your name, phone number, and fax number along with your message so that the doctor can either reply directly or designate someone in his office (usually one of the nurses) to reply with recommendations. Doctors are usually extremely busy, so don't expect a reply that same day — you'll probably hear something within a week or so. (After a week, you can try faxing the note again, or you can move on to other doctors.)

Searching academic centers

Many men search for doctors at academic centers. A majority of urologists who subspecialize in genitourinary cancer work at these centers. An advantage of an academic training center is that usually you can find all the highly trained specialists you might need (not only urologic oncologists, but also medical oncologists and radiation oncologists) gathered together in one place. Still, most urologists who work outside academic centers are well-trained and excellent physicians, and although they practice more general urology, they know a lot about taking care of men with prostate cancer. Many men go to academic centers to get a second opinion, and then they go back to their original urologist, reassured that they are in good hands, and relieved that they can get good care closer to their homes.

Surfing your way to a specialist

In today's high-tech world, one good way to identify a specialist is to do some research over the Internet. You can find physicians online, or you can find information about doctors who have been recommended to you. If you don't know how to use the Internet, ask a friend who's adept at using computers. Or ask your local public or university reference librarian to help you.

To find out if a doctor has a Web site, use a search engine (such as www.google.com) to search by the doctor's name, specialty, and city and state. If the doctor has a Web site, the site probably has a "contact us" icon to click on, enabling you to e-mail him. The site may list the doctor's fax number, as well. Some doctors are great about replying to e-mail, while others may ignore it completely. So e-mail the doctor a brief note *and* fax him.

You may be very impressed by a physician's Web site, but a great-looking Web site doesn't automatically mean that the doctor is the best one for you. (It doesn't cost much to hire someone to create a dazzling site.) Be skeptical. Also, make sure that the doctor provides his own personal results with potency and incontinence on his Web site. If he does nerve-sparing prostatectomies, and he doesn't have results that are equal to or better than 40 to 50 percent potency, cross him off your list. If he claims results with incontinence, he should have at least a 90 to 95 percent success rate. Of course, Dr. Internet could be lying or exaggerating. How could you tell? That's a hard one! One good clue is that the doctor has published his results in reputable journals, which should also be noted on the site.

What's Up, Doc? Questions to Ask When Considering a Specialist

Whether the doctor you're considering is a urologist or an oncologist, it's a very good idea to ask him some basic questions in person before signing up. Some men who've had prostate cancer say that they wish they would've asked more questions before agreeing to treatment, because they believe that a more experienced doctor might have preserved their sexual potency or provided them with better treatment. Learn from their mistakes and ask questions. You're making a pivotal decision, because the treatments the doctor provides will have a significant effect on your life — hopefully, a significantly positive effect!

You generally need to make an appointment to see the doctor and ask her questions, and you have to pay an office visit fee, but it's usually well worth it.

Here are some questions to consider when talking to a urologist, radiation oncologist, or medical oncologist, as well as any other specialists you communicate with:

> ✔ **Have you treated many cases of prostate cancer?** This question is more tactful than asking directly how many cases of cancer the doctor has treated. But you may prefer the direct approach, and that's okay, too.

The answer will usually generate a number (such as, "I've treated over a thousand cases since 1990") or some other answer. Seek someone with experience. If the doctor is a surgeon, he should perform at least 15 prostatectomies a year and have several hundred or more under his belt.

- ✔ **About what percentage of your prostate cancer patients are around my age?** This is important, because if you're 50 years old, for example, and nearly all the doctor's patients have been older than 70, he may be less knowledgeable about preserving your sexual potency or your urinary continence than a doctor who treats patients closer to your age.

- ✔ **What are the possible side effects of the specific treatments you recommend?** The doctor should talk to you about possible problems with impotence, mood swings, and other side effects. If the doctor waves away your questions or tells you to ask the nurse to explain everything, he's not the right doctor for you.

- ✔ **What is your success rate with the preservation of potency and continence?** If he cites "the literature," tell him that you want to know about his results, not the general results for all doctors.

- ✔ **Do you see prostate cancer as a treatable illness?** The answer should at least be a qualified "yes," because you want to be treated by a doctor who's going to fight for you, even if your case is a difficult one. Of course, you need to accept what he tells you, as well.

Talking Effectively with Your Specialist

When you find a specialist you want to work with, it's vitally important that you understand what the doctor proposes to do, as well as what he wants *you* to do, and that you feel comfortable conveying concerns and questions to him. You need to establish a basic trust level and feel confident enough to ask the doctor about worrisome issues.

You, like many people, may fear that you're "bothering" the doctor when you ask him questions. Or you may worry that the doctor will think that you're stupid or annoying if you ask questions. This is rarely true! To communicate effectively with your doctor, follow these basic hints:

- ✔ If you don't understand what your doctor says, don't say that you do. If possible, rephrase what you think he said, and then ask if you understand him correctly. ("Doctor Digital, you're saying that I need to lose weight before surgery, correct? If so, how much weight, and how fast do I need to lose it?")

- ✔ If you really don't get anything that your doctor says, ask him to explain it again, but in very simple (non-doctorish) terms. It's also a good idea to ask him to explain any words or phrases that you don't understand.

- ✔ Tell your doctor that you're upset, and it's hard for you to grasp what he's saying (assuming this is true). Ask if he can explain it again at your next appointment.

- ✔ Bring your partner or a friend with you when the doctor explains his treatment plan. They may be upset, because they care about you, but they'll probably be able to listen better than you can.

- ✔ Take notes when your doctor talks to you. Then ask him about any points that are unclear to you.

- ✔ Ask your most important questions first. Don't ask major questions last, when the doctor is walking out the door to see other patients.

- ✔ When you start your treatment, be sure to tell your doctor if you have problems. Listen carefully to his suggestions on how to resolve them.

Testing, Testing! Important Tests the Specialist May Order

To help determine whether you have cancer, and if so, how bad it may be, the specialist may order a variety of important tests, including a blood tests, a rectal examination, an ultrasound, and a biopsy. If you have prostate cancer, you may have a bone scan and/or a computerized tomography (CT) scan or magnetic resonance imaging (MRI) scan. You may also have a cystoscopy. I cover all of these tests in this section. I also provide a brief description of the biopsy, another test that's used to detect cancer. (You can read more about biopsies in Chapter 7.)

PSA and rectal examinations

When you go to Dr. Specialist, he may order or reorder a PSA blood test. Don't be upset if you already had a PSA test; often, rechecking the PSA is a good way to double-check your condition. The specialist may also perform a rectal examination even if your primary care physician has already performed one. The specialist really needs to feel the prostate for himself so that he can give you the best advice and care possible.

Utilizing the ultrasound

If you're going to a specialist to see if you have prostate cancer, and the PSA test and/or rectal examination suggests a possible problem, the doctor will probably want to do an ultrasound examination to get a better impression of your cancer.

The *ultrasound* test uses sound waves to form images of your internal organs. The specialist may use an ultrasound probe, called a transrectal ultrasonography (TRUS), to perform an internal ultrasound to check for prostate cancer. By gently inserting the TRUS into your rectum, your doctor may identify potential sites of cancer. He can then take tissue samples (biopsies) from these suspicious areas and from other areas of your prostate.

Briefly regarding the biopsy

A *biopsy* is a tissue sample that's taken from the body and analyzed to determine whether a person has cancer. Specialists may want to administer a biopsy test if the PSA test and the digital rectal examination suggest a possible problem.

In the case of prostate cancer, the tissue samples are extracted from the prostate gland and then examined by a *pathologist,* a doctor who's an expert at identifying cancer and how serious it is. *Staging,* the process by which physicians determine how advanced the cancer is, helps doctors determine what treatment to recommend. Read more about the staging of cancer in Chapter 8.

Boning up on scans

If prostate cancer migrates beyond the localized area of the prostate gland, as it often does with advanced cases, it usually spreads to the bones. In fact, prostate cancer, more than any other form of cancer, is likely to invade the bones if its progression isn't halted and confined to the prostate, either with surgery, radiation treatments, or hormone shots (treatments I discuss in Part III). Doctors often use bone, CT, and MRI scans to determine if cancer has spread to your bones.

Bone scans

Doctors differ on when to order a bone scan. Some doctors order a scan in almost all of their patients who have prostate cancer, while other doctors only order a scan when they think that the prostate cancer may be advanced. So don't worry if your doctor orders a bone scan: It doesn't necessarily mean that you have an advanced case of cancer.

When the doctor performs a bone scan, which usually lasts about a half-hour or so, several hours before you have the procedure, the doctor will inject a radioactive fluid into your arm vein. This fluid bathes the bones so that he can check them for cancer. This radioactivity is virtually harmless and quickly passes from your body once it has done its job. If the cancer has invaded your bones, this cancer is usually found in your ribs, pelvis, or your spine. With a bone scan, the *nuclear medicine specialist* (a doctor who's an expert at performing and reading a variety of tests that involve radioactive materials) takes pictures of you as the radioactive fluid passes through your body. If cancer is present, the fluid acts as a sort of visual Geiger counter. When cancer has invaded the bone, it leaves a characteristic "signature" on the bone scan in the form of a dark lesion.

If your doctor schedules you for a bone scan, he may encourage you to drink plenty of fluid before the outpatient procedure. He may also encourage you to drink a lot of fluid after the procedure, to wash out the radioactive tracer that is injected.

CT and MRI scans

If the doctor sees an indicator (like the dark lesion) on the bone scan, he may decide that it means the cancer has spread to your bones and he will recommend treatments for advanced bone cancer. However, he may decide that the spots on the bone scan need further investigation, because sometimes bone scan spots just mean that you have some arthritis in that area or an old injury. In this situation, the doctor may order a CT scan or an MRI for further clarification, because these scans can often tell if the bone scan lesion is arthritis rather than cancer (although you may still have prostate cancer in the prostate). CT and MRI scans are also used to determine if the cancer has spread to the pelvic and/or the abdominal lymph nodes. The doctor may order these scans even if the bone scan is okay, because prostate cancer can spread first to the lymph nodes in the pelvis before traveling to the bone. Read more about how CT scans and MRIs are used to stage your cancer in Chapter 8.

Fantastic voyage into your bladder: The cystoscopy

About 30 years ago, a popular movie, "Fantastic Voyage," featured a plot where scientists were shrunken to a microscopic size and injected into a man so that they could find out what was wrong with him. Science has made amazing strides since then, but it's still not possible to shrink your doc and send him on an expedition inside your body (even though you may find the idea appealing sometimes). However, some of the diagnostic tests performed today can provide important details about your inner world that are almost as good as what those injected scientists were able to obtain.

One tool that can provide important details about your inner world is the *cystoscope,* a thin instrument that urologists use to inspect the inside of your bladder. It can also be used to check your prostate. The procedure that is performed with the cystoscope is called a *cystoscopy.* With this procedure, the cystoscope is inserted gently into your urethra and maneuvered into your bladder. This device provides an internal view that can show your doctor if you have any swelling or rough spots that shouldn't be there, such as bladder tumors or spread from prostate cancer. He can also search for kidney stones or any other problems that may be impeding your urine flow. The cystoscopy is not always used by the urologist in deciding if you have prostate cancer and/or how far it has spread, but sometimes this test is very important.

The insertion of the cystoscope can be a little uncomfortable, as can the movement of the instrument through your urethra, but when it's in your bladder, you usually don't feel any discomfort. If a larger cystoscope is necessary for a better view, your urologist may give you a general anesthesia.

After the procedure, your doctor may want you to take a precautionary dose of an antibiotic, in case any bacteria that were lying around in the bladder vicinity become excited and start to multiply themselves, causing an infection. The cystoscopy usually takes about 15 minutes or so and is usually an outpatient procedure.

Chapter 7

Understanding the Biopsy

· ·

In This Chapter

▶ Figuring out what the biopsy means

▶ Understanding how biopsies are performed

▶ Deciphering the biopsy report

· ·

*H*earing that you need a prostate biopsy to test whether you have prostate cancer can be pretty staggering information to take in. Actually *having* the biopsy is a pivotal event — not because you have a lot of pain (you shouldn't have much pain at all), but because if the test is positive, the cancer treatment process will be set in motion. Working with your specialist, you'll need to make tough decisions, such as what types of treatment to consider, which treatment is best for you, when treatment should occur, and who'll provide your treatment (a local physician, or a doctor at a more distant location).

I devote an entire chapter to the prostate biopsy because it's such an important topic. In this chapter, I talk about what the biopsy is and what it can tell you, how it's performed, and how to determine the meaning behind your biopsy report. I also discuss the minor discomfort that may result from the biopsy, when anesthesia medications have worn off. Finally, I give you advice on what questions you should ask your doctor about your biopsy results.

So What Is a Prostate Biopsy, Anyway?

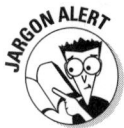

A *prostate biopsy* involves removing tissue samples from the prostate gland for the purpose of determining whether you have prostate cancer. The samples taken from your prostate are just a sliver of tissue; these slivers of tissue are called *cores*. Most often, the tissue core samples are taken from different sections of the *peripheral zone* (the outer part) of the prostate gland, because the peripheral zone of the prostate gland is where cancer is most likely to be found (if it's found at all).

The doctor (almost always a urologist) removes a series of 6 to 14 samples of tissue to be analyzed by a pathologist (this team of specialists is introduced in Chapter 6). If your prostate is very large, the doctor may take more than 14 samples to avoid missing any areas that may have cancer cells. Most doctors lump all the samples together in their mind and refer to them collectively as "the biopsy," even though at least 6 samples are taken.

The pathologist thoroughly examines the samples under a microscope, and then provides the findings to the physician. This process usually takes a week or two. Next, the physician explains the results of the biopsy to you.

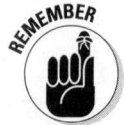

Some men worry that having a biopsy for cancer may make any existing cancer cells spread throughout the body. Studies have shown that the biopsy doesn't arouse cancer cells and make them grow out of control. So you don't need to fear that a biopsy may make things worse: It won't.

Understanding Information Biopsies Can Provide

The biopsy provides two types of information. First, the biopsy results tell you whether you have prostate cancer. Next, if the biopsy reveals cancer, the tissue samples can help the pathologist classify the cancer and determine how aggressive it is. (For more detailed information on the grading and staging of prostate cancer — the key ways doctors classify the status of your cancer — check out Chapter 8.)

Determining whether you have cancer

The key piece of information that you gain from the biopsy is whether you have cancer. Without a biopsy, your doctor really won't know for sure if you have prostate cancer, no matter how strongly he may suspect that you do.

But some margin of error is present in all biopsies, and sometimes biopsies miss cancers that are really there. In general, biopsies capture about 80 percent of all cancers. If your initial biopsy comes up free of cancer, but your doctor thinks that your prostate specific antigen (PSA) blood level is suspiciously high or you have other indicators or symptoms of the possible presence of prostate cancer, he may order another biopsy in a few months, just to be safe. (You can read about the PSA blood test in Chapter 5.) In nearly all cases, the follow-up biopsies capture information on cancer, which may have been inadvertently missed during the first go-around.

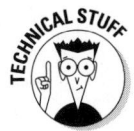

In some cases, pathologists identify *prostatic intraepithelial neoplasia (PIN)*, which are precancerous cells that may indicate that cancer is present or may be developing. PIN is either low-grade or high-grade. PIN 1 is a low-grade PIN, and PIN 2 and PIN 3 are categorized as high-grade. You only need to be concerned about high-grade PIN because it's a potentially precancerous condition. Low-grade PIN doesn't carry any risk, as far as is known. Unless you are positively identified as having prostate cancer, your doctor usually will decline to treat you for PIN alone. But if your biopsy shows high-grade PIN, your doctor will either request another biopsy (biopsies only require a small sliver of tissue, so prostate cancer can sometimes be missed) or pay close attention to your next PSA blood level. If your PSA blood level rises significantly (in your physician's opinion) or registers a worrisome measurement (usually above 4) a year after you have your biopsy, you may need to have another biopsy.

How advanced the cancer is

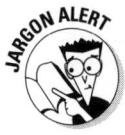

If your doctor diagnoses cancer, the biopsy can provide important information on how advanced the cancer is. Not only do you need to know that you have cancer but you also need to know if the cancer is just starting, is an intermediate case, or is an advanced case. Your doctor also needs to know if the cancer is *localized,* or confined to your prostate, or if it has *metastasized,* or spread beyond it. This information will help your doctor determine the best treatment for your illness.

Looking at How Biopsies Are Performed

In the not-so-distant past (about 20 years ago), doctors didn't have the equipment to view the prostate when they did biopsies. Doctors literally had to grope around with their fingers for the tissue that they'd subsequently remove with a special needle. They were basically flying blind compared to the sophisticated biopsy procedure that's performed now, complete with ultrasound and special probes.

Thanks to the advances of modern medicine, most physicians today use a *transrectal ultrasound probe* to perform a biopsy. This probe, which is inserted into the rectum, shows pictures of the inside of your prostate on an ultrasound. This device allows doctors to carefully sample tissue from specific standard areas of the prostate and also from areas that may look suspicious on the ultrasound, or feel suspicious in the rectal examination.

The *biopsy gun* is the other important piece of equipment used along with the ultrasound probe. Don't worry, it doesn't shoot bullets into your private parts. Instead, the biopsy gun is a special needle that's placed through the end of the transrectal ultrasound probe. The biopsy gun is spring-loaded to respond to the physician's touch. When the doctor sees that the probe is in an area that he wants to test, he puts the biopsy needle gun through the probe and presses the button on the biopsy gun. The needle then moves in and out in less than a second to quickly extract a tissue sample.

Preparing for and Having a Biopsy

A biopsy is an invasive procedure in the sense that the doctor is taking something from inside your body, even though it's only microscopic tissue. But having a biopsy is not nearly as big a deal as having surgery. The biopsy is only a little more risky than getting a cavity filled or having a mole removed. Most biopsies are performed on an outpatient basis. The biopsy takes about 15 minutes from start to finish.

Even though the biopsy is not a major procedure, you have certain actions that you need to take before undergoing the biopsy. Your doctor also warns you about what to watch out for several days after the procedure.

Before the biopsy

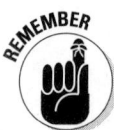

You need to take some simple actions to prepare for your biopsy. For example:

- ✔ Your urologist may want you to give yourself an *enema* (a liquid forced into the colon through the anus as a purgative) the night before the procedure. Enemas are available at virtually any drugstore and most supermarkets. The purpose of the enema is to clean out your colon so that it doesn't interfere with the ultrasound picture. Don't make any major plans after giving yourself an enema: Diarrhea may be your main partner for the evening.

- ✔ Your doctor may want you to take antibiotics before having the biopsy to prevent the risk of infection during the procedure. Some doctors prescribe antibiotics to be taken after the procedure is done, also for the purpose of avoiding infection.

- ✔ Your doctor also advises you not to take any blood-thinning medications (for example, aspirin, herbal supplements such as ginkgo biloba, very high doses of Vitamin E, and especially Coumadin) for at least a week before having your biopsy. These drugs can complicate your procedure, which is why they're best avoided before having a biopsy. Consult with your primary care physician (especially in the case of Coumadin) to determine when you can start taking blood thinners again after the procedure.

You may be really scared the night before you're scheduled to have a biopsy. You may not necessarily be worried that the biopsy will hurt (although some men may be concerned about the pain possibilities). Instead, you may be concerned about the broader ramifications and the overall sense that the test results may change your life. If you're nervous about having the biopsy, it's not unmanly to ask your doctor for some medication to take the night before the procedure. If your anxiety level is sky-high, your doctor may prescribe an anti-anxiety medication, such as Valium (generic name: diazepam), ahead of time. Your doctor will probably only give you enough pills for one day. Don't worry, one day's worth of pills isn't habit-forming.

If your anxiety level is building up before the biopsy, and your doctor hasn't given you a prescription for Valium or another anti-anxiety drug, call the office and ask for one. Your doctor can call such a prescription in to the pharmacy. (Try not to wait until the day before your procedure — give your doc as much time as possible.)

When the biopsy is performed

On the day of the biopsy (which is usually performed at an outpatient surgery center, a hospital, or your doctor's office), you come in, get undressed, and put on a hospital gown. You're positioned on the table so that you're lying down on your side with your knees slightly bent. The doctor then gently inserts a lubricated ultrasound probe into your rectum and looks at your prostate on the ultrasound screen. (Don't worry — you can't feel the ultrasound waves, and they're harmless.)

The ultrasound shows your doctor how large your prostate is and helps him identify any potential trouble spots that he needs to explore with the biopsy. Using this information, he can map out your prostate and determine where to take tissue samples from.

After your urologist maps your prostate, he places the biopsy needle gun into the probe and starts taking biopsies. You may hear a snapping sound and feel a twinge of pain with each biopsy. Most doctors give you a local anesthetic or an intravenous anesthetic, which drastically cuts down the pain. If you're nervous the anesthetic won't help you manage the pain, you may wish to ask your doctor to put you totally out during the procedure. Some doctors may not like the idea, believing that this high level of sedation is not necessary, but many physicians will often respect your wishes. If your doctor does agree to sedate you, he may use a light form of sedation that induces a *twilight sleep,* a form of sleep that is deep enough to prevent you from being bothered by the procdure but light enough to wear off in just a few hours. (You may have heard your doctor say that something doesn't hurt when it really does. I had a biopsy, and it really isn't that bad.)

If your doctor uses any form of sedation, you absolutely must not drive yourself home (or anywhere else) after the procedure. Instead, recruit your significant other or someone else to drive you home after the procedure. When you get home, rest for the remainder of the day. Before you have your biopsy, make sure that you have a way to get home: Doctors often refuse to do the biopsy if you don't have a designated driver available to take you home after the procedure.

After the procedure, your doctor generally gives you an antibiotic. Of course, if your doctor gives you one before the procedure, he may forego this step. (Don't worry. antibiotic is a precautionary step against possible contamination from bacteria in the colon. The risk of infection is usually only about 1 percent.)

Following the procedure

You should be able to go back to work right after the procedure (provided you weren't sedated before the procedure), although you may prefer to take the rest of the day off. Either way, you'll likely experience little discomfort and notice few side effects after the biopsy. If anything, you may notice a little blood in your urine or coming from your rectum shortly after the procedure — on the same day and possibly the next day. (It's usually not much, maybe a few drops, so don't worry.) You may also have some blood in your *ejaculate* (the fluid that comes out during a sexual orgasm) during the next few weeks. This side effect is common. I advise my patients to abstain from sexual activity for 72 hours after the biopsy.

If you notice what seems to be more than just a little blood coming from your rectum or in your urine for several days after your biopsy, let your doctor know about it. You really don't need to worry unless the blood is profuse. A few drops now and then are within the normal range of what's expected after a biopsy for prostate cancer. Of course, if you experience fever and/or chills, contact your doctor immediately.

Acetaminophen, aspirin, or ibuprofen can help take care of any minor pains you may experience as an after-effect of having the biopsy. These drugs are all over-the-counter (OTC) drugs, so you can pick them up in a pharmacy or supermarket. (You probably already have at least one OTC painkiller in your medicine cabinet already.) If the pain becomes severe, which usually doesn't happen, be sure to tell your doctor. Also, make sure that you drink plenty of fluids (ideally water) after your biopsy to wash out or prevent any possible blood clots. You should strive to drink at least ten glasses of water on the day that you have your biopsy. You can cut back to about eight glasses of water per day after you have the procedure.

 Avoid riding vehicles such as motorcycles for a few days after your biopsy, because the bouncing around can aggravate your pelvic area. Right after a biopsy also isn't a good time to try out that new off-road vehicle or tank you just purchased. You need to avoid heavy lifting for a few days after your biopsy, as well — don't suddenly decide that you really need to help your friends move their grand piano up to the 11th floor of their new apartment building! Give your pelvic muscles a little rest instead. Wait at least five to six days after the biopsy before doing any work that requires heavy lifting or muscle straining, such as lifting weights or performing any strenuous exercises (or helping lift pianos, for that matter).

Waiting for your results

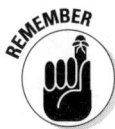 It'll be at least two to three days, and sometimes as long as ten days, before your doctor receives the pathology report from your biopsy, so don't call your doctor the day after the procedure to get your results. And if your biopsy was performed before a holiday weekend, you need to allow a few extra days for the results. If you don't hear anything from your doctor after two to three weeks, call your physician and explain that you're concerned, and you'd really like to know if the results of your biopsy are in yet.

Your doctor and his staff will do their best to try to expedite the findings of your biopsy. They do have other patients, and sometimes information may be delayed for other pressing concerns. If you waited long enough, and you still haven't heard anything, be sure to call.

Understanding the Biopsy Report

If the biopsy shows cancer, your doctor should explain your biopsy findings in very clear terms. If the results are negative, all you need to know immediately is that no cancer was found, but later (as I explain subsequently) you need to talk with your doctor about a follow-up plan.

 If your biopsy is positive, arrange to talk with your doctor about the biopsy report in person when you're more calm. Don't try to get all the details in one hurried phone call. If you feel that you must talk about the details of your diagnosis right away over the phone, and your doctor is willing and able to provide the information at that time, jot down notes and then repeat what you think he said. By repeating the information back to him, your doctor can then make sure that you understand him.

Requesting a clear explanation, not a lecture

When you meet with your physician to discuss your biopsy, he may explain the results to you in his own words rather than go over the paperwork with you. Most doctors realize that simple terms are better than confusing medical terminology when describing the results of a biopsy. But every once in a while, your doctor may forget to keep things simple and lapse into what sounds like medical jargon.

If your doctor starts to describe your biopsy results with language you don't understand, politely interrupt him when he stops to take a breath (although some doctors can say an awful lot with one breath) and ask him to please give you the straight skinny on your biopsy findings with plain and simple words.

Asking your doctor questions

If you have any questions about the results of your biopsy, whether it's positive or negative for cancer, be sure to write them down so that you can remember to discuss them with your doctor.

If the biopsy is positive for cancer

Here are some questions to ask your doctor in the event that the findings are positive for prostate cancer:

- **What is the *stage* of the cancer?**

  The urologist will assess how far the cancer has extended, and whether it has spread beyond the prostate gland or is still localized to the prostate. Most doctors use the Tumor Node Metastasis (TNM) system to determine the stage of the cancer. (I describe staging in more detail in Chapter 8.) The doctor may have to do more tests before he can tell you the correct stage.

- **What is the *grade* of the cancer in the biopsies?**

  The grade of the cancer is determined by the pathologist, who looks at the biopsies through a microscope. He uses a special scale (usually the Gleason scale) to determine the grade. (You can read more about grading cancer in Chapter 8.) Grading is basically a process that provides an estimate of how chaotic or aggressive the cancer is.

✔ **What is the *amount* of cancer in the biopsies?**

The amount of cancer in the biopsies can give your doctor some indication of how much space or volume the cancer takes up inside your prostate. Tumor volume has some importance in estimating how serious the cancer is, although it's not as important as stage, grade, or PSA level.

The doctor can't obtain an exact reading on the volume of the cancer in your prostate with a biopsy. To obtain an exact reading, the doctor needs to remove your prostate. When the prostate is removed with surgery, the pathologist calculates the actual cancer volume in the removed prostate. However, before surgery or any other type of treatment, your urologist can get a better idea of how big your cancer is by looking at how many biopsy cores are positive and/or how much of each core contains cancer.

✔ **How much time do I have before I need to start getting treated for prostate cancer?**

Using the grading and staging information as well as other basic information, such as your age and your overall health, your doctor gives you a recommendation for what treatment you should receive for your prostate cancer (whether it's surgery, radiation, hormone therapy, another form of treatment, or even a combination of several treatments) and when you should receive it.

In some cases, the doctor may recommend no current treatment, which is also referred to as *watchful waiting*. This approach is generally advised when a person has less than a ten-year life expectancy or is in poor health, or the cancer is very low risk. You can read more about watchful waiting in Chapter 9.

If the biopsy is negative for cancer

You're much more likely to have many questions if the biopsy is positive, but you may also have some questions if the test comes out negative. For example, you may wonder if a negative test means that you're safe forever from the scourge of prostate cancer. Sadly, the answer isn't always yes. A negative biopsy means that you don't have cancer or that you don't have a very big cancer — but biopsies are only slivers of tissue, and sometimes cancer can be missed.

Whether to biopsy you again is a very complicated issue that has to do with family history (you have a greater chance of having prostate cancer when you have relatives with it, as I explain in Chapter 3), the level of your PSA and whether it's rising, and what your prostate feels like in a rectal examination. Your urologist knows about all these issues, so he can form a follow-up plan with you.

Chapter 8

Staging and Grading the Cancer

*S*taging and grading are important concepts that you need to understand if you have prostate cancer, because your doctor uses the information to recommend specific treatments for your cancer.

In this chapter, I describe the Gleason system of grading prostate cancer, which is used to denote how aggressive your cancer is based on a pathologist's evaluation of cancer cells that were taken during your biopsy. (Read more about biopsies in Chapter 7.) I also cover the TNM tumor classification system, which is used by your doctor to evaluate the stage of your cancer, and whether it's a localized, regional, or advanced case. In addition, I describe certain tests your urologist may order to help stage your cancer, including the CT and MRI.

Staging and Grading Basics

Keep the following points in mind about staging and grading cancer:

✔ The grade tells you how aggressive the cancer cells are, which also gives some indication of how advanced the cancer is. To determine the grade of the cancer, the pathologist looks through a microscope at the cancer cells from the biopsy that the physician has extracted from your prostate. She compares the sick cells to the healthy, normal-looking cells to determine how close or how far afield the cancer cells look. She then grades the cancer cells using the Gleason score (described later in this chapter).

✔ The stage tells you how extensive or advanced your cancer is, and whether it has *metastasized,* or spread, beyond the prostate gland or it's still *localized,* or confined to the prostate. To stage the cancer, your doctor (usually your urologist) performs a rectal examination and, sometimes, also orders other tests, such as having a radiologist do CT scans or MRIs with or without endorectal coils (these options are discussed later in this chapter). He then uses the TNM system to stage your cancer (this system is also discussed later in this chapter). Doctors perform two types of staging: clinical staging and pathological staging.

- Clinical staging is where urologists can evaluate the cancer before you have any treatment.

- Pathologic staging (or surgical staging) is reserved for patients who have a radical prostatectomy. This staging provides much more precise information about the status of the prostate cancer because the pathologist is looking at the entire excised prostate.

Making the Grade with the Gleason Score

When men who have prostate cancer talk to each other, they sometimes exchange their Gleason scores or their cancer stages with an intensity that two combat veterans might use when exchanging the name of a battle they both served in. They say such things as "I'm a Gleason 6," or maybe "I'm a Gleason 4" — rather than saying that they were at the battle of Khe San in Vietnam or in the Gulf War. This new prostate cancer identity is now more important than where these cancer veterans are from, how much money they make, or even what type of job they have. Cancer trumps everything.

"So what is the Gleason score, and how does it work?" you ask. Read on!

Getting the scoop on the score

The Gleason score was invented in 1966 by Dr. Donald Gleason, a pathologist. He based the score on information derived from studies of the biopsies of nearly 3,000 patients who had been diagnosed with prostate cancer. Pathologists worldwide rely on the Gleason score. The score provides an effective measurement that helps your doctor determine how severe your prostate cancer is, based on the appearance of the cancer cells when viewed under a microscope. All cancer looks abnormal to a pathologist, but low-grade cancers have cells that often look similar to healthy cells from the gland or organ that has been affected by the cancer. As a result, the pathologist can recognize that she's looking at prostate cells under the microscope. But when the cancer is aggressive, the cancer cells look less and less like normal prostate cells (or any other kind of cells).

Pathologists find the Gleason grading system to be very reliable. For example, if the Gleason score indicates that the cancer is an intermediate risk cancer (a Gleason score of 7) it nearly always *is* an intermediate risk. (Read about low-, intermediate- and high-risk cancers later in this chapter in "Grouping Stage, Grade, and PSA Together.") As a result, doctors can make predictions from Gleason grades. The more distorted and aggressive the cancer looks, the higher the Gleason grade, and the more aggressive the cancer behaves in the body.

Understanding how it works

The lowest number on the Gleason grade scale is 1, and the highest is 5. *Two* Gleason grade numbers are actually determined and then added up to get the final Gleason score.

Here's how it works: The pathologist looks at the biopsied tissue samples through a microscope to determine where the cancer is the most prominent (the primary grade) and then where it's next most prominent (the secondary grade). Next, he assigns a score from 1 to 5 to each area: one score for the primary grade and one score for the secondary grade. The *Gleason score* is the sum of the primary and secondary grades. As a result, the total score can be anything from a 2 (1 + 1) to a 10 (5 + 5).

Take a look at Figure 8-1 for a visual depiction of primary cancer cells, from grades 1 through 5, and compare how radically different grades 3 through 5 are from grades 1 and 2, as well as from each other. Notice that when the cancer is grade 5, the cells look pretty wild and don't resemble each other at all, unlike in earlier stages.

Interpreting the results

The lower the score, the better. A combined Gleason score of 10 is very bad (although there are still many treatments that doctors can offer men with high Gleason scores). Here's how the scores break down:

- Scores from 2 to 4 are very low on the cancer aggression scale.
- Scores from 5 to 6 are mildly aggressive.
- A score of 7 indicates that the cancer is moderately aggressive.
- Scores from 8 to 10 indicate that the cancer is highly aggressive.

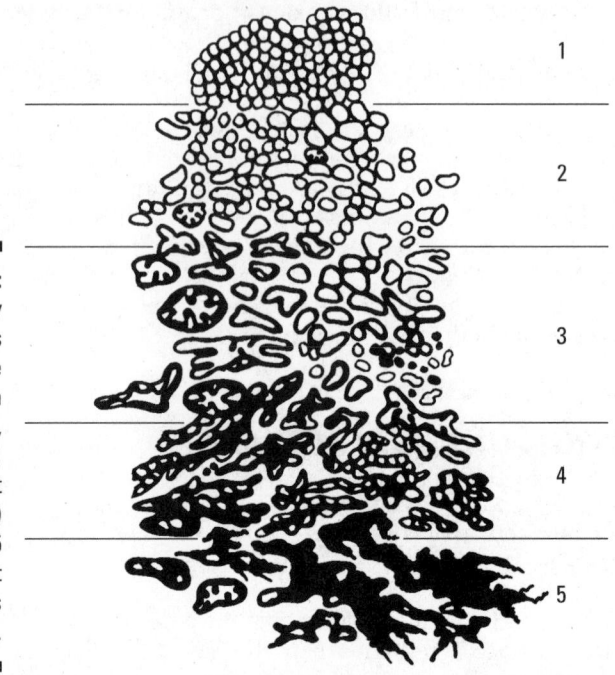

1

2

3

4

5

Figure 8-1:
Primary
cancer cells
on the
Gleason
grade scale,
from grade 1
(least
cancerous)
to grade 5
(most
serious
cancer).

Here's a tricky little feature of the Gleason score for you to keep in mind: The Gleason score usually is reported with the primary cancer number given first, and the secondary cancer number reported second. For example, if Jack Sprat's Gleason score is reported as a 4 + 3 = 7, the primary cancer number is a 4, and the secondary cancer number is a 3. Add them up, and they equal a total Gleason score of 7. But remember, not all Gleason scores are equal.

It may sound strange, but if the pathologist classifies Clark Kent with Gleason scale numbers of 3 and 4, which gives him a Gleason total score of 7, Clark is actually in a little better shape, cancerwise, than Jack. Here's why: When the primary grade (the first number) is 3, it means that the cancer has not advanced as far with cellular deterioration as cancer with a primary grade of 4 (such as is the case with Jack's score). Even though their total scores still equal 7, Jack and Clark's Gleason scores aren't exactly the same.

So if you want to know the real deal on your Gleason score, get a breakdown of the two numbers that comprise the score. Ask your doctor for your Gleason score, starting with the primary grade first, followed by the secondary grade and then the total.

Grading and staging before and after surgery

If you're going to have a prostatectomy (the surgical removal of the entire prostate), it's important to understand that there's a difference between the grading and staging that occurs before and after surgery. The clinical staging before surgery relies on the results of your rectal examination, as well as on tests your doctor orders, such as a CT scan or MRI. The grading before surgery (performed by a pathologist) relies on only the slivers of tissue taken during the biopsy. But when the entire prostate is removed, it's a whole new ballgame, because the entire gland can be evaluated and staged by the pathologist. When the gland is removed, the staging of the localized disease is generally more accurate, because the pathologist has the entire gland to work with, instead of just the few tiny bits of tissue taken during the biopsy. If you don't have a prostatectomy, the pathologist won't be involved in the staging process; he will only do the initial Gleason grading based on an analysis of the biopsy.

Also, if an MRI or CT scan is obtained before surgery, it may show if the pelvic lymph nodes are enlarged and this could mean they are cancerous. But sometimes cancerous nodes are missed when the cancer is not very large and the lymph nodes don't appear bigger than normal. After you have a prostatectomy, the lymph nodes around the prostate in the pelvic area are actually removed and (not just viewed on films) examined under a microscope to determine whether cancer has spread to them. Because the prostatectomy gives the doctor a much better idea of the true stage of the cancer, it can help him advise you a little better about how well you'll do from now on. If more treatment may be needed, he can discuss your options with you.

One warning is in order: Even if the grading and staging after surgery look good, it's still possible that small amounts of cancer cells have escaped and lodged somewhere. These cancer cells may become visible and cause symptoms later on. Therefore, your prostate specific antigen (PSA) blood levels should be monitored after your prostatectomy (or radiation therapy) to make sure that the cancer really is gone. Your doctor will determine how often your PSA levels should be tested. (Check out Chapter 11 for more about prostatectomies, and Chapter 5 for information on the PSA blood test.)

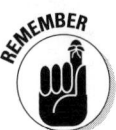

The Gleason score from the prostate biopsy (which is just a few slivers of tissue from the cancer) may not be exactly the same as the score the pathologist calculates after surgery, when he's able to look at all the cancer in the entire prostate. Sometimes the score goes up a little, and sometimes it goes down a little. See the "Grading and staging before and after surgery" sidebar in this chapter for more information on the differences between these scores.

Staging with the TNM System

Several different methods for staging prostate cancer are available to your doctor, including the older and less commonly used Jewett-Whitmore system (developed by the American Urological Association), which classifies cancer into A, B, C, and D levels, with D being used for the worst cases. (D1 is used when the lymph nodes are positive for cancer, while D2 refers to a metastatic spread to bones or other organs.) Some doctors and hospitals continue to use this older system. However, most doctors in the United States, Canada, and other countries rely instead on the *Tumor Node Metastasis (TNM) system* to stage prostate cancer.

The TNM cancer classifying system was developed by the American Joint Committee for Cancer (www.cancerstaging.org), and has recently been updated for 2003. TNM provides doctors with key pieces of information on how advanced the prostate cancer is. The TNM system is considered so effective that it's also used to stage all the other forms of cancer that people may be diagnosed with, including bladder cancer and colon cancer.

With the Gleason scale (see "Making the Grade with the Gleason Scale," earlier in this chapter), the pathologist grades your cancer by analyzing your biopsy. With staging, your urologist relies on his findings in the rectal examination, which is sometimes also followed up with imaging tests (such as the CT scan, MRI, or bone scan).

Staging tests your doctor may use

When your doctor diagnoses cancer (with your biopsy results, your PSA test, and other tests that he may have ordered), it doesn't necessarily mean that you're all done with testing. The doctor may also order a few other imaging tests (scientific ways to take pictures of internal structures so that disease is more apparent), including a CT test, an MRI, or a bone scan, to help clinically stage your cancer. These tests may help your doctor determine the presence, location, and size of the tumor.

If your doctor determines that your cancer isn't very serious, based on your PSA level, your grade, and your stage, he may not order an MRI, CT scan, or bone scan. These tests rarely provide any useful information when the cancer is at a very low level, and sometimes they may lead doctors to order needless additional tests, such as more x-rays and biopsies that probably won't provide any different results. However, some doctors are extra cautious, so don't assume that your doctor thinks that you may have advanced cancer just because he orders a CT scan or MRI.

In addition to the imaging tests, your doctor will also perform a digital rectal examination (DRE), which I describe in Chapter 5. Although DREs are often performed by your primary care physician — it may be the test that raised suspicion about your having prostate cancer in the first place — your urologist may want to perform one, as well. This test helps your urologist determine the presence and status of the tumor, and he then uses his findings to help stage your cancer.

CTs

Your doctor may also order a *computerized tomography (CT)* test to help stage your cancer. This special imaging test is noninvasive and painless. Before the test, your doctor may ask you to drink a lot of fluids so that you have a full bladder. The amount of time necessary for performing the test varies, but the procedure usually only takes about 20 minutes from start to finish. When the test is finished, the radiologist evaluates the results and gives your doctor a written report. Your doctor then conveys the results to you.

When you arrive for the test, you're given a hospital gown to wear, and you're instructed to lie down on the table that's connected to the machine. The equipment operator does all the work, so all you have to do is lie back and relax.

When performing a CT test, when possible, doctors use contrast dye to help better identify any abnormalities that may be tumors and to screen out your intestines, other organs, and blood vessels, so that they won't show up erroneously on the scan as a possible cancerous mass.

If your doctor wants you to give you a CT test, be sure to tell him ahead of time if you have any kidney problems or if you ever had an allergic reaction to the dye. If you don't know whether you're allergic to the dye, let your doctor know whether you ever had an allergic reaction to iodine or shellfish like shrimp, which contains iodine. If you had a bad reaction to the dye, iodine, or shellfish, your doctor will either use another type of dye or give you a medication (such as antihistamines) before the test to prevent an allergic reaction.

The dye is administered in two ways: It is given to you in a drink and it's also injected into your system through an intravenous needle in your arm.

If the CT scan shows the possibility of cancer in the lymph nodes, the doctor will withdraw some tissue from the suspicious lymph node by inserting a skinny needle into your abdomen. (Of course, the doctor will numb the area before inserting the needle.) The extracted tissue will then be evaluated for cancer. This needle procedure is called a *percutaneous fine needle aspiration.*

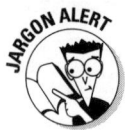

You may be wondering, "What are lymph nodes, anyway?" *Lymph nodes* act as filter stations within the lymph system, working to rid the body of toxins and dangerous substances. The cancer cell is one of the dangerous substances that the lymph nodes try to filter out. If cancer gets into the lymphatic system, it may spread to the rest of the body, although the lymphatic system will do its best to destroy the cancer. Your body has many lymph nodes. So taking some of them out as a part of your cancer treatment won't cause you any harm.

MRIs

Magnetic resonance imaging (MRI) is another test that is often used for staging prostate cancer. MRI is a noninvasive imaging test that uses magnetic waves to provide a picture of the internal organs. The test can also help detect localized prostate cancer as well as tumors that have spread.

Most doctors still use closed MRIs, in which the patient is placed in a small chamber. This chamber can feel like the inside of a tomb to some people, so if you have *claustrophobia* (a fear of enclosed spaces), you may want to ask your doctor to give you a mild sedative, such as Valium (generic name: diazepam), before the test. You may also request to have your MRI in an open facility that's designed especially for claustrophobic patients. Be aware, though, that many doctors don't have access to open MRIs, and your insurance company may not be willing to pay for this extra expense.

MRI machines are very noisy. Because loud noises can be very aggravating to some patients, many MRI facilities provide earphones to help mask the sound of the MRI machine.

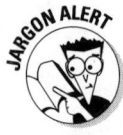

Endorectal coils can be used with an MRI to help your doctor evaluate how advanced your cancer is and determine what treatment to recommend. The coils are inserted into your rectum during the MRI. The procedure lasts about 30 to 45 minutes. Studies have not been able to definitively prove the value of the endorectal coil (results have been mixed). Many doctors don't use the coils at all, but some doctors believe that they give some valuable additional information about the extensiveness of the prostate cancer.

Bone scans

In addition to other tests, your doctor may also want to order a bone scan. In particular, he may want to order a bone scan if the cancer seems to be serious, as shown by your PSA level or the stage or grade of your cancer. (The bone scan is described more completely in Chapter 6.) Basically, the bone scan is a test that uses a relatively harmless radioactive fluid, which acts a sort of visual Geiger counter, to help the doctor determine if the prostate cancer has spread to your bones.

Referrin' to the Partin tables and other key charts

A variety of charts and tables are available to help you and your doctors find out a little bit about the severity of your cancer. With one such table, the Partin tables, you can look up your clinical stage, your pre-treatment PSA level, and the grade of your tumor on the biopsy and then find the "probability" that the pathologist will find an extension of the tumor beyond the prostate capsule — whether it extends into the seminal vesicles, or whether it has spread to the pelvic lymph nodes — if a radical prostatectomy is performed.

Other types of charts take your stage, PSA level, and grade and tell you what the chances are that your PSA level will stay low and steady over the next five years if you have surgery or radiation therapy. A new type of chart or table (with more and more factors that can better tell doctors and patients what may happen with cases of prostate cancer) becomes available almost every month.

These increasingly sophisticated tables and charts are very helpful to doctors who are planning for clinical trials. (Read more about clinical trials in Chapter 15.) However, for the individual patient, I'm not sure that they help very much, because the numbers are only probabilities, not certainties. (If your chance of having a little extension outside the prostate is 30 percent, how does that help you?) Knowing the odds that your cancer may spread through the prostate capsule or your PSA may go up in five years does not, in my opinion, help you decide on the right treatment option.

However, more information is better as long as you don't endlessly accumulate facts and needlessly delay your treatment decision. Maybe someday these tables and charts will be so accurate that doctors can tell their patients exactly what's going to happen and what treatment option will be most effective.

Deciphering the results

The *T* in the TNM system refers to the tumor itself. The doctor classifies (stages) the tumor based on the size of the lump, whether it's on one or both sides of the prostate, and whether it has gone beyond the prostate. The T can be either T1, T2, T3, or T4 — T1 is the least dangerous category, while T4 is the worst. Your doctor uses the findings from your rectal examination to help her determine which T to choose when classifying the tumor.

Basically, any form of T1 (T1, T1a, T1b, or T1c) or T2 (T2, T2a, T2b, or T2c) refers to localized cancer, while any form of T3 (T3a or T3b) refers to *regional cancer* (cancer that has spread just outside the prostate, but not too far). T4 (which has only one category) refers to the most advanced tumor (cancer that has spread to your bladder or other surrounding organs).

The *N* part of the TNM system refers to whether the cancer has spread to the nodes in your pelvis. N0 means that the cancer hasn't spread to the pelvic lymph nodes; N1 means that the cancer has spread to the lymph nodes in the pelvis. If the doctor suspects that cancer has spread to the lymph nodes, based on the rectal examination, PSA level, and sometimes other factors, he'll order a CT scan to further check for any spread. (But surgery is the most surefire way to determine whether the cancer has spread to the nodes.)

If the cancer spreads beyond your prostate and migrates into the lymph nodes of your pelvic area, it can develop into a serious problem for you and your doctor. The reason: When cancer spreads to the lymph nodes, it's more likely to move beyond the nodes and into the rest of your body, making it harder to treat.

The *M* in the TNM system refers to whether the tumor has spread or metastasized beyond just the lymph nodes in the pelvis. M has four ratings: M0, M1a, M1b, and M1c. M0 means zero metastasis. M1a means that the cancer has spread into the lymph system outside the pelvis. M1b means that the cancer has spread to the bones. M1c refers to when the cancer has spread beyond the lymph nodes and bones, to other organs. The M rating is determined mostly by imaging studies, such as bone scans.

Check out Table 8-1 for further information on the different aspects of the TNM system.

Table 8-1	The TNM Classification System (2003 Standards)
Stage	**Indications in This Stage**
T1	The doctor feels nothing in the rectal exam, but cancer is present.
T1a	The tumor is often discovered when the doctor performs surgery to correct benign prostatic hyperplasia (BPH). It's not a major problem, and the tumor takes up less than 5 percent of the prostate at this point and is a low grade.
T1b	The tumor may be found when the doctor does BPH surgery and finds more cancer than in the T1a stage and/or it's a high grade (a Gleason score of 7 or more).
T1c	The tumor is often detected by an abnormal PSA, causing the doctor to order a biopsy to confirm that cancer is present.
T2	At this stage, the doctor can feel a hard lump on the prostate, and the biopsy shows it's cancer, but it seems localized to the prostate, and it hasn't spread beyond it.
T2a	The doctor feels a small lump on one side of the prostate.
T2b	A larger lump is present on one side of the prostate.

Stage	Indications in This Stage
T2c	Cancer is present on both sides of the prostate.
T3	The doctor feels a lump that extends beyond the prostate and may go into the seminal vesicles.
T3a	The tumor feels like it's extending a little beyond the prostate on one or both sides, but not into the seminal vesicles.
T3b	The tumor goes into the seminal vesicles.
T4	The doctor feels a massive tumor with extension into the bladder, and/or other adjacent areas of the pelvis.
N0	The cancer hasn't spread to the nodes in the pelvic area.
N1	The cancer has spread to pelvic nodes.
M0	The cancer hasn't advanced or metastasized beyond the prostate.
M1a	The cancer has spread into the lymph nodes beyond the pelvic area.
M1b	The cancer has spread to the bones.
M1c	The cancer has spread to other parts of the body besides the lymph nodes and bones.

Source: "Cancer Staging Manual" and "Comparison Guide: Cancer Staging Manual," both published by the American Joint Committee on Cancer.

Grouping Stage, Grade, and PSA Together

Having a lot of information about the status of your prostate cancer — in terms of PSA, Gleason grade, and TNM stage — can be great, but it can also be confusing. You may wonder, "What do I *do* with this information, and what does it all mean in my particular case?" This section explains how doctors sometimes group PSA, Gleason grade, and TNM stage to determine your prostate cancer's risk factor.

High PSA levels by themselves can indicate that the cancer isn't good, but this isn't always the case. Instead, your doctor may find it helpful to consider your PSA in context with your Gleason score and your tumor stage. These groupings are most valuable when you have localized cancer, that is cancer in the T1 to T2 stage that hasn't spread to the lymph nodes, bones, or other organs. Experts have worked out many different groupings for this information. I offer my favorite common-sense grouping in the following list. These groupings help doctors advise patients on what therapies they may need.

✓ **Low risk:** PSA less than 11, TNM classification between T1 and T2a, and Gleason score between 2 and 6

✓ **Intermediate risk:** PSA between 11 and 20, or TNM classification of T2b, or Gleason score of 7

✓ **High risk:** PSA greater than 20, or TNM classification of T2c, or Gleason score between 8 and 10

If you fit into the low-risk category, you'll generally do well if you have a prostatectomy or radiation therapy. Doctors usually don't find any spread of the cancer to the lymph nodes in patients who are low risk.

With the intermediate-risk category, the chances of a cure aren't as good as they are with low-risk patients. If you fit into the intermediate-risk category, and you're going to have radiation therapy with seeds (called brachytherapy, which I describe in Chapter 12), then you usually should also have external beam therapy. Another option is to have external beam radiation only.

If you're at the intermediate-risk level and you're going to have a prostatectomy, the doctor will strongly consider *not* sparing the nerves that control erections so that he can be more confident about getting all the cancer out. The doctor will also check the lymph nodes for cancer very carefully after surgery. Some doctors who treat patients at intermediate risk order a bone scan and CT scan *before* surgery to make sure that the cancer hasn't spread too far beyond the prostate. (If it has, the surgery will be cancelled.)

If the PSA, TNM staging classification, and Gleason score indicate that you are in the high-risk category, the doctor will have other treatment choices for you to consider. Your doctor may want you to consider, hormones plus radiation therapy, surgery plus hormones afterwards, or a clinical trial.

Part III

Getting to Wellness: Treating Prostate Cancer

The 5th Wave
By Rich Tennant

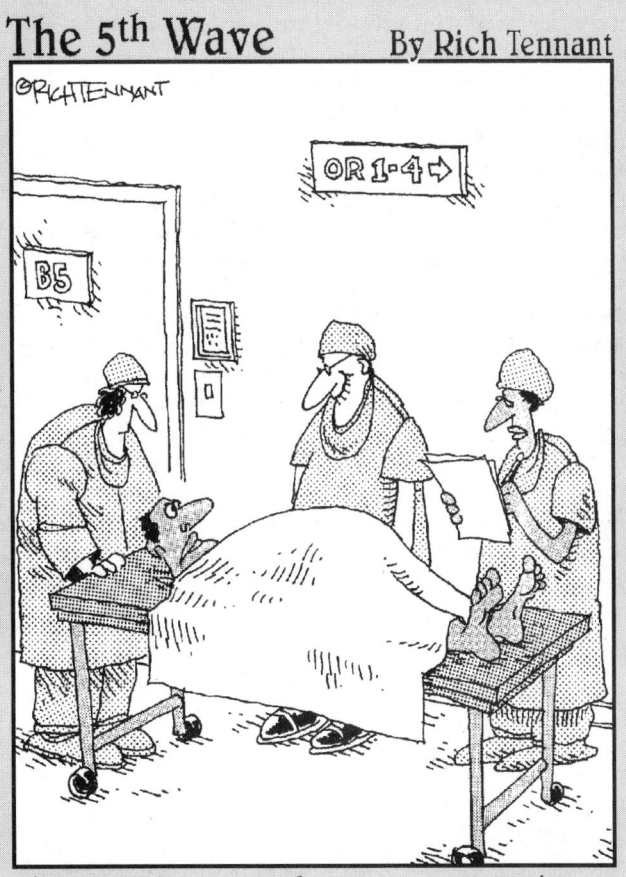

"Included with today's surgery, we're offering a manicure, pedicure, haircut, and ear wax flush for just $49.95."

In this part . . .

This part is all about getting well. It can be tough to decide whether you should have surgery, radiation treatments, or some other form of treatment for your prostate cancer. For this reason, this part helps you evaluate different treatment options. I offer you decision-making advice in Chapter 9. In Chapter 10, I cover the major fears that so many men experience when they're first diagnosed with prostate cancer. I talk about the fears of death, incontinence, and impotence, and I discuss ways to overcome your fears and take charge of the situation.

Chapter 11 covers everything you need to know about the *radical prostatectomy* (the complete removal of the prostate gland), including the nerve-sparing option that often preserves sexual potency as well as the non nerve-sparing surgery. Chapter 12 focuses on radiation therapy, which includes *brachytherapy* (radioactive seeds implanted in the prostate) and *external beam radiation therapy* (where beams of radiation are focused on the prostate externally).

You may need additional treatment to shrink the tumor before surgery or radiation, or to prevent the cancer from spreading. In Chapter 13, I provide an overview of hormone therapy. You may also want to consider experimental therapies, especially if your cancer is advanced. Chapter 14 talks about some cutting-edge therapies, such as cryosurgery, microwave therapy, and genetic therapy. Chapter 15 discusses treatment options for very advanced forms of prostate cancer.

Chapter 9

Making a Treatment Plan

Gloria says that her husband Joe was so shell-shocked by his diagnosis of prostate cancer, and so immobilized with his terrible fear and anxiety, that he asked *her* to make the treatment choice for him. This initial reaction is not unusual among men diagnosed with cancer, but in most cases, men prefer to make their own treatment decisions — with the assistance of their physician.

Choosing a treatment plan that you can live with is a crucial part of coping with your prostate cancer. It can be a difficult decision to make, because your doctor may urge you toward surgery while others may try to pull you toward radiation or some other form of treatment. Complicating the whole decision is the fact that after you make your choice and have the treatment, you can't go back and select the choice you rejected. For example, you can't undo surgery if you're unhappy with the results, nor can you change the effects of radiation therapy if it doesn't work out for you. (Radiation therapy damages the prostate, making subsequent surgery difficult to perform without complications.)

I can't tell you which treatment is the one true path for you, but I can try to help you sort it all out. In this chapter, I talk about the therapies you need to consider when your cancer is *localized* (hasn't spread outside the prostate). I also talk about the options you need to think about when your doctor tells you that the cancer has *metastasized,* or become more advanced. Even with advanced cancer, you still have treatment decisions to make, such as whether you should have hormone therapy, chemotherapy, or newer treatment options like *cryosurgery* (freezing the cancer) or *microwave therapy* (heating the tumor).

You may need a combination of treatments; for example, some doctors order hormone therapy to shrink the tumor *before* you have surgery or radiation therapy. Your doctor may recommend another form of treatment if he considers it necessary, or if he just wants to be on the safe side. After surgery, hormone therapy or other treatments sometimes are required. In this chapter, I cover the bare bones of your treatment options.

Considering Your Own Personal Situation

Your doctor will perform a careful evaluation of your test results, including your biopsy, your prostate specific antigen (PSA) blood test, your rectal examination, and imaging studies (such as an ultrasound, computerized tomography test, or bone scan). After he considers the results of the tests, as well as how your cancer's seriousness is classified by grade and stage (topics I cover in Chapter 8), your doctor will often look at several additional factors before recommending a course of treatment. These factors include

- ✔ **Your life expectancy:** This factor is also tied to your health and your age. Your doctor evaluates whether he thinks you have at least ten years left to live. If, by his estimation, you're likely to be good for at least ten more years, he'll be more likely to recommend aggressive treatment to combat your prostate cancer, even if the cancer is in an early stage.

- ✔ **Your race:** If you're black, you may need a more aggressive form of treatment. Some studies suggest that American blacks are at a greater risk than other races for developing an aggressive form of prostate cancer.

- ✔ **Your age:** Many doctors are reluctant to pursue aggressive cancer treatments with older men (older than age 70 or 75 — different doctors have different age cutoffs). These doctors believe that the surgery, radiation, or hormone shots may have a worse effect on older men than the prostate cancer itself, especially if the cancer is not growing quickly. I think that this perspective is somewhat discriminating, so I concentrate instead on using life expectancy as a key factor to consider. Some men who are in their early 70s are robust and healthy. If your doctor refuses to treat your prostate cancer solely because of your age, even though you're in otherwise good health, consider getting a second opinion. (See Chapter 6 for suggestions on how to find a good doctor.)

- ✔ **Your general health:** If you have one or more serious health problems, such as diabetes, heart disease, or extreme hypertension — or maybe a combination of serious illnesses — your doctor will need to keep your health problems in mind when considering how to treat your cancer.

✔ **How fast your PSA is rising:** If your PSA (prostate specific antigen) level is rising fast, you should begin aggressive treatment soon — unless your age or health problems make aggressive treatment a bad idea.

Table 9-1 compares treatment options according to a variety of different personal situations and the severity of the cancer. As I discuss in Chapter 8, cancer severity can be described in a variety of ways, including *low risk* (most patients will do well with a prostatectomy or radiation therapy, and the cancer is more likely to be curable than with intermediate- or high-risk cancer), *intermediate risk* (chances of cure aren't as good as with low risk, and you may be able to have a nerve-sparing prostatectomy), and *high risk* (you may need hormone therapy, chemotherapy and other treatments). Please keep in mind that I can't possibly consider every ramification of treatment that may come up in different cases. For example, because of your excellent heath, you may still be a great candidate for surgery even though you're older than age 70 — although many doctors advise against a prostatectomy on the basis of age alone. (I'm not one of them.) Use this table only as a guideline and a basis for discussion with your physician.

Table 9-1	A Simple Comparison of Treatment Options by Situation
The Situation	*Possible Treatment Options (in order of my preference)*
You're younger than 70, your cancer is localized, and you have an intermediate to low risk.	Surgery (Chapter 11) or radiation therapy (external beam or brachytherapy; see Chapter 12)
You're 70 or older, your cancer is localized, and you have a low or intermediate risk.	Watchful waiting, radiation therapy (external beam or brachytherapy), or less likely, surgery
You're younger than 70, and your cancer is high risk but still confined to the prostate.	External beam radiation with hormones, or less likely, surgery or clinical trials
You're 70 or older, and your cancer is high risk but still seems confined to the prostate.	Hormone therapy, or external beam radiation with hormones
You're younger than 70, and your cancer has spread beyond the prostate.	Hormone therapy and/or clinical trials
You're older than 70, and your cancer has spread beyond the prostate.	Hormone therapy or clinical trials

Analyzing Your Doctor's Recommendations

If you're diagnosed with prostate cancer, your physician will offer you his best judgment about what you should do about the problem. Many men pretty much follow whatever treatment their doctor recommends. In most cases, the treatment works. But cancer is not like a minor infection that can be treated with another antibiotic if the first one doesn't work. The treatment choice you make is very important; you need to be able to live with it later on. Some men end up wishing that they would've done much *more* investigating before leaping into a decision about which treatment to have. Make sure that you consider all the possible options before deciding which treatment is best for you.

Because you likely have several months or more before you must decide what to do about your prostate cancer, take the time to gather information. Ask a close friend or family member to help. Talk to other men who have undergone a prostatectomy, radiation therapy, hormone therapy, or any other treatments your doctor tells you may be appropriate for your situation.

Consider all your options. For example, if your physician says that either surgery or radiation will work, but he favors one over the other, investigate both options. On the other hand, if your physician says that the cancer has definitely spread, and you need hormone therapy or chemotherapy, don't bother wasting your time amassing data on surgery and radiation therapy.

Even if your doctor offers you only *one* option, you should still investigate that one choice. Knowledge is power.

You should always consider a second opinion, no matter how wonderful and smart your doctor is. Don't worry about your doctor feeling horribly insulted if you say that you want to get a second opinion. Doctors know that talking to more than one expert about a serious problem like cancer is a good idea. But don't make a career out of going from doctor to doctor. See several specialists, read about prostate cancer, talk to others (such as friends and family members), and then make up your mind about which treatment to have.

Thinking about Short- and Long-Term Plans

If you have localized cancer or advanced cancer that has spread beyond your prostate, create both a short- and long-term plan for combating the cancer. Your first choice of treatment (which may also be the only treatment you need) is the short-term plan. If you have localized low risk cancer that can be cured by surgery or radiation, your short-term plan will be either surgery or radiation.

Even if your short-term plan provides you with a cure, you still need a long-term plan. Your long-term plan should be to have regular checkups with your doctor, which includes periodic checks of your PSA blood levels to verify that you're still fine. If you have localized high risk cancer, you may still opt for surgery or radiation, but your long-term plan is to anticipate that you may well need additional treatments, such as radiation and/or hormones.

If you have advanced cancer, your first treatment (and your short-term plan) needs to be either hormone therapy or chemotherapy — or in some cases, both. Your doctor will help you make a long-term plan if your PSA levels indicate that more treatment is needed. At that point, you may wish to join a clinical trial.

Some doctors don't want to talk about any treatments beyond what they're recommending to their patients right now. These doctors concentrate solely on the short-term, even when their patients also want to know about long-term treatments. They may think that you're better off concentrating on the therapy you're going to undergo first (or have just undergone), and that you shouldn't worry about possible future treatments. Yet many men say that they can't avoid thinking about these what-if scenarios. They also say that they feel much better when the doctor is completely candid about what's likely to happen in the next year or so. If your doctor won't tell you what's going to happen if your first treatment doesn't work, get tough with him and politely but firmly insist that you really must know what lies ahead (for your own peace of mind). If the doctor still resists, think about consulting another doctor who will give you the answers you seek.

Information can be liberating

Dr. Overprotective told Jim, after his surgery, that the pathologist discovered that some of the cancer penetrated through the prostate capsule and, therefore, may have escaped from his prostate. Dr. O said Jim probably still would be okay, but he'd need to have more frequent PSAs and monitoring than if he had been deemed completely cured. Jim really wanted to know what treatments he would need if his PSA levels started to go up. Dr. O. told him not to worry about it, and that they'd cross that bridge when they came to it. "Be happy that you're well and free of symptoms now, Jim," said Dr. Overprotective.

But Jim *did* worry about what was going to happen to him, and about what treatment he'd need if there was any evidence that the cancer had spread. Jim spent many nights losing sleep, worrying about what was going to happen to him and how long he had to live, until his wife demanded that he go back to the doctor and get some answers. So Jim went back to talk to Dr. Overprotective. Unfortunately, Dr. O was *still* vague, saying that other treatments would be needed, and that it would all "depend." (He didn't say *what* it would depend on, though.)

Finally, Jim told Dr. Overprotective that the lack of information and his own fears were driving him crazy. At last, Dr. O told Jim that if his PSA started going up again, he would probably need hormone therapy. That's all Jim wanted to know. He slept much better with this new information under his belt.

Planning Treatment for Localized Cancer

Most people still mistakenly believe that any diagnosis of cancer is a death sentence, but this belief just isn't true when it comes to prostate cancer (or to many other forms of cancer). In many cases, the prostate cancer is still localized to the prostate when first detected. Localized prostate cancer is often not only treatable but curable, as well.

Your *Gleason grade* (the pathologist's measurement of how aggressive your prostate cancer cells are) and the *stage* of your cancer (how advanced it is, and whether it has spread outside the prostate) are important for determining which treatment (surgery, radiation, or watchful waiting) is right for you. I describe the advantages and disadvantages of each treatment option in the following sections. See Chapter 8 for more about grading and staging, and Chapters 11 through 14 for details about each treatment option.

Sorting out specialists' biases

When it comes to localized cancer, the two broad categories of treatment choices are either surgery or radiation. These two choices can be broken down into subcategories. For example, if you're going to have surgery, and your cancer is not too aggressive, you can have a nerve-sparing radical prostatectomy to help preserve your sexual potency (see Chapter 11), or you can have the simpler prostatectomy where the nerves aren't spared. Both of these surgeries can be done with or without *pelvic lymphadenectomies* (removal of the lymph nodes in the pelvis). And you can choose the surgery that's done *laparoscopically* (with a small incision in the abdomen), or the you can choose more invasive surgery. (Of course, whether you may be a candidate for the laparoscopic surgery is really up to your physician; few physicians perform that kind of surgery.)

With radiation therapy, you also have choices, such as whether you should have external beam radiation therapy or brachytherapy (implanted radioactive seeds). Or maybe you can try both, if your doctor recommends it. (See Chapter 12 for more info on radiation therapy.)

Choosing between surgery and radiation can be tough. And your decision is complicated further by the reality that specialists generally recommend the procedure that falls within their own specialty.

Another problem is that no studies have been able to definitively determine whether surgery or radiation is better. Surgeons often urge patients with localized cancer to have surgery, because they don't believe that any other "real" choices are available. On the other hand, *radiation oncologists* (radiation cancer doctors) generally believe that radiation is the best choice for most patients with non-advanced cancer. Some radiation oncologists may even denigrate the prostatectomy as a treatment for prostate cancer and, conversely, some urologists may denigrate radiation therapy. I'm a surgeon, and I try very hard to counsel patients without bias, but it can be very difficult for surgeons or radiation therapists who treat prostate cancer regularly not to have strong feelings toward their specialty.

When you're not a physician (and even when you *are* a doctor who's just been diagnosed with prostate cancer), it can be hard to sort out these sometimes unconscious medical biases (doctors don't always realize that they have them) and cut to the chase of what's best for your situation. One option that may help you is to locate a *medical oncologist* (a doctor who treats cancer patients with medications). When you have localized cancer, you won't need drugs. Some medical oncologists, especially those who specialize in prostate cancer, are very familiar with treatments. They generally don't favor one treatment over the other (surgery or radiation), so they may be able to give you an unbiased opinion about what you should do.

In addition, you may want to keep in mind the surgeon's bias for surgery and the radiation oncologist's bias for radiation treatments. When you realize that doctors often have these biases, you may have an easier time sorting out the facts.

Polling John Q. Public about treatment

In 1999, Roper Starch Worldwide, the prestigious polling firm, polled 627 U.S. men ages 50 and older, asking them what factors would affect their decisions about the treatments they'd choose if they had prostate cancer. This poll elicited some very interesting information; however, the poll had one major drawback: The men who were polled didn't actually have prostate cancer (as far as they knew), and no one knows for sure if they would behave the same way that they think they would.

The researchers found that 74 percent of the men said that they thought that the key factor in their decision would be the treatment's effectiveness. This response was followed closely by what their doctors would advise them to do (73 percent). More than half of the men (51 percent) said that they'd consider the potential side effects of the treatment.

Age seemed to have an effect on the responses among the men. For example, men ages 65 and older were less concerned with how the treatment might affect their sex life than younger men were. Only 29 percent of the older men said that a treatment's potential effects on their sexuality would affect their choice of treatment, versus 42 percent for men who were 50 to 64 years old.

Another interesting finding was that the majority of the men surveyed said that if the treatment they chose wasn't covered by their insurance, they'd probably stick with it anyway. Apparently they'd be willing to go into debt if necessary. This response seems to be supported by a 2002 article in the *Wall Street Journal,* in which some men actually *did* go into debt when their insurance companies refused to cover their nerve-sparing prostate cancer surgery.

Keep in mind that even if your doctor is biased toward the prostatectomy or radiation therapy, it doesn't necessarily mean that he's not recommending the best treatment for you. But you still need to check out the other options before deciding.

To help screen out any biases, ask your doctor the following questions:

- ✔ "If I choose another therapy, other than the one you're recommending, what will happen?"

  If the doctor says that you'll die if you have radiation instead of surgery for your localized cancer, he's reflecting his bias. In this case, you should also consult with a radiation oncologist.

- ✔ "What are the main disadvantages of having the therapy you recommend?"

  If the doctor says that the therapy doesn't have any disadvantages (or hardly any), or if he brushes the question aside, he's too biased. All therapies have some downsides, and you need to know what they are.

- ✔ "Can you recommend a radiation oncologist or surgeon to give me a different point of view?"

  If the doctor can't (or won't) give you a name, or if he dismisses your request, he's too biased.

- ✔ "Can I have about a month or two to make up my mind about treatment."

  If he says no, and that you'll die or get worse if you take that much time to decide, he may be pushing his approach too hard. Prostate cancer doesn't escalate that quickly.

Thinking about surgery

If you're thinking about surgery for your prostate cancer, you're thinking about the *radical prostatectomy,* or the removal of the entire prostate gland and the accompanying seminal vesicles. (See Chapter 2 for some basic anatomy info and an illustration of the prostate gland and the surrounding area.) This procedure is a good idea for many men with localized cancer. With surgery, you get a better idea of how much and how aggressive the cancer is, and you find out whether the cancer has spread. When you have surgery, all the removed tissue is examined by the pathologist under a microscope. This tissue helps the pathologist determine whether the cancer is localized (or whether it has spread).

Of course, as long as the cancer truly is localized, it isn't likely to recur after your prostate is removed.

Some studies also indicate that even if the cancer has spread beyond the prostate, surgery, along with other treatments, may still be effective at delaying any further spread. But many doctors won't perform surgery on a patient whose cancer seems likely to have spread beyond the prostate, because such surgery is still considered controversial.

The main disadvantage of surgery is that it requires a lot of recovery time (at least four weeks). After the surgery, you have to spend a few days in the hospital — if you're hospital-phobic, this thought may be quite unappealing. During your recovery, you may have some temporary problems with incontinence. And if you don't have nerve-sparing surgery, you'll be permanently impotent.

Surgeons perform prostatectomies in several different ways, including

- **Retropubically:** The prostate is removed through an incision in the lower abdomen. (Read Chapter 11 for more details.)

- **Perineally:** The prostate is removed through an incision between the scrotum and rectum. (Chapter 11 offers more info.)

- **Laparoscopically:** The prostate is removed through tiny holes in the lower abdomen. This recent advance in surgery uses a telescopic device with a small TV camera to guide the physician as he removes the prostate. This procedure results in smaller incisions and a more rapid recovery when compared to the other procedures. However, few physicians perform this surgery, because it's new and technically demanding.

Discovering basics about radiation therapy

Radiation therapy is another option to consider for treating localized prostate cancer. With radiation therapy, radiation is used to zap the cancer. Radiation therapy can be performed externally, with *external beam radiation therapy (EBRT),* or internally, with *brachytherapy* (a procedure where radioactive seeds are either permanently or temporarily inserted into the prostate).

Some men, especially those with advanced cancers, are treated with *both* external beam radiation therapy and brachytherapy — first one form of radiation, and then the other. (When men have both types of radiation, the external beam radiation therapy is usually performed first.)

Radiation offers a faster recovery period than the prostatectomy — a great benefit to many men. You may need to take time off for radiation therapy, but you don't have to take four to six weeks to recover, as may be necessary after a prostatectomy. In addition, radiation therapy isn't as painful, and you don't have to be hospitalized.

Many men opt for radiation therapy because they believe that it brings a lower risk of serious side effects (such as impotence and incontinence) when compared to the prostatectomy. Radiation can also cause impotence and incontinence, but in general, these side effects are not as common as they are with surgery. However, with radiation, the buildup of scar tissue can cause impotence a year (or more) after treatment. Radiation can also cause other problems with the bladder and rectum. (I describe these side effects in detail in Chapter 12.) Don't assume that radiation treatments have no side effects.

Wondering about watchful waiting

Your doctor may tell you not to have surgery, radiation treatments, hormone therapy, or any other treatment. Instead, he may advise you to just come back in three to four months for another PSA blood test (to see if your PSA levels are higher). If your PSA levels haven't increased over that time, he may tell you to come back again in three to four months for another PSA test and maybe even another prostate biopsy. This form of therapy is called *watchful waiting*. It may be a good form of therapy if you're older, you're in poor health, or you have a small amount of low-risk cancer (check out Chapter 8 for more details on low-risk cancers). If any of these situations apply to you, a prostatectomy or radiation therapy may not be advisable, and you don't need hormone therapy. The doctor will monitor your condition and, if your PSA starts going up, will usually recommend some form of treatment.

In the United States, watchful waiting is generally favored for men who have a life expectancy of less than ten years, either because of their advanced age or because of some very serious health problems. However, in Europe (especially Britain and the Scandinavian countries), watchful waiting is also a popular treatment for younger men with prostate cancer.

In North America, doctors are much more aggressive when it comes to treating prostate cancer. Interestingly, a study released in 2002 compared European men who were treated with prostatectomies to men who were monitored with watchful waiting. The men who had the prostatectomies had a significantly lower rate of death from prostate cancer. A similar study is taking place in the United States, but the results aren't available yet. I don't know if these studies will cause experts to rethink the benefits of watchful waiting in younger men, but I'm guessing that they will.

Don't get me wrong! I believe that watchful waiting has a legitimate place in treatment options, even for the younger man (younger than age 70) who makes that choice. For example, if the cancer seems very small in a rectal examination and on the biopsy results, the cancer is a low grade (see Chapter 8), and the patient has a very low PSA and is very hesitant to have any aggressive treatment, then just keeping a very close eye on him with semi-annual PSA tests, rectal examinations, and periodic prostate biopsies is a definite option. If the cancer progresses under these circumstances, surgery or radiation may still be an option later on.

Analyzing initial treatment decisions

When you make the initial decision on how to treat your localized cancer, you need to consider the potential outcomes of your treatment choice. Your decision-making process should also include an analysis of what's most important to you. Ask yourself the following questions:

✔ Is having more information about the severity of your cancer (as you get with a prostatectomy) the most important priority for you?

For some men, knowing the severity of the problem is very important. If you have a prostatectomy, the pathologist will stage the excised organ, and you'll know if the cancer has been cured or there's any spread. If you don't have a prostatectomy, you won't know for sure how severe the cancer is.

✔ What options is the doctor offering you?

Some doctors perform surgery when the cancer is severe but localized, while others only perform surgery if the cancer is localized and low risk. You can't really weigh your options until the doctor shows you his cards.

✔ Do you want to get back on your feet as soon as possible after the treatment?

Prostatectomies require some downtime — at least four weeks, and sometimes longer. If you feel that you can't be out of work for that long, you may have to forego this treatment choice.

Pondering the Options for Advanced Cancer

If the cancer has spread beyond the prostate gland itself (maybe to the bones or elsewhere, as indicated by rising levels of PSA and a biopsy of your prostate), it can't be cured, but it can be controlled usually for many years.

If you have advanced cancer, your doctor won't wait until the cancer causes you to have symptoms. Instead, he'll come up with a treatment plan to stop your cancer in its tracks right away. (You can read about treatment options for very advanced cases of cancer in Chapter 15.) His plan may include hormone therapy as well as some newer treatment options, such as chemotherapy, immune therapy, or gene therapy.

You need a short-term plan and a long-term plan when you have advanced cancer. The short-term plan is the treatment you choose for beating back the cancer right away. The long-term plan covers what you're going to do when that therapy isn't working for you anymore.

Talking about hormone therapy

When you receive hormone therapy, your doctor gives you hormones to suppress your natural *testosterone* (a male hormone). Testosterone can make cancer grow faster, so suppressing it helps slow down the rate of cancer growth, at least for awhile. The types of hormones that are used vary depending on how advanced your cancer is and whether you have tried hormone treatments in the recent past.

Hormone therapy is usually administered and managed by urologists, but medical oncologists or radiation oncologists can also prescribe hormone therapy.

Hormone therapy is generally used when the cancer is considered initially to be in an advanced stage, or when it has come back after other initial therapies. Some doctors also use hormone therapy as a supplemental treatment to radiation therapy when the cancer is advanced but still localized to the prostate. (For a more detailed discussion of hormone therapy, see Chapter 13.)

Considering other options

Another treatment option is *chemotherapy,* which refers to taking cancer-killing drugs. Chemotherapy is often combined with hormone therapy. Chemotherapy has mixed results with advanced prostate cancer. Some doctors believe that chemotherapy doesn't work well at all, while others (including me) believe that it may be effective in helping prolong patients' lives. You can read more about chemotherapy in Chapter 15.

Before you try chemotherapy (or if chemotherapy isn't working for you), you may also want to ask your doctor about joining a clinical study that offers experimental treatments. (See Chapter 21 for more info on joining a clinical study.)

You may also want to consider *cryosurgery* (freezing the cancer) or *microwave therapy* (killing the cancer cells with high heat), two new options for treating localized cancer. Both options are meant as sorts of search and destroy treatments. They can be considered for initial local therapies, or if the cancer comes back after radiation treatments. For more info on cryosurgery and microwave therapy, see Chapter 14.

Asking your doctor treatment questions

Finding out that you have advanced cancer can be pretty shocking. Here are some questions to ask your doctor when making treatment choices for an advanced case of prostate cancer:

- ✔ "What will I gain from treatment?"

    For example, will you live a longer life or feel better?

- ✔ "What are the disadvantages of each possible treatment?"

    For example, will you feel sicker or have a worse quality of life?

- ✔ "What will happen if I don't have treatment?"

- ✔ "How should my family be involved in my treatment decision?"

- ✔ "What can I gain from joining a clinical study? What are the downsides of joining a clinical study?"

    The main disadvantage of joining a clinical study is that you may be in the group that doesn't get the medication or therapy. The main benefit is that the medication or therapy may work for you. Whether you receive the new therapy or not — your medical care is carefully monitored by a large group of expert doctors. In addition, your participation in a clinical study can help future generations of men, including your sons and grandsons.

Chapter 10

Mastering Your Fears

· ·

· ·

*W*hen the doctor tells you that you have prostate cancer, a series of panicky fears start to dart around inside your mind like hyperactive hummingbirds. Before the biopsy, when you knew that you *might* have cancer, you were plenty frightened. But now the diagnosis has been confirmed, and the whole situation is more terrifyingly real.

These fears generally start with the fear of death and then move on to other common fears that men with cancer must deal with. For example, you may wonder if your masculine identity will become compromised; you may suffer from various subsets of basic identity issues, such as questioning whether others, especially your partner, will continue to value you; or you may agonize about whether you can do anything to protect your future sex life from being destroyed forever.

In this chapter, I provide an overview of the major fears most men experience after being diagnosed with prostate cancer, including the fears of death, impotence, incontinence, and disability. I also provide you with basic information on the realities of these feared situations and what you can do about them.

I dedicate entire chapters to the problems that are particularly distressing to men with prostate cancer, including *erectile dysfunction,* which is also known as impotence (Chapter 19), loss of bladder control, which is known as *incontinence* (Chapter 20), and dealing with the workplace (Chapter 22) and the emotions of your family (Chapter 23).

Fear and Frustration Are Normal — It's How You Handle Them that Counts

If you say that you have no fears after being diagnosed with prostate cancer, you're either lying or you have some interesting psychological problems. The reality is that fear is a normal reaction to hearing that you have a very serious illness. This fear can be greatly compounded by a lack of knowledge about the prostate gland. In fact, many men never even know that they have such an organ until they have a problem with it. Knowledge truly is power, and the more you know about prostate cancer, the more empowered you'll be.

Fear often turns into frustration. The pervasive loss of control that cancer brings to your life is one of the hardest parts — if not *the* hardest part — of coping with a cancer diagnosis. Maybe you've always been great in the boardroom (or the bedroom, or both arenas), and now this insidious medical problem is taking away your control. This loss of control is not something the average man can accept easily. You may feel very angry that your body is sick with cancer through no fault of your own. Maybe you exercise, eat right, avoid cigarettes and alcohol, and do everything *right,* and yet somehow you still developed prostate cancer. It's not fair. (But you probably know by now that life often isn't fair.)

You need to face your fear and frustration and deal with the anger, depression, and stress. You can't eradicate the emotions that you're feeling — you shouldn't even try. But you can use certain methods and therapies to help manage your emotions (see Chapter 16). Use your powerful emotions to propel you toward working with your doctor to develop the best treatment plan.

Dealing with the "D" Word: The Fear of Death

I was going to finish this chapter with the most common fear that men have when they're first diagnosed with prostate cancer: the fear of death. But this fear looms so large for most men, that it just can't be ignored or delayed. So I'm going to jump right into a discussion of this fear first.

From Mr. Do-Nothing to Mr. Action

Everybody gets upset and stressed-out when they find out that they have prostate cancer. Not everyone reacts to the news exactly the same way, but some common personality types can be found among men diagnosed with prostate cancer. Here are some examples of these different personality types:

✔ **Mr. Do-Nothing:** He takes no action, convincing himself that whatever happens, happens. He doesn't follow up with his doctor, and he delays making any treatment decisions. He acts like the problem is totally out of his hands. Through his inaction, Mr. Do-Nothing has defaulted to a do-nothing decision. As a consequence of this behavior, Mr. Do-Nothing's cancer may start growing beyond the localized area. Because he doesn't act, his do-nothing attitude may end up killing him.

✔ **Mr. Worrier:** He agonizes endlessly about the what-ifs of his prostate cancer. "What if I die?" "What if I become impotent or incontinent, or both?" Mr. Worrier also worries about many unrelated details; for example, he may worry that he hasn't accomplished enough in his life, that he has missed out on many important things, or that he's too young to die.

Actually, excessive worry is normal for most men when they're first diagnosed with prostate cancer, but they eventually move on. Mr. Worrier is paralyzed with fear. He isn't nonchalant like Mr. Do-Nothing, but the end result of his behavior is often the same; because he's afraid to make the wrong choice, Mr. Worrier doesn't make any choices at all. His behavior is not at all conducive to a good outcome. By not acting at all, Mr. Worrier sinks into his own quicksand of indecision.

✔ **Mr. Needmore:** He always needs more information, no matter how much he obtains from his doctors and gathers on his own. A second or even a third opinion isn't enough for him — he still seeks more options to consider. This type of personality is most commonly found among control freaks. The real problem with Mr. Needmore is that he delays making a decision as he continues to seek a never-ending source of information.

✔ **Mr. Action:** Like every other man who finds out that he has prostate cancer, Mr. Action is initially very upset about his diagnosis, and he may feel a little (or a lot) helpless and hopeless. He's worried about what's going to happen to him, and he isn't eager to have surgery, radiation treatments, or hormone shots. But Mr. Action's doctor has told him that he *must* make a choice soon. So he's determined to get as much information as he can so that he can make an informed choice. Mr. Action gives himself a deadline for selecting the best possible treatment. He doesn't want to get trapped in an endless cycle of worrying (like Mr. Worrier). He then makes his choice and doesn't look back. For him, there are no wouldas, couldas, or shouldas.

Realizing that your fear is natural

The fear of death is a normal reaction to the diagnosis of prostate cancer. In fact, this reaction is actually a good reaction, because it can encourage you to discover everything you can about your prostate cancer, so that you and your doctor can work out the best possible treatment plan (see Chapter 9). Your fear of death may temporarily paralyze and shock you, preventing you from acting for awhile. You may imagine that your situation is hopeless, but this is rarely the case.

Most people recover from the initial shock of a prostate cancer diagnosis fairly quickly. Reality hits you over the head, and you know that you need to get moving. Of course, the fear of death may be hiding in the corner of your mind. This fear is often accompanied by other negative thoughts, or thoughts about what you should have done to prevent the prostate cancer. Shrug them off and keep moving ahead.

You may also find a considerable amount of solace by talking to a member of the clergy or to people in your faith group. You may want to ask them to pray for you. Chapter 16 offers additional ways to help you overcome the stress of a cancer diagnosis.

Understanding that prostate cancer isn't an automatic death sentence

Many people mistakenly think that cancer equals death. If you tell these people that cancer is survivable, they may give you condescending or pitying looks, and say, with exaggerated patience, "Oh sure, it doesn't always cause death." Or they may say nothing and give you a look that suggests, "I know what's going to happen, but you, poor thing, don't realize it yet." No matter what you say to such people, they still often think that they *really* know the truth of the situation.

Prostate cancer is generally a slow-growing form of cancer, which makes it highly treatable. However, even though prostate cancer is usually slow-growing, it doesn't mean that you can just do nothing and let nature take its course. Sometimes prostate cancer is very aggressive. So unless your doctor recommends that you do absolutely nothing (and if he does, you may want to get a second opinion, just to be on the safe side), you need to select a treatment plan and do everything you can to either cure or get your cancer under control.

Coping with Fears of Impotence

The next most common fear after the fear of death (or for some men, sometimes even before it) is the fear of impotence, which is also often referred to by doctors as *erectile dysfunction*. (Doctors like to make everything sound fancy and hard.) Your sexual abilities are probably very important to you; they may play a key role in your life and identity.

When it comes to choosing a treatment option for cancer, it can be difficult to identify the option that is least likely to cause impotence later on. Most men are primarily concerned with staying alive, but after that, they are concerned about retaining their sexual abilities. However, for some men, potency factors can be the driving force behind treatment decisions. For example, they may find that surgery is a better choice for prolonging life, but they may choose radiation therapy instead, if they think that it will allow them to continue having sex for a few more years.

You may get treated for your cancer and not lose your sexual prowess. But the reality is that many men have potency problems after any form of prostate cancer treatment, including surgery, radiation, and hormone therapy. One way to try and avoid impotence is to have nerve-sparing surgery. This procedure has proven effective at retaining potency in more than half of the men who undergo it. (For a more detailed discussion of nerve-sparing surgery, see Chapter 11.) Nerve-sparing surgery may not be an option for you, so I devote an entire chapter (Chapter 19) to overcoming erectile dysfunction.

Another common fear that comes with erectile dysfunction is the fear that your partner will reel back in horror and leave you after hearing about your cancer diagnosis, because she may think that you'll somehow be less of a man. This situation is rare, but it does occasionally happen. When it does occur, it generally is the result of a lack of information and education. Your partner may not realize that prostate cancer is often curable and nearly always treatable, and she may have unrealistic thoughts of having to care for an invalid. She may believe that your disease means giving up sex with you forever, which often is not true. One good way to combat a lack of information is to read up on the subject. You can suggest that your partner read this book. (Or leave it lying about in a prominent place in your home, turned to this chapter.)

Your fears of being abandoned may also be totally in your mind. Many men feel very insecure when they're diagnosed with prostate cancer, and they imagine that their wives or significant others are going to quickly replace them. Don't worry — the person you love isn't going to leave you.

And if she does leave you, tell yourself that she wasn't worthy of you. Of course, prostate cancer causes a great deal of stress, and being abandoned by someone you live with further magnifies the stress. Read my suggestions for coping with stress in Chapter 16, and consider talking to a therapist or a clergyperson; he or she can help you master the difficult emotions you may be feeling.

You can help counter your fears and your partner's fears by exploring the many options for solving your erectile dysfunction problems. The reality is that even after you're treated for prostate cancer, you can still have a satisfying sexual relationship, and you can still have sexual orgasms — and so can your partner. "It ain't over 'till it's over," as baseball legend Yogi Berra once said.

Dealing with Fears of Urinary Incontinence

The fear of *incontinence* (loss of control over the release of urine) is a common fear among men diagnosed with prostate cancer. In fact, for some men, incontinence seems worse than impotence. Treatments for prostate cancer can sometimes cause temporary or long-term incontinence. (I cover incontinence in more detail in Chapter 20.) But you may be comforted to know that the majority of men with prostate cancer overcome all or most of their incontinence problems within a year or so of receiving treatment. In fact, most men overcome their problems with incontinence much sooner, and some men don't experience any problems.

If you're worried that people will find out that you're incontinent (maybe you're afraid they'll see an accident, smell it, or somehow just *know*), make sure that you wear absorbent products sufficient enough to handle any leakage you may experience. Most absorbent products are deodorized, so you don't have to worry about smelling bad. Nobody will know you have an incontinence problem.

Fearing Infertility

Prostate cancer treatments can eliminate or severely impair your fertility. If you and your partner want children, the prospect of infertility may be a major fear of yours. Most men facing prostate cancer have no interest in fathering a child. But fertility may be a concern for you.

Prostatectomies always cause infertility. Radiation treatments also usually cause problems with infertility. If you want to father a child after your treatment for prostate cancer, you have a couple of options:

✔ You can freeze your sperm before your surgery, radiation treatment, or hormone therapy. That way, your sperm will be available if you want to father a child later on.

Be sure to clearly spell out — in a written contract drawn up by an attorney — what should happen to the sperm in the event of your death. Make it known whether you want it destroyed, donated, or to go to a specific person. Some women have actually found themselves in battles over frozen sperm that was donated by their husbands before they were married.

✔ After chemotherapy, your doctor may be able to extract sperm from your testicle (unless you have been on long-term hormone therapy). The sperm can then be externally combined with a woman's egg to create a fertilized egg that can be implanted in your partner, and hopefully, a child will be born.

Take action to lower stress

In an intriguing study reported in a 2002 issue of *Cancer,* researchers studied psychological distress in about 100 men with prostate cancer. Before the men had a biopsy, the researchers analyzed their style of coping with a test that asked numerous questions about how they reacted to problems in their lives. The questions measured the levels of optimism, pessimism, and coping styles that they experienced when problems occurred in their lives. The researchers then measured the participants' distress levels after the results of their biopsies were revealed.

Of course, the men with negative biopsies experienced a decrease in distress because they didn't have cancer. But the researchers made one key finding about the distress levels in the men whose biopsies proved that they were positive for prostate cancer: The researchers found that optimism or pessimism didn't affect their distress levels significantly. (Many people

suspected that optimism and pessimism would be key factors in predicting distress.)

A sunny or sour disposition didn't make these men more or less resilient when they discovered that they had cancer. Instead, an avoidant coping style predicted high levels of distress when a biopsy came back positive. (Men with avoidant coping styles do things like deny that a problem exists or fail to act.) The men with avoidant coping styles were more stress-prone.

Avoidant people do not engage in active coping or planning. So, the bottom line is, hiding your head in the sand until you're no longer able to do so (because your symptoms force you to go to the doctor, or because someone insists that you get a biopsy) can make you escalate your own distress. In contrast, people who regard themselves as active players in the game of life (rather than as bystanders) have lower levels of distress.

If your partner is still in her childbearing years, ask her how she feels about your fertility. If you both decide that you want to explore one of the options I mention in this section, be sure to talk to your doctor right away, before you begin treatment for prostate cancer.

Worrying about Change at Work and Home

If you're like most men, work is important to you. You may gain a substantial part of your personal identity from your work achievements. If you don't believe that this is true, think about how you define yourself when someone asks you to describe who you are. You probably state your name and then go on to say that you're an accountant, a mechanic, a teacher, or whatever. In this section, I talk about fears that may loom large at work and home when you're diagnosed with prostate cancer.

Handling fears about work

If you have to miss days, weeks, or months from work because of treatments for your cancer, you may worry that these absences will negatively affect your upward climb on the corporate ladder. Federal and state laws are in place to protect your employment. But maybe you're concerned that, despite the numerous laws that cover workers who are sick or disabled, you may get passed over for a promotion because of your illness. Sometimes it can be hard to determine whether this kind of fear is valid or whether it's all in your mind. If your boss actually does discriminate against you because of your illness, you may be able to take legal action.

You can read about both the Family and Medical Leave Act and the Americans with Disabilities Act in Chapter 22. These laws were made to protect your rights in the workplace.

Providing support for your family

You may be concerned about whether you'll be able to earn enough money to support your family. Or, in a worst-case scenario, you may worry about how your family is going to manage, both emotionally and financially, in the event that they lose you.

Communicating through family meetings

Often family counselors can help you and your loved ones deal with the fears associated with prostate cancer and the idea of losing you. If you don't want to hire a family therapist to help, you may want to hold a family meeting to discuss your family's concerns. Bring your family together at one time so that you can address issues once and avoid saying the same thing over and over to each family member. If you can't get everyone together, maybe you can set up a telephone conference call.

Before you start your family meeting, set some basic ground rules (and be sure to follow them yourself). The following list offers some good ground rules for a family meeting:

- Don't monopolize the discussion — everyone gets a chance to talk. Shy members are encouraged to speak up.

- Don't make sarcastic or mean remarks. Family members must be respectful to each other.

- Eliminate distractions, such as a blaring TV or radio. Family members aren't allowed to read the newspaper or a book during the meeting.

- Don't let the meeting last longer than an hour. Most people, especially children, can't pay attention longer than that and will resent being held "captive."

Open the meeting by explaining that you want to discuss your prostate cancer and what you may need from the family. Let your family know that they can also ask you questions. If the questions get too personal, don't answer them. Whether you'll become impotent or incontinent is none of your son's business — but don't worry, he's unlikely to ask you about these issues, anyway. The questions are more likely to be about whether you're going to live, how you're going to treat and beat the cancer, and what you need from them.

You may not need that much from your family members — just their love and support. Maybe you need them to drive you to treatments. Maybe you need them to temporarily take over the household jobs you normally do, such as taking out the trash or cleaning the garage. Tell your family what you need from them, and don't be afraid to ask for suggestions. You may be surprised when your daughter offers to take over a chore she doesn't like, just to help you.

When you have a family meeting, you may feel very awkward; you may feel like it isn't going to work. And afterwards, you may think that it was a failure. Give the family meeting a chance, even if you don't notice results right away. Who knows, you may overhear your daughter telling your son that she was wondering if you were going to be all right, and now she's relieved to hear that you're going to be just fine.

Addressing financial concerns

What about the financial security of your family? Even if you don't have advanced prostate cancer, you may want to do some basic financial planning periodically.

Getting your personal and financial affairs in order involves telling your loved ones about what bills need to be paid, showing them where your will is (or drawing up a will if you don't already have one), and providing adult family members with a complete rundown of all your financial assets and liabilities.

If you're not sure where to start when it comes to straightening out your financial affairs, check out *Estate Planning For Dummies,* by Jordan Simon and Brian Caverly (Wiley Publishing).

Seeking Support from Support Groups

If you're like many men, you may look down on support groups as organizations for people who are whiners and losers, or you may think that support groups are for women. In reality, support groups have real men as members. They're a place where you can gain information, morale-boosting, and recommendations regarding doctors and treatments. They can also help you gain information to counteract your fears about prostate cancer. (I include additional information on support groups in Appendix B.)

Groups to consider

Man to Man is a support group for men who've been diagnosed with prostate cancer. It was adopted by the American Cancer Society in 1993. Hundreds of Man to Man chapters can be found nationwide. Some chapters welcome wives and girlfriends, while others prefer that women and men meet separately. The group provides information on prostate cancer as well as opportunities to discuss issues related to cancer. To locate the Man to Man chapter nearest you, call your local chapter of the American Cancer Society or contact the national American Cancer Society office at 800-227-2345.

For information about prostate cancer support groups in Canada, contact the Canadian Prostate Cancer Network's (CPCN) national office in Ontario. The CPCN was launched in 1995. Today, 125 different support groups are located throughout Canada (in all the provinces).

Meetings are usually held monthly, and in most cases, women are invited to attend. For more info, contact: The Canadian Prostate Cancer Network, P.O. Box 1253, Lakefield, ON K0L 2H0, Canada; phone 705-652-9200; Web site www. cpcn.org. (The CPCN Web site features a map of Canada where you can click on your provincial location to receive an alphabetical list of support groups.)

US Too! International is an international support group for men with prostate cancer. The organization was launched in 1990. Chapters are located in many parts of the United States, Canada, and other countries. For more details, contact: US Too! International, 5003 Fairview Avenue, Downers Grove, IL 60515; phone 630-795-1002 or 800-808-7866 (toll-free support hotline); Web site www.ustoo.org.

Looking at the benefits

A good support group (whether online or in your local community) can provide you with an opportunity to talk about issues that concern you, and to discover ways that others have resolved the problems and fears you currently face (or may face in the near future).

Support group members can also often provide very practical assistance and information. For example, if you plan to travel out of state for surgery or other treatments, members of your support group may be able to recommend good hotels. They may know, for example, which hotels have *medical rates,* or nightly rates that are lower than the regular fee charged to most guests. They may also be able to recommend items that you may need after your surgery — items that may be easier for you to buy at home before leaving on your trip (such as pads for incontinence).

Being wary of the problems

Support groups aren't perfect organizations, no matter how effective they are. Some members of support groups may become very entrenched in their position, and they may think that *only* surgery or *only* radiation is the one right way to deal with prostate cancer. They may believe that anyone who takes another view or questions their position is flat out wrong. You need information and support, not arguments or cheerleading for a particular treatment that may or may not be the best one for you.

Another problem that sometimes occurs with support groups is that some members may be very closely affiliated with other organizations, companies, or even physicians who promote particular drugs or treatments that may or may not interest you. Obtaining financial funding from corporations isn't necessarily bad, as long as the organization is completely upfront about any of its ties to pharmaceutical companies, doctors, or other organizations.

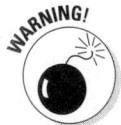

One major drawback to support groups is that some people, especially those who've never been to a support group before, may become very frightened by what they hear. Keep in mind that support groups are filled with prostate cancer patients in many stages of the disease, ranging from those who have localized cancer that can be cured (or has been cured) to patients whose cancer has spread and is controlled but not curable. Support groups may also include patients who are dying. When all these different types of patients talk about their cancer at a meeting, they may not have the insight to know that they're not talking about your stage of cancer. Take everything that's said with a grain of salt until you have a chance to talk with your physician.

Finding and evaluating groups

You may be wondering how to tell if a support group may be helpful to you. One way to find out is to actually attend at least one or two meetings of the support group. Listen and observe what's going on. Ask yourself what the goals of the group seem to be. After you attend a support group meeting, ask yourself the following questions:

- ✔ Do the members or attendees of the group seem to be mostly upbeat and hopeful people — or is the atmosphere more of a "woe is me" kind of doom-and-gloom aura, with people who concentrate on complaining about how bad they feel rather than on discussing possible solutions? You shouldn't walk out of every meeting feeling far more depressed than you felt before you went into the meeting.

- ✔ Do you feel like you can learn something from other members — or do you think that you probably know more about cancer than they do? You want to find a group that can help you gain information. If you know more than the group's members, maybe you should think about starting your own group.

- ✔ Do people who wish to say something at meetings get a chance to speak, or is the meeting instead dominated by a few people who apparently love to hear the sound of their own voices? Although some people are more talkative than others, support groups work better when every member in the group can speak up if he wants to.

✔ Does the group ever have expert guest speakers, such as physicians, social workers, or others, who may have helpful and important information? Ask the leader of the support group if it has guest speakers, and if so, how often. Also ask what types of topics are discussed by guest speakers.

✔ Does the group allow family members to attend meetings? If you think that you may feel inhibited by wives or others attending meetings, and you go to a meeting and see that many women are there, it may not be the right group for you. On the other hand, if you're looking for a group that both you and your family members and/or partner can go to, it may be a good group for your needs.

Your partner may also benefit from what a support group has to offer. Some groups include or center on women who have partners with cancer. You may be able to find these support groups locally or online. (The Circle is one such online group; see Chapter 24.)

Working with informal networks

You may benefit by talking to your own friends about the problems you face with prostate cancer. When talking to your friends, you may find that they know other people who are also dealing with prostate cancer. If you're open to discussing the problem, you may want to get together with these men and talk about their questions and concerns. You should emphasize that you can only speak to the experiences that you have had, and that what was right for you may not be the best treatment for them. At the same time, you can empathize with the shock, anger, fear, and general aggravation they may feel.

If you think that you may benefit from an informal network, where two or three men meet and exchange opinions over a beer or lunch, start your own group. Let it be known at work, your house of worship, or clubs you're a member of that you have prostate cancer and you'd like to meet with other men who also have it (or have had it).

Share your phone number with others who have prostate cancer, and don't be surprised if you get a few phone calls now and again. You probably won't be overwhelmed with calls, because many men are reticent and embarrassed about having prostate cancer. But if the shy guys out there know that men like you (people who are willing to be candid and open about cancer) are available to help, they may be more inclined to open up. You can gain (and give) a lot of helpful information within informal networks.

Chapter 11

Prostatectomy: A Mainstay Treatment for Prostate Cancer

· ·

· ·

I'm a surgeon and an expert on the *radical prostatectomy* (complete removal of the prostate gland), and I've actually had a prostatectomy to cure my own prostate cancer. When the prostatectomy is performed by a skilled and experienced surgeon, it offers a very good chance for a cure.

Urologists often perform prostatectomies on patients with *localized cancer* (cancer that's confined to the prostate). Some urologists also perform prostatectomies on patients who have a slight spread of cancer. If your doctor tells you that you should consider having a prostatectomy, you need to read this chapter.

In this chapter, I talk about the radical prostatectomy. I also discuss the nerve-sparing radical prostatectomy procedure, where the surgeon (in addition to removing the prostate) attempts to save the nerve bundles that control erection, and thus preserve the patient's sexual potency. Only about half of all men in the United States who have prostatectomies have the nerve-sparing procedure. The other half who have prostatectomies don't have nerve-sparing surgery either because they don't know about it, don't want it, their doctors don't perform this technically demanding procedure, their cancer is too advanced for it, or other reasons. The nerve-sparing prostatectomy allows as many as 40 percent to 75 percent of patients (younger than 70 years old) to retain their sexual potency.

Examining the excised prostate

Did you ever wonder what happens to organs doctors remove during surgery? Maybe you imagine that the surgeon simply throws them out with the trash. Eventually, excised organs *are* destroyed, but first they're studied, because they provide valuable information.

With prostate cancer, the pathologist studies the excised prostate, including many tissue samples taken from it, and produces a final pathology report. At some academic centers, the excised prostate is taken to the laboratory and used in research after the pathologist has thoroughly studied it. Of course, doctors must seek your permission before using the excised prostate in research. (However, the research is very important, and I urge you to agree, if asked.)

In addition to both the non-nerve-sparing prostatectomy and the nerve-sparing prostatectomy, I discuss a procedure, performed by several doctors in the United States (including me), in which a nerve is grafted from the leg to try to preserve sexual potency when nerve bundles around the prostate can't be saved.

I describe the best candidates for a prostatectomy, provide basics on the different ways the surgery can be performed, and describe the recovery period. I also talk about the decisions you may have to make if surgery alone doesn't improve your condition, because the cancer has spread outside the prostate. (See Chapter 15 for info on what you can do if your cancer is very advanced.)

Defining Radical Prostatectomy

If you have prostate cancer that's localized to your prostate, your doctor may recommend that you have a *radical prostatectomy,* which is surgery to remove the entire prostate gland and the adjacent seminal vesicles.

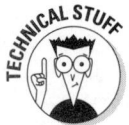

The radical prostatectomy surgery is different from the *simple prostatectomy,* which removes just the inside of the prostate and is sometimes performed when men have troublesome benign prostatic hyperplasia (BPH). (See Chapter 4 for details on BPH.)

The main benefit of the radical prostatectomy is that it often stops the cancer cold in its tracks. If the cancer hasn't spread beyond your prostate, and the cancerous prostate is removed, the cancer cells will no longer be around to grow and attack the rest of your body. As a result, the prostatectomy cures your prostate cancer.

If cancer *has* escaped your prostate, the prostatectomy can no longer cure you. Your doctor won't know for sure how far the cancer has spread until after he performs surgery. If cancer has spread beyond your prostate, the procedure may still prolong your life by removing most of the cancer. (See "Deciding If Surgery Is Right for You," later in this chapter, for more on the pros and cons of surgery.)

Understanding the Reasoning Behind Your Doctor's Recommendation

After you're diagnosed with prostate cancer, your doctor evaluates you and tells you if he thinks surgery is the best answer for you. In general, a prostatectomy is ideal if you have cancer confined to the prostate (staged at T1 or T2), a PSA (prostate specific antigen) blood test level less than 20, and a Gleason score under 8. (Read about the PSA test in Chapter 5, and the Gleason score and staging in Chapter 8.)

If your cancer has some more severe characteristics, surgery is not necessarily out of the question. Some doctors (including me) believe that surgery is still a very good option when certain combinations of severe factors are present. Be sure to consult your doctor for more info.

Other factors that affect whether surgery is the best treatment include:

- ✔ **Your age and life expectancy:** No, your doctor isn't practicing age discrimination when he considers your age and decides whether to advise you to have a prostatectomy. In general, men over age 75 are advised against having this procedure, because in many cases prostate cancer is slow-growing. Consequently, it can take ten or more years for the disease to spread enough to possibly kill you. So if your life expectancy is less than ten years, your doctor will probably advise against having surgery.

- ✔ **Your general health:** If your overall health is poor, surgery may be too dangerous for you. The procedure is not really considered risky, but when a person is sickly, even minor surgery can be a bad idea — and the prostatectomy is a major operation. Also, if you're in poor health, your life expectancy may not be more than ten years.

If your urologist feels that a prostatectomy is the right treatment for you, he should thoroughly discuss the surgery with you. Make sure that he describes the advantages and disadvantages of the surgery in your case, as well as

Processing the stats

You may be wondering if the radical prostatectomy is an effective surgery and if many men have had this operation. Here's what is known:

- According to a study released in 2002 by researcher Gerald W. Hull and his colleagues, the radical prostatectomy is an effective solution for men with localized prostate cancer, and even for men with high risk cancers whose cancer had spread beyond the prostate. Hull and his colleagues looked at nearly 1,000 patients who had undergone prostatectomies between 1983 and 1998 at the Baylor College of Medicine in Houston, Texas (all performed by Dr. Peter Scardino), and checked how they were doing. In most cases, the patients were doing very well, and of those with localized cancer, 92 percent were cancer-free ten years later. Only about 1 percent died from prostate cancer, while 4 percent died from other illnesses. The prostatectomy was also found to be successful ten years later (based on measures such as the Gleason scale and their PSA scores before surgery) in the majority (53 percent) of men with high risk cancers.

- Many men undergo radical prostatectomies every year. According to the National Center for Health Statistics, 192,000 men in the United States had prostatectomies in 1999. The prostatectomy is almost always performed to treat prostate cancer, so it's logical to assume that nearly all of these 192,000 men also had prostate cancer.

- A study reported in a 2002 issue of the *New England Journal of Medicine* showed that the risk of cancer death in prostate surgery patients is significantly reduced when compared to deaths among similar patients who receive *watchful waiting* (skipping treatment but having a doctor monitor the condition). This doesn't mean watchful waiting is always less preferable. For older men or men with low-risk cancers, watchful waiting may be best. (Read about low-, intermediate-, and high-risk cancers in Chapter 8.)

what may happen to you if you don't have the surgery. He should also let you know how soon you need the surgery. Prostate cancer is usually slow growing, so don't rush into a decision. At the same time, don't wait forever, either. Make your treatment decision in one to three months.

Deciding If Surgery Is Right for You

Deciding whether to have surgery can be difficult, especially when it comes to an area of your body you'd prefer to keep away from a surgeon's scalpel — your sex organs. Of course, no procedure is risk-free, but prostatectomies provide several advantages, as well, including a possible cure. If your doctor recommends surgery, do a sort of personal cost/benefits analysis, taking into account the risks that the surgery may present to you personally, as well as the benefits it may provide you.

Considering the risks

Life comes with many risks, and surgery for prostate cancer presents another major risk. At the same time, surgery also offers you hope for an extended life and even a cure.

The major risks that you may face when having a prostatectomy are as follows:

- ✔ **Incontinence:** Incontinence (the loss of control over the release of urine) is usually a temporary problem for men after undergoing a prostatectomy. (See Chapter 20 for info on what you can do about incontinence.)

- ✔ **Impotence:** Impotence is the inability to get or sustain an erection. The main reason men have a nerve-sparing prostatectomy (which I discuss later in the chapter) is that they hope the doctor will be able to preserve the nerve bundles (located near the prostate) that control erections. (See Chapter 19 for more info about impotence and what you can do about it.)

- ✔ **Significant blood loss that requires a transfusion:** Don't be too alarmed by this risk; only a minority of patients require transfusions, which are relatively safe.

- ✔ **Pain from surgery:** Physicians normally prescribe painkilling medications after surgery, so the suffering should be minimal.

- ✔ **Blood clots in the legs:** Blood clots are the number-one cause of death from prostate cancer surgery, but they happen very rarely. To greatly reduce this risk, doctors often insist that you wear special support stockings after surgery. (I discuss blood clots in more detail in the section, "What you can expect right after surgery," later in this chapter.)

- ✔ **Lymphoceles in the pelvis:** This problem, which refers to a large collection of lymph fluid that must be drained, occurs rarely and only if pelvic lymph nodes are removed during surgery. (See "Undergoing a pelvic lymphadenectomy," later in this chapter, for more information.)

- ✔ **Infection in the incision or pelvis:** Infections can form *abscesses* (swollen, inflamed areas in which pus gathers) that must be drained. This complication is very rare.

✔ **Miscellaneous surgery-related problems:** With major surgery, all kinds of unusual things may happen, such as nerve damage from lying on the table in the wrong position, swelling in your legs from the removal of lymph nodes, injury to the rectum or ureters, and so on. These complications are very rare.

Focusing on the benefits

As you make up your mind about whether to have a prostatectomy, you need to also consider the benefits of the procedure. The following list discusses the key advantages of having a prostatectomy:

✔ It often cures the cancer.

✔ You get a better idea of how serious your cancer is than you do with radiation treatments, because the pathologist evaluates your prostate after it's removed. If the pathologist finds that your cancer has spread even a little, you and your doctor can decide what to do next.

✔ The bladder and colon almost always remain unharmed during surgery. With radiation therapy, damage to the bladder and colon is possible.

✔ It can help you retain your sexual potency (assuming you have successful nerve-sparing surgery).

Some of your friends and relatives may urge you away from having a prostatectomy, telling you, "Your Cousin Bill had radiation treatments, and they worked great for him, so you should have radiation, too." Or they may tell you, "Your Uncle Frank had radiation treatments, and his life has been a living hell since then, so *you* should have surgery." You aren't your Cousin Bill or your Uncle Frank. Their situations may have been very different from yours. It can be tough to sort out all the information you receive. In the following section, I give you several major points to consider when making a decision about treatment. (You can also check out Chapter 9 for more information about the factors you should consider when selecting the right treatment for you.)

Asking yourself the tough questions

When weighing the pros and cons of a prostatectomy, ask yourself the following questions:

✔ "Have I talked to my doctor about all other possible treatment options, such as radiation therapy, hormone therapy, or watchful waiting?"

If you're younger than 50, some doctors (including some radiation oncologists) believe that the prostatectomy is clearly best because the long-term results of modern radiation therapy are not as well-known as those of modern surgery. Alternatively, if you (and your doctors) conclude that either treatment is acceptable, and you absolutely can't take time off to recover from surgery because of your active business or personal life, radiation therapy or even careful watchful waiting may be a better option for you.

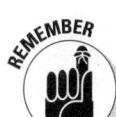

No one knows for sure which treatment — radiation or surgery — gives a better chance for a cure or a better quality of life, and each has different side effects. The one undeniable advantage to surgery is an emotional one: When your prostate is out, you and your doctor will know how bad the cancer really is; you'll also know whether you can sigh in relief or you need to get an early jump on having additional therapy.

✔ "Am I healthy enough to withstand surgery?"

If you have serious illnesses that may make it hard for you to withstand surgery, or if you have good reason to believe that you don't have a ten-year life expectancy, then radiation therapy is probably a better treatment option than the prostatectomy. After carefully evaluating you, your doctor can advise you on this issue.

✔ "Can I accept that I may become impotent after surgery?"

Even with *nerve-sparing surgery* (the procedure surgeons perform during a prostatectomy to attempt to save the nerve bundles that control erections), you still have a risk of losing your sexual potency. Of course, radiation therapy can cause impotence, too (see Chapter 12); but even in expert hands, a radical nerve-sparing prostatectomy is slightly more likely to cause impotence (about 10 percent or so more) than radiation therapy — at least in the short term. Radiation therapy can cause impotence gradually over several years. With nerve-sparing surgery, the impotence is immediate, and it improves later. (If you don't have the nerve-sparing procedure during your prostatectomy, however, you'll almost certainly be impotent after your surgery.)

Medicines and devices are available to help correct impotence (see Chapter 19), but some men consider the maintenance of natural potency to be their number-one concern.

✔ "How scary is incontinence to me?"

To most men, incontinence is very scary (perhaps even more so than impotence). But in expert surgical hands, bad incontinence is very rare (less than 2 percent). If bad incontinence does occur, it can often be fixed with minor surgery (see Chapter 20). Some incontinence after surgery is common, but it usually lasts only a few days or weeks and then becomes a few drops that require a small pad or nothing at all. Yet to some men, even the possibility of a small amount of leaking is too much.

If you and your doctor decide that a prostatectomy is right for you, you'll want to go over the basic information I provide in the next section.

Basic Info on the Prostatectomy Procedures

Doctors can perform prostatectomies in one of three different ways: perineally, retropubically, or laparoscopically. Nerve-sparing prostatectomies, which are procedures that are performed during prostatectomies to save the nerve bundles that control erections, can be performed with any of these approaches.

Even if you decide to forego the nerve-sparing procedure (or your doctor says that it's not indicated because of the spread of cancer within your prostate), you still need an experienced surgeon to perform your prostatectomy. Nearly all urologists can capably handle this surgery, but you'll be better off working with a doctor who has performed at least 50 of these surgeries, and who does at least 15 of them per year. If your physician doesn't perform that many prostatectomies, seek a more experienced doctor.

Performing the prostatectomy

Surgeons (urologists) perform prostatectomies perineally, retropubically, or laparoscopically. Not all urologists are comfortable with the different types of surgery, so don't assume that your urologist will, for example, want to remove your prostate gland laparoscopically through your belly.

With the *perineal* surgery, the doctor makes an incision between the patient's anus and scrotum. He then removes the prostate through the small incision. Today, very few surgeons perform this operation. However, perineal surgery does have its advantages: It usually results in less blood loss, it generally doesn't take as long, and, when compared to the retropubic method, the patient feels better during the first few days after surgery.

I performed prostatectomies perineally for years, but I now find that making the incision in the lower abdomen (*retropubically*) works better for me and my patients. (The retropubic procedure is also referred to as the *radical retropubic prostatectomy,* or RRP.) I think the retropubic method enables me to do better nerve-sparing surgery because it helps me to see the area better. And if I'm doing nerve-sparing surgery, I can save the nerve bundles that control erection more easily with the retropubic method, unless the cancer has spread too far. The retropubic method also enables me to remove not only the prostate but also the surrounding lymph nodes, so I can tell if the cancer has spread to them. Other doctors prefer the perineal surgical approach. They believe that nerve-sparing is just as feasible with perineal surgery.

Lymph node removal isn't possible with perineal surgery, but doctors who use this method either don't believe in removing lymph nodes in most candidates for radical prostatectomies or they remove the lymph nodes through another abdominal incision at the same as they do the prostatectomy or at another time.

In both of these *open operations* (operations made through a 4- to 6-inch incision in the perineum or abdomen), the prostate and adjacent seminal vesicles are detached from the bladder and urethra and removed, and the bladder opening is sewn to the end of the urethra so that urine can again pass from the bladder and out the penis. This sewing is called an *anastomosis.* When performing this operation, the surgeon must be careful to remove the entire prostate (and the cancer) without damaging the bladder or, more importantly, the urethral sphincter. This sphincter is located just inside the end of the urethra that joins with the prostate. If the sphincter gets damaged, urinary control can be a problem.

The newest method for performing prostatectomies is to remove the prostate *laparoscopically.* With this method, the surgeon removes the prostate with a telescopic device called a *laparoscope.* He makes a very small incision near or at the belly button and inserts the laparoscope. A camera connected to the laparoscope allows the surgeon to see inside the abdomen so that he can perform the surgery. Next, more small incisions are made in the lower abdomen to fit long thin surgical instruments through. This procedure doesn't require a large incision as with the open surgeries, and the patient may heal faster and experience less pain than with the perineal or retropubic procedures.

Laparoscopic prostatectomies are very technically demanding; most surgeons don't yet perform them (so you may need to search to find appropriate facilities and surgical expertise if you're considering a laparoscopic prostatectomy). This procedure may become more popular when surgeons begin using robots to assist in visualizing and cutting. I'm still not completely sure that the laparoscopic radical prostatectomy is as good as the open approaches, but I think it's very close. However, I believe that the laparoscopic approach may soon become the preferred, and perhaps superior, approach.

Nerve-sparing prostatectomies

Nerve-sparing prostatectomies save the bundles of nerves (one on each side of the prostate gland) that are involved with getting and keeping erections. Many men are interested in the nerve-sparing prostatectomy, because without the procedure, the risk of becoming impotent after the standard prostatectomy surgery is very high: Nearly all men will lose all sexual potency after the standard surgery. If both sides of the nerve bundles can be saved, potency is about 40 percent to 85 percent likely, depending on which expert is consulted and the patient characteristics. If only one side of the nerve bundles can be saved, the potency probability drops to about 25 percent to 45 percent.

To spare the nerves, surgeons must take the prostate out without leaving any behind, and yet they must also get close to the nerves on the right and left side facing the rectum. Many surgeons use microscopic glasses so that they can get just far enough away from the prostate without getting too close to the nerves and damaging them. However, if the nerve-sparing procedure isn't performed, surgeons can take out the prostate with a wider margin. If nerve-sparing surgery can't be done, some surgeons will use a nerve graft procedure (see Potency-preserving nerve grafts," later in this chapter).

If, in the process of doing nerve-sparing surgery, the doctor suddenly realizes that the cancer has spread beyond the prostate, he will remove the prostate, along with the nerve bundles on one or both sides, to make sure that he gets all the cancer.

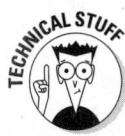

The nerve-sparing prostatectomy was developed in 1984 by Dr. Patrick Walsh at Johns Hopkins in Baltimore, Maryland, after he discovered the location of the nerve bundles. Since then, many doctors have learned to perform the procedure. No one knows for sure how many men in the United States have nerve-sparing surgeries for their prostate cancer, but experts and publications like the *Wall Street Journal* have estimated that nerve-sparing prostatectomies are performed in about 50 percent of all prostatectomy surgeries.

If you want to have the nerve-sparing prostatectomy, make sure that the physician you're considering is experienced and skilled in the procedure. However, until the doctor actually performs your surgery, he won't know whether he can save the nerve bundles; if the nerve bundles can be saved, you'll be better off working with a surgeon who is skilled at saving them.

Questioning your doctor about nerve-sparing surgery

Before deciding if you want a doctor to perform your nerve-sparing prostatectomy, ask him the following questions:

- ✔ "About how many nerve-sparing prostatectomies have you performed?"

  It should be at least 50.

- ✔ "How many of your patients have positive margins — that is, how many have cancer right at the edge of the excised prostate when the pathologist examines it?"

  The types of patients urologists operate on vary (some doctors operate on men with only very favorable cancers, and others do surgery on men with more severe cancers). If the urologist's positive margin rate is more than 35 percent, you should think about getting another opinion.

✔ "About what percentage of the men you perform prostatectomies on are sexually potent a year after the procedure?"

Ask the doctor for *his* statistics, not "what studies say." If his personal success rate is lower than 40 percent, consider seeing another urologist. But remember, success rates are not only related to surgical skill and experience but also to a patient's age and preoperative sexual function. If your urologist operates on many older patients, he may have a lower success rate than a urologist who only performs nerve-sparing surgery on younger patients, yet both doctors may be equally skilled.

✔ "About what percentage of the men you perform prostatectomies on have incontinence a year later?"

Ask specifically what the urologist means by incontinence. I believe that it means never having to wear a protective pad — or at most, you shouldn't have to wear more than just a small underwear-liner occasionally. If a patient needs to wear one or more true incontinence pads, he's incontinent. The urologist's percentage of incontinence should be no more than 5 percent to 10 percent. If his percentage is higher, find another surgeon.

✔ "What percentage of your patients need a blood transfusion?"

If the percentage is higher than 40 percent, it's too high.

Keep in mind that some patients aren't good candidates for nerve-sparing surgery, because their cancer is too large or they're not sufficiently potent to begin with. For example, if John says before surgery that he takes Viagra but it only works occasionally, he isn't a good candidate for nerve-sparing surgery. On the other hand, if Jim says before surgery that he has an active sex life and he doesn't need any extras to get him started and keep him going (and assuming Jimmy's cancer hasn't spread to the nerve bundles), he's generally a good candidate for nerve-sparing surgery. Your doctor can help you decide if you're a good nerve-sparing candidate.

Factors against having nerve-sparing surgery

Maybe you're not sure whether you should have a nerve-sparing prostatectomy or a traditional prostatectomy (one that doesn't spare the nerves). To help facilitate your decision, you need to know that two erection nerves (a right and a left one) travel from the spinal cord to the penis. These nerves run very close to the right and left side of the prostate. There is a slight risk in saving the nerve bundles, which is that surgeons must get very close to the prostate in this procedure, and in attempting to save the nerves, may miss some cancer cells. This risk is low in carefully screened patients, but I always alert patients about the risk and some men, especially those who aren't that worried about continued sexual activity, will tell me to get all the cancer for sure, and not worry about the nerves.

Your doctor may think that the nerve-sparing procedure isn't a good idea if your cancer is very severe. If, during a rectal examination of the prostate, the cancer feels close to the edge of the prostate, or the amount of cancer on the biopsy is large or of a high Gleason grade, then nerve-sparing surgery on one side or both sides may not be advisable. Also, if you're already impotent, saving the nerves won't be useful, and it will probably be best to avoid the risk (very slight as it may be) of getting too close to the cancer. Additionally, nerve-sparing surgery is often not effective for men older than 70. If you're older than 70, you need to ask your doctor if the procedure is worth having. Finally, you should also talk to your significant other. If she's not interested in continuing sexual relations, a nerve-sparing prostatectomy may not be worth having.

In 2002, the *Wall Street Journal* published an article about men whose insurance companies had denied them coverage for nerve-sparing prostate cancer surgery performed by doctors who weren't local. In some cases, the men had to cash in their lifetime assets to pay the entire cost of the surgery themselves. (In some prominent places, the cost of the surgery can be $30,000 and up, not including travel costs.) For these men, their potency was worth the price, although they didn't understand why their insurance companies refused them coverage. (Maybe their insurance companies denied coverage because nerve-sparing prostatectomies cost more than standard prostatectomies.) Check with your insurance company as soon as you decide that you may be interested in nerve-sparing surgery (even if you're not sure you want it), so that you'll have the insurance information if you need it to help you decide.

Keep in mind that even the most talented doctor on the planet may not be able to save your nerve bundles. If the cancer has spread too far, the doctor's primary concern is to save your life, so the nerve bundles may have to be removed.

Potency-preserving nerve grafts

Several surgeons (and I'm one of them) use *potency-preserving nerve grafts* to repair injured nerves that, when working properly, enable erections. The procedure uses grafts of the sural nerve, an expendable nerve near the ankle. This procedure must be performed at the same time as the prostatectomy, and it's only done if the doctor can't save the nerve bundles. I usually can't tell for sure if the graft will be necessary until I look at and feel the prostate during the surgery to see if I can safely save the nerve bundles. So I prepare ahead of time by asking a neurosurgeon or plastic surgeon to be ready to assist me. I make sure that the patient's leg is prepared, and I also make sure that the patient knows all the details and wants to proceed. If the procedure works, patients should see an improvement in their potency within a year or two.

During the procedure, the surgeon uses the graft to connect the two ends of the potency nerve that remain after a segment of the nerve has been taken out along with the prostate. This sural nerve segment, which bridges the gap, actually dies (but not in vain). The hundreds of channels (or conduits) that surround the grafted nerve survive. The potency nerves in the pelvic area that come from the spinal cord use these channels to find their way toward the penis where they can start working.

When successful, this regrowth takes about a year or two. A small area around the ankle from where the sural nerve was taken will become a little numb, although this rarely is a problem for patients.

Sural nerve grafts have been used by neurosurgeons and plastic surgeons for a long time. Dr. Peter Scardino first performed the sural nerve graft procedure (for repairing potency nerves) when he was at Baylor Medical Center in Houston in 1998. I started doing the procedure in 2000. But not all urologists believe that these grafts are necessary, because saving the nerve bundles on one side can preserve potency in 25 percent to 45 percent of men who are ideal candidates for sural nerve grafts. Also, if both nerves have to go, radiation and/or hormone therapy are often necessary and no potency-saving procedure should be considered. Some experts aren't sure that grafts work well. Studies to prove their usefulness are now underway. I believe that the procedure will become increasingly popular over the next few years, as more surgeons learn to perform it, and the results become more mature.

Undergoing a pelvic lymphadenectomy

With many radical prostatectomies, the doctor removes a portion of the lymph nodes near your prostate. This procedure is usually performed at the same time as the prostatectomy. If you're having a retropubic prostatectomy, the lymph nodes are removed through the same incision that the prostate is removed through. With a perineal prostatectomy, the lymph nodes are removed through a separate abdominal incision.

Lymph node removal is done so that doctors can better determine if the cancer has spread from the prostate to the lymph nodes, to better stage your cancer (see Chapter 8 on staging). If the removed lymph nodes look or feel suspicious for cancer, the doctor may send them immediately to the pathologist for pathologic staging. The pathologist analyzes the lymph nodes and tells the surgeon, during the operation, if they contain cancer. The surgeon may then decide to remove more lymph nodes from the area. Some surgeons believe that if the pelvic lymph nodes contain cancer, taking out the prostate is not going to help, so they'll stop the operation without removing the prostate. Instead, these doctors will recommend treating you with radiation and/or hormones.

Other surgeons (and I'm one of them) believe that taking out the prostate when the tumor has already spread to the lymph nodes (provided there is not too much spread) can be helpful. Also, patients who are going to have radiation therapy for their prostate cancer are sometimes advised to have a lymphadenectomy first. If the lymph nodes are cancerous, the radiation oncologist may decide to radiate a wider area to make sure she gets as much cancer as possible. The doctor may also recommend hormone therapy alone (rather than radiation plus hormone therapy).

The pelvic lymphadenectomy usually adds 15 to 30 minutes to the time it takes to perform a radical prostatectomy. Removing these lymph nodes causes little harm; the body has plenty of lymph nodes, so it won't miss them. The operation usually causes no additional side effects. Rarely, this procedure can cause some nerve damage or a collection of lymph fluid that can lead to leg swelling or an infection and have to be drained. Some doctors believe the lymphadenectomy can be avoided in some patients — generally, patients with low-risk cancers. Ask your doctor for his particular philosophy regarding pelvic lymphadenectomies, and find out whether he's planning to perform one on you.

Scheduling and Preparing for Surgery

You may wonder how fast you need to decide whether you want to have surgery. And if you do decide to have surgery, you may wonder how soon it should be performed. These questions don't have one right answer, but remember that prostate cancer, even the severe localized kind, is slow-growing. Waiting three months because you or the surgeon is too busy is okay from a cancer-control angle. However, I find that most patients don't want the stress of waiting around. Generally, I try to do the surgery six weeks or so from when the patient says "go;" however, other surgeons may feel comfortable with longer waiting times. Alternatively, waiting for some time after the prostate biopsy to let things settle down inside is a good idea. I believe that one month is enough time to wait unless there are significant problems with the biopsy, in which case waiting several months is better. Also, if the patient recently had a transurethral resection of the prostate (TURP) to treat benign prostatic hyperplasia (BPH; see Chapter 4), I wait at least three months before attempting a radical prostatectomy. If your doctor says that you need the operation as soon as possible, be a little skeptical.

After the operation is scheduled, what's next? Preparation! Before undergoing any new experience, you need to plan ahead. If you're going to Alaska in January, for example, you'll want to pack snowshoes and skis rather than your surfboard and swim trunks. Maybe you'll also want to turn the heat down at home for a few days to help accustom yourself to cooler tempera- tures. When it comes to surgery, you need to take some actions beforehand, too. Some actions should be taken weeks or days before, while others can be taken the day and night before. Your doctor will go over exactly what you need to do, but the following sections offer some basics.

Actions to take weeks before your surgery

To get ready for the surgery, as well as for your own safety, your doctor will advise you to stop taking some medicines about five to ten days before the procedure — especially aspirin or Coumadin (generic name: warfarin). These drugs can thin out your blood, and you don't want your blood to be thin when you're going to have an operation, because it can cause any bleeding that occurs to be more profuse than necessary. Some herbs, like ginkgo biloba, should also be avoided before surgery, because they also act as blood thinners.

If your doctor recommends that you donate blood in case you need a blood transfusion, set up the donation with the Red Cross or another blood-donation facility in your area. I don't advise my patients to donate their blood, but some doctors do. Allow at least a month for setting up your donation. Ask your doctor who to contact as well as what forms are necessary.

If you're having a doctor in another area perform your surgery, and you need to fly there, make your airline reservations at least a month before the surgery date. Last-minute reservations can be pricey. In some cases, you may not be able to get a ticket at the last minute. Make hotel reservations for the night before surgery. In general, I advise my out-of-town patients to stay close to my office for at least two days after they leave the hospital.

You may need to make plans regarding your work. (I cover work issues in more detail in Chapter 22.) You should arrange to take at least two to six weeks off from work. If your job entails significant physical exertion or mental stress, you should take six to eight weeks off. Make some basic arrangements for your recovery. Make sure that someone will be nearby (in the house or next door) during your first several days at home to assist you if you need help. Make sure that your bed isn't too far away from the kitchen, bathroom, and other areas you need to get to (and doesn't require you to climb a lot of stairs). You'll need to get a lot of sleep during the first week of your recovery.

Readying yourself for surgery the day before

The day before surgery, your doctor may want you to consume only clear fluids, such as broth and water, for your evening meal. This dietary restriction helps keep the formation of stool at a minimum in case the surgery involves your rectum. (It almost never does, but the dietary restriction is still a good precaution.) Don't eat or drink anything at all (including water) after midnight. Your fast should continue all the way up until your surgery. If you urgently need to take a medication, such as insulin, tell your doctor ahead of time, and he'll advise you on what to do.

Your doctor may have you take medicine to clean out your bowels (giving you diarrhea) the night before surgery. (So stick close to home or the hotel, and don't stray too far from the bathroom.) Your doctor may also want you to give yourself an enema on the morning of your surgery. Follow your doctor's recommendations.

The day of surgery

You'll be admitted to the hospital on the day of your surgery. Your doctor's office should help you take care of all the forms and insurance permissions ahead of time so that you won't have to worry about them right before your surgery.

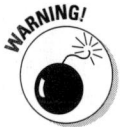

Your doctor will tell you what time you need to be at the hospital. Be sure to get there on time. Your doctor may have other surgeries scheduled, and if you're late, he may skip ahead to the next patient.

Just before the surgery, the surgical nurses will give you a hospital gown (a very skimpy little thing that usually ties in the back and doesn't close that well — don't worry, the nurses and doctors have seen many male bodies before). The *anesthesiologist* (the doctor responsible for giving you anesthesia and making sure that you're okay during the entire operation) will talk to you about the last time you ate and drank, and ask you basic questions about whether you have any allergies, what medications you take, and so on. You'll likely see an anesthesiologist weeks before in preparation for the surgery, but repeating at least part of the process with the same or another anesthesiologist just before surgery is a good idea.

If you've ever had a problem with blood clots, tell the urologist and the anesthesiologist ahead of time so that they can be prepared if they encounter any problems during your surgery. You also need to tell them if you've ever had any trouble with anesthesia, and if you've ever had any trouble with swallowing. The more information your doctors and nurses have about you upfront, the better they can treat you.

After the anesthesiologists and nurses are satisfied, you're good to go. They begin by inserting an intravenous needle in your hand, forearm, or arm. This needle is your hookup to anesthesia for the surgery as well as for the pain medication and any other drugs that you may need after surgery. It will stay in you for at least one day after the surgery.

You'll start to feel a little drowsy just before it's time to go to the operating room, because you'll have been given a sedative before then. Your bed will be wheeled into the operating room and placed right next to the operating table. The nurses will help you move from one bed to the other. The anesthesiologist will then tell you that he's going to administer the medication — and very soon afterward (seconds), you'll be unconscious and in a deep sleep, feeling no pain at all.

In most cases, the anesthesiologist will use an *amnesiac* (a drug that causes you to forget what happens just before, during, and after surgery). When I had surgery for prostate cancer, I was given such a drug: I can't remember the move into the operating room. (Most people consider this a good thing, and I am one of them!)

Recovering from Surgery

No one leaps out of bed and sprints down the halls of the hospital the day after surgery. It doesn't matter how healthy and fit you are: You're going to feel worse after the operation than you did before it. This doesn't mean that you'll be in terrible pain: If you are, complain immediately and loudly. (The doctor will give you pain medications to help deal with the pain.) You also need to let your doctor know if you feel feverish or very ill after surgery. Surgery is a trauma to your body. Your body needs time to recover from being drugged, cut open, and having your prostate removed. Even though the surgery was performed to protect your body from the cancer spreading further, it still needs time to recover.

What you can expect right after surgery

After your surgery, you'll still be hooked up to the intravenous (IV) tubes that the surgical staff put in you before the surgery. The IV supplies painkilling medication, saline solution to keep you from becoming dehydrated, and any other drugs that you may need. The IV stays in for about a day or two after surgery. Many doctors also order a special pump that dispenses pain medication. With this device, you press a button when you start to feel pain, and the drug is then released into your IV. (You can't overdose on the drug, because the machine is programmed to dispense only a certain amount.)

Don't wait until you're in sheer agony before pressing the button on the pain pump. Patients heal faster and better when their pain is under control. If you're not hooked up to a pain pump, ask the nurse to give you a pain shot when you start feeling bad. Some doctors may also give other pain medications, instead of or in addition to the pump, during the hospital recovery period. Ketrolac is one such pain reliever. The physician will likely give you a prescription for painkilling medications that you can take at home.

You'll have to keep an *abdominal drain* (a drain that removes the lymph fluid or urine that may temporarily leak in your pelvis) in for at least one to three days. Doctors usually remove this drain before you leave the hospital. Occasionally, they may want you to keep it in for some time after your return home.

Your legs will be encased in supporting socks, which you keep on for at least a day or two after the surgery. (Of course, you remove them to take a shower, and then put on a clean pair afterward.) I usually allow patients to bathe within two to three days after surgery, but follow your own doctor's orders. Support socks help prevent blood clots from developing right after surgery; moving your legs around after surgery can also help prevent blood clots. Some physicians may ask you to wear support stockings for as long as a week, although I don't do that with my patients. However, it's very important for patients to follow their doctor's recommendations.

You'll also be hooked up to a *catheter* (a small tube that's inserted into your bladder through the urethra and used for draining urine). The catheter is connected to a urine bag that's taped to your leg. And yes, catheters are inconvenient and sort of aggravating. But you probably will only have to wear one for about a week or two. (At the most, it's three weeks, but that's not the usual.) The catheter makes it easier for urine to get out of your body when you recover; it also helps the anastomosis heal (see "Performing the prosta-tectomy," earlier in this chapter). While you're in the hospital, the nurses will show you (and your significant other, if appropriate) how to manage your catheter. They will show you how to disconnect it when showering, how to clean it and the area around your penis, and how to change the bags. (You wear a small bag on your leg when walking, and a large bag when you sleep at night.)

You need to keep your legs moving after surgery, because blood clots can form in your legs and pelvic veins as a result of relative immobility. Some people have a tendency to form blood clots; if you're one of these people, make sure your doctor knows about your condition before he performs your surgery. (If you have a blood clot tendency, your doctors will probably put you on a blood-thinning medicine before, during, or after surgery — an exception to the rule that you should avoid blood thinners before surgery.) Doctors want to avoid blood clots, because they can break off and travel to your lungs (referred to as *pulmonary embolus*). This problem can be lethal, so if you have blood clots, your doctor will put you on blood thinners immedi-ately and watch you closely. He may also want to rehospitalize you.

Walking is an excellent exercise that can help you prevent blood clots after surgery. When you're fully recovered from surgery, continue walking. (I talk about the benefits of walking in Chapter 17.) When you're not walking or moving about, for at least a week after surgery, sit with your feet propped up (rather than flat on the floor) to decrease the risk of blood clots.

Sometimes blood clots form even after you and your doctor have followed all the precautions. If you have any of the following signs of a blood clot, call your doctor immediately. Blood clots can be a factor for weeks or months after surgery, so be alert.

- ✔ Leg swelling — especially if the swelling is sudden, significant, or limited to one side

- ✔ Pain, tenderness, or redness in your leg, especially around your calf muscle

- ✔ Sudden chest pain, shortness of breath, cough, or bloody saliva and mucus

Don't be alarmed if your urine is somewhat bloody right after surgery. This is normal. It may continue to be at least pinkish in color for several days, and then it should go back to a yellow or clear color. (The more water you drink, the better, because water helps clean out your system and rid it of any bacteria.)

Contact your doctor immediately if the blood in your urine is bright or dark red and/or if you find any clots in it. After surgery, you may also find that your urine is a little bloodier after you have a bowel movement the first few times (don't strain!). As long as there aren't any blood clots in your catheter bag, this blood is usually not a cause for concern.

If all goes well with your surgery, you should be able to resume a regular diet a day or two after surgery. Expect to stay in the hospital for two to three days, after which you'll go home to recuperate for at least three to six weeks.

Post-surgery take-home tips

Surgeons often provide detailed written instructions on what to do and not do after your surgery. Here's a quick summary of the key points to keep in mind when you return home after your prostatectomy:

- ✔ Empty the urine bag connected to your catheter before it gets to the overflow point. Always empty the bag before you go to bed, because you'll probably sleep for at least six to eight hours. (You may want to use the large urine bag, rather than the smaller one that may be provided to you.)

✔ If your catheter falls out (which rarely happens), don't panic — just call your doctor right away. You need a urologist to put it back in again. If urine doesn't come out spontaneously, or you can't urinate, see a doctor immediately. You need to get help before your bladder feels like it's going to burst. Waiting too long to get help may jeopardize your ability to get over your incontinence.

✔ During the day, tape the urine bag to your leg so that you don't step on it or trip over it. To keep your penis from getting sore, make sure that the bag is stabilized.

✔ Buy pads to handle any problems with incontinence that may occur after the catheter is removed. Buy them even if you don't think that you'll need them. Better safe than sorry.

✔ Take regular walks to keep your blood flowing well.

✔ Check your wound at least once a day (such as when you're in the shower). Call your doctor if you notice that the wound is very red or something is coming out of it — you may have an infection.

✔ Call your doctor if you develop a fever of 100 degrees or more, *or* if you have chills. These symptoms may signal a bladder infection, and you'll need antibiotics to treat it.

✔ Avoid constipation. Pain medications may make you constipated. If they do, take stool softeners. (You don't have to have a bowel movement every day, but if you haven't gone for two days or more, you're considered to be constipated.) An oral laxative is the next thing to try. Enemas may be useful, too, but check with your doctor first. Some doctors worry about rectal injury with enemas.

✔ After the catheter is removed, do *Kegel exercises* (bladder-sphincter strengthening exercises that can help you avoid incontinence problems). Your doctor or nurse will show you how to do these exercises and tell you how often to do them. (See Chapter 20 for more on Kegel exercises.)

Some men experience bladder spasms after having a prostatectomy. If your catheter is still in, and you feel like you're passing urine or you need to pass urine, *or* if you notice urine coming out from around your catheter, you may be experiencing bladder spasms. When you have a catheter inserted, your urination habits are very different from your normal pattern of urination. With a catheter, you experience a continuous flow of urine. You never feel like you have to go, because you don't have to go — the catheter is doing the job for you. But if you feel pressure or pain, or if you feel like you have to urinate, tell your doctor. These symptoms may be a sign of bladder spasms, which can impair your healing. Your doctor can give you a bladder-relaxing medicine to help calm the spasms down.

What you can expect two to three weeks after surgery

Your catheter will be removed one to two weeks after your surgery (three weeks at the most). The procedure requires a visit to your urologist's office. After the catheter is out, you'll be able to urinate normally again, although you may experience a little hesitancy with urination the first few weeks after surgery. If you're like many men, you may worry that the removal of the catheter will be painful. In reality, it rarely hurts. When the doctor or nurse removes the catheter, it feels like a little pinch for just a second or so. After the catheter has been removed, you can urinate the way you always have before. Your stream may be a little halting at first, but don't worry; it nearly always comes out fine in short order. (If it doesn't, tell your doctor immediately so that he can advise you about what to do.)

Later in the healing process, be alert to a sudden or gradual weakening of your urinary stream. This symptom may be a sign of a *bladder neck contracture,* or excess scarring at the anastomosis (see "Performing the prostatectomy," earlier in this chapter) that can narrow the opening and weaken or (rarely) shut off the urinary stream. Alert your doctor if you notice that your urine stream is getting weaker. A simple five-minute dilation (widening) that can often be done without hospitalization may be all you need to get going again.

Initially, incontinence is common, but the problem usually resolves gradually, becoming inconsequential in days, weeks, or (rarely) months. For most men, normal urination eventually resumes. Most men find that their urinary problems have completely disappeared by six months after surgery. Kegel exercises can often speed up the process.

You should avoid heavy lifting for about six weeks after surgery — anything more than 20 pounds is too much. Don't make yourself have a relapse because you want to show everyone what a macho man you are.

You can usually drive about a week after surgery. But you'll have to hold off on sex for about three weeks or so. You probably won't feel very sexy until then, anyway.

Feeling like your old self

After your prostatectomy, you may be eager to feel "normal" again, which is understandable. The problem is, surgery is a trauma to your body, and it needs time to heal and recuperate. The recovery time can be very hard to accept. After all, you may be accustomed to moving at a fast pace. You can withdraw money at an ATM, go to a drive-through restaurant to buy some fast food, return to work, eat your food, and maybe fax or e-mail notes to your co-workers all on your lunch break. You're used to working quickly and efficiently. But you can't put your recovery period on the fast track, reducing it to only a few days or weeks.

You're going to need at least four to six weeks (or more) to fully recover from the surgery. Less time is just not enough.

After I had a prostatectomy, I was back to playing tennis in about a month — but I was definitely not at my best. Everyone's recovery period is different, so you shouldn't expect to be up to speed in a month.

By the three-month point after surgery, you may be feeling normal or close to normal. If you had initial problems with erections or incontinence, these problems are usually resolved after six months, although it can sometimes take longer than six months to really feel okay. (It may take a year or longer to regain full sexual potency.) If you're still having problems after a year or so, it's probably permanent. (See Chapter 20 on incontinence solutions, and Chapter 19 on potency solutions.)

If you don't start having spontaneous erections about one to two months after nerve-sparing surgery, your doctor will likely recommend that you try potency aids, such as Viagra, a vacuum device, or penile shots. (See Chapter 19 for more info about potency aids.)

If the surgery is successful, and your doctors don't discover after the operation that your cancer has spread, your follow-up plan will require you to see your urologist on a regular basis (twice a year or more, depending on the doctor) and have a regular PSA test. (Your urologist determines how often you need to have a PSA test.) You should also continue to have routine rectal exams.

When Surgery Isn't Enough

When you undergo a prostatectomy, you and your doctor hope that the surgery is going to cure you. But when the pathologist examines the removed prostate after surgery, he may find that the cancer is more serious than anticipated. The pathologist may find that the cancer has spread outside the prostate. This happens in about 15 percent to 30 percent of cases.

If the pathologist finds that the cancer has spread, the urologist needs to determine whether further treatment beyond surgery is necessary. For example, if the cancer spreads to the seminal vesicles or the lymph nodes, the doctor may recommend radiation (see Chapter 12) or hormone therapy (see Chapter 13). Or he may recommend *combination therapy* — radiation treatments and hormone therapy. He may also want to follow you especially closely with check-ups and PSA tests.

You may have to play a waiting game, using the PSA test as your barometer of continued health or a developing illness. After surgery, your PSA level should be at or less than 0.1 ng/ml (nanograms per milliliter). Because of laboratory variations, your PSA level may go as high as 0.4 ng/ml, but in most cases, anything above 0.2 is worrisome. However, if your PSA level climbs to 0.5 ng/ml or higher, your doctor needs to discuss additional therapy with you.

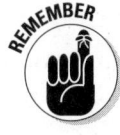

When cancer is found, after surgery, to be more serious than expected, or the PSA level immediately or gradually becomes abnormal, many men rely heavily on what their doctors recommend as the next step in fighting prostate cancer, while others prefer to do heavy-duty research on all the treatment options (or ask their partners to do the research). At some point in time, however, you must make a choice. Even doing nothing is a choice. (Read more about making treatment choices in Chapter 9.)

Chapter 12

Destroying the Cancer with Radiation Therapy

*T*he idea of obliterating your cancer with radiation has an appealing, almost vengeful sort of *rightness* to it. That cancer has threatened your life, and its continued existence torments you: It's a no-brainer that it deserves to die, preferably as soon as possible. Sometimes radiation therapy really *is* the best attack plan for you. But to make a reasoned decision, you need facts.

In this chapter, I talk about what radiation is and what it does. I also discuss the best candidates for this form of treatment, as well as the risks and benefits. And finally, I cover the options of radiation therapy that are available today, including brachytherapy and the various types of external beam radiation therapy, and the side effects you may experience.

Defining Radiation

Radiation throws cancer cells into a tailspin of death. When you receive radiation, your radiation oncologist targets the part of your body where the cancer is located to destroy the cancer cells. Carefully delivered radiation can effectively kill cancer cells without usually causing too much damage to the nearby healthy cells or to your healthy tissues, thus minimizing the radiation to the adjacent organs, such as the rectum, bladder or urethra. In this way, radiation is often an effective method for treating prostate cancer.

Radiation therapy often can be used to effectively treat men who have the whole spectrum of localized prostate cancer, including low-risk and intermediate-risk cases of cancer, and even high-risk cases of prostate cancer, as long as the cancer is still localized (confined to the prostate) or at most regional (outside the prostate but still confined to the immediate regions around it). If the cancer has spread, such as to the pelvic area, it's far less likely that radiation can cure you. In these circumstances, at best radiation therapy can only delay the continued spreading of the cancer and prevent the local cancer from blocking urine coming from your kidney into your bladder, or from your bladder to the outside. Thus, your urologist may want you to consider radiation when he has ruled out surgery because your cancer has advanced beyond the prostate, or when he thinks that you'd have trouble with surgery because of your age or health.

Radiation treatments are relatively painless, but they can cause some side effects (see "Considering the risks you face," later in this chapter). Don't worry, you won't glow in the dark. Your spouse or partner won't be harmed by close contact with you, either.

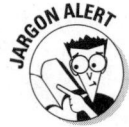

Two types of radiation therapy are used to destroy the cancer cells:

- **External beam radiation therapy (EBRT):** With this therapy, machines focus radiation beams (which go into your body from the outside) on your prostate gland, where the cancer is located.

- **Brachytherapy:** With this therapy, radioactive seeds are implanted directly into the prostate and used to steadily destroy the cancer. *Note:* The *brachy* part of the word *brachytherapy* is pronounced "bracky," which rhymes with "wacky" or "tacky." But brachytherapy is far from wacky or tacky. Instead, it's an extremely effective form of cancer treatment.

Doctors sometimes use both EBRT and brachytherapy, but they usually only combine them if the cancer is intermediate- or high-risk. Generally, when radiation is selected to treat localized low-risk cancers, either brachytherapy or EBRT alone is used.

You may wonder how the radiation the doctor administers to kill your prostate cancer is different from the radiation used to take x-rays of broken bones. These two forms of radiation have several differences. The anti-cancer radiation is much higher energy than an x-ray, which uses just enough radiation to take a picture; it's also far more targeted than the radiation you receive during an x-ray. In addition, radiation treatments are given for therapeutic treatment, while diagnostic x-rays are usually used to identify broken bones, arthritis, or other illnesses.

People sometimes confuse radiation treatments with chemotherapy, but they're actually very different treatments. Chemotherapy refers to anti-cancer drugs that travel through the whole body and kill cancer cells, whereas radiation, which involves no drugs at all, is carefully aimed at specific areas of the body. Radiation therapy is normally used for localized cancer, but it's also used to relieve bone pain in men with advanced prostate cancer. Chemotherapy, which is normally used to treat advanced cancer, is almost never used to treat localized cancer. I discuss chemotherapy in detail in Chapter 15.

Understanding the Reasoning Behind Your Doctor's Recommendation

With radiation, the goal is not to merely wound the cancer cells, but instead to wipe them out completely. The means for achieving this goal can vary. Your radiation oncologist will evaluate your situation and recommend the treatment that offers you the best chance to either get rid of the cancer or, if it has advanced beyond the prostate gland, contain it and prevent you from developing problems with urinary blockage or pain.

In general, if you're a good candidate for surgery, you may also be an ideal candidate for radiation therapy. Radiation is often the better of the two options if, because of your age or health, it would be difficult for you to withstand surgery. Similarly, if your age or health is such that your life expectancy is greater than five years but less than ten years, radiation is probably the better choice. Almost all radiation and surgery experts (even those who favor surgery) believe that surgery offers no advantage over radiation if a man doesn't have a life expectancy greater than ten years.

Prostatectomy versus radiation

I'm a surgeon, so my first choice for treating localized prostate cancer is to is to remove the prostate with *radical prostatectomy* (the surgical removal of the entire prostate gland). But there's no question that radiation therapy cures many prostate cancers and has few side effects. Thus, radiation oncologists would select radiation therapy as their first choice for treating localized prostate cancer. Not enough information is presently available to determine whether surgery or radiotherapy (radiation therapy) is the better treatment.

At the University of Washington, my colleagues and I are currently leading an international study comparing the outcomes for men who have radiation treatment to the outcomes for men who have prostatectomies. The study, which is focusing on thousands of prostate cancer patients in the United States and Canada with low-risk disease (which I explain in Chapter 9), will take about ten years to complete. The results of the study will help doctors and their patients get a much better idea of which treatment may be the most beneficial for men with localized cancer.

If you have extensive localized cancer that isn't curable, radiation therapy may be given to control some of the symptoms that may develop.

Your doctor will base his recommendation on several factors, including

- ✔ **Your age and life expectancy:** If you're 75 to 80 years old or older, and you also have other health problems (as many older men do), you may not be a good candidate for any form of radiation therapy. (You're certainly not a good candidate for surgery, either.) Even if you're in great shape for your age, your life expectancy may be considered to be less than five years, and it may be hard for you to cope with the side effects that can come with radiation treatments. Watchful waiting (see Chapter 9) or hormone therapy (see Chapter 13) usually works just as well in these cases.

- ✔ **Your overall health:** Your radiation oncologist will take into account whether you have any medical conditions that make radiation inadvisable for you, given that the treatments themselves have temporary and some-times long-term side effects. Your doctor also will consider what other health problems you may have (such as diabetes, hypertension, and heart disease) before deciding whether to recommend radiation therapy.

- ✔ **Problems with nearby organs:** Radiation therapy may not be a good option for you if you already have an irritable bladder or your prostate is significantly blocking your urine flow, making it hard to urinate. (Sometimes that problem can be fixed with a six-month course of hor-mone therapy.) Radiation treatments can make these symptoms worse. If you're unhappy with your urinary problems now, surgery may be the better option. Also, if you're already having rectal or intestinal problems, such as chronic diarrhea or chronic inflammatory diseases of the bowel, radiation therapy may make them unacceptably worse.

Deciding If Radiation Is Right for You

When you have prostate cancer, you may feel like you have a ticking time bomb inside your prostate, ready to explode at any moment. But unless your doctor has specifically told you that your cancer is a very aggressive form, you should have at least a month or two (maybe longer) to make the decision about your prostate cancer therapy. So don't let yourself get panicked into making an immediate decision.

On the other hand, don't go off and forget about your problem, assuming that somehow everything will all turn out for the best. Think about the pros and cons of radiation compared to other forms of treatment, talk to your doctor, talk with other doctors, do research, make an informed decision, and then act.

Considering the risks you face

Wiping out cancer cells with radiation therapy can cause some side effects. Nature really didn't intend for you to get continuously bombarded with radiation, so your body may struggle for awhile to cope with the after-effects of radiation therapy. But the good news is that most of the side effects of radiation therapy are temporary; your body will return to normal within weeks of your last treatment.

Possible side effects to radiation treatments include

- **Impotence:** Although the risk of impotence is generally lower initially with radiation than with surgery, the risk of permanent impotence may still be as high as 20 percent to 40 percent.

- **Urinary incontinence:** With radiation therapy, urinary incontinence may result from a damaged urinary sphincter. With radiation therapy, significant urinary incontinence (requiring one or more pads daily) occurs in 1 percent to 3 percent of all patients. Only rarely (less than 1 percent of cases) is it permanent.

- **Severe urinary frequency or urgency:** These symptoms result from irritation to the bladder, which is so close to the prostate that it invariably gets some radiation. Usually, the symptoms are temporary and can be controlled with medication. Permanent urgency (having to go to the bathroom every hour, and needing to get there fast) occurs in less than 5 percent of patients, but it's more likely to be experienced by patients who have bladder problems before radiation treatments.

- **Rectal problems:** You may experience a flare-up of hemorrhoids, rectal burning with bowel movements, diarrhea, or bowel urgency. These symptoms are often temporary and controllable with medications. Permanent rectal problems, which aren't common (occurring in less than 5 percent of cases), are more likely to occur if you have bowel problems before radiation treatments.

- **Hair loss:** Radiation treatments can cause some pubic hair loss, but not any hair loss outside the radiation field. If you experience pubic hair loss, the good news is that it's usually only temporary — when the radiation treatments are finished, your hair will grow back. However, you may experience permanent hair loss in the areas that were zapped — just remind yourself it's a very small price to pay for the cancer-killing benefits you gain.

- **Weakness and tiredness:** You may feel exhausted after your EBRT treatments, especially toward the end of the eight-week course. Usually, taking a short nap solves the problem.

✔ **Severe tissue damage:** Radiation oncologists do their best to target only the cancer cells, but sometimes radiation therapy causes some damage to the bladder, the rectum, or other surrounding tissues. Severe tissue damage is not a common side effect, but it can happen, especially if the cancer is widespread and your doctor is trying to target the radiation on a large area. If tissue damage does occur, you may possibly develop incapacitating problems with burning urination, bladder irritability, or a loss of bladder control (urinary incontinence). Additional surgery may be necessary to help control the incontinence. (You can read about incontinence in Chapter 20.) You may also experience bladder or rectal damage and may need surgery. Severe tissue damage is extremely rare (less than 1 percent of all cases) but can be very distressing to the patient and hard to correct.

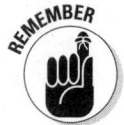

When you're undergoing radiation therapy, you can expect to easily continue your everyday work schedule, unless you have a particularly strenuous work requirement. If you feel tired, remind yourself that the cancer cells are getting killed, and they're not going down without a fight. You and your doctor are giving the cancer cells one heck of a fight, and it's a showdown that you intend to win.

Focusing on the benefits

Some of the side effects of radiation therapy can be intimidating, but there are many benefits to radiation therapy as well:

✔ Overall, it's easier on you than a prostatectomy.

✔ You don't have to deal with a long recovery period like you do with a prostatectomy.

✔ During your radiation treatments, you can continue to work.

✔ If your prostate cancer is localized, radiation may be able to cure you without you having to undergo surgery.

Asking yourself the tough questions

Before you decide whether to have radiation treatments, ask yourself several key questions, such as

✔ "Is it important for me to know as much as I can about how severe my cancer is, or would I rather not know so much, to cut down on any stress or worry?"

If knowing the severity of your prostate cancer is paramount to your decision, you should choose surgery over radiation, because surgery can give you the most definitive results about how much the cancer has spread (after the pathologist analyzes your excised organ). Keep in mind that surgery doesn't necessarily provide a better opportunity for a cure, it just gives you more information about the status of your prostate cancer.

✔ "Do I want to make sure that I only miss a week or so of work after receiving treatment?"

If you don't want to miss a lot of work, radiation may be a better choice, because you miss at least three to six weeks after having a prostatectomy.

✔ "Do I have an especially unusual fear of radiation?"

Most of the time, the fear of radiation is without foundation, but it can still legitimately influence your decision.

✔ "How do I feel about the doctor who's treating me?"

This question may sound silly, but it's an important issue. If you don't have any emotional trust in your radiation oncologist or urologist, your decision may be affected.

Considering questions to ask the radiation oncologist

Just as I've advised you to talk to a urologist and ask questions before deciding upon having a prostatectomy, I also think it's important to talk to a radiation oncologist before you're convinced that radiation is the best therapy for you. Although your urologist may thoroughly discuss the relative benefits and side effects of radiation therapy with you, a radiation oncologist can better explain the facts associated with the treatment. You need to go into this treatment with a good understanding of what's going to happen.

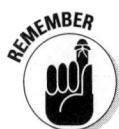

Ask the radiation oncologist the following questions (in addition to any others you may have):

✔ "What are the approximate odds that radiation will work for me?"

If the odds are less than 50 percent, ask if any other options have better odds.

✔ "Do you regularly treat prostate cancer? If so, what method do you use, and how many cases do you treat per year?"

If you're considering EBRT, the radiation oncologist should have treated at least 50 cases overall and 15 EBRT cases per year. If you're thinking about having brachytherapy, the radiation oncologist should have experience with at least 30 cases, and treat at least 15 cases per year.

✔ "What are the main side effects of radiation, and how long will they last?"

The doctor should give you an overview of possible side effects. If she says there are no side effects, consider consulting with another doctor.

Basic Info on Radiation Procedures

This section offers you a general walk-through of the two types of radiation therapy, external beam radiation therapy and brachytherapy, so you can consider both and work with your doctor to determine which type is right for you

Getting beamed up with external beam radiation therapy

If you receive external beam radiation treatments (EBRT), the radiation will be beamed into you by external machines. The doctor uses computers to help aim the radiation beams with precision, and focus as much radiation as possible on the prostate gland, and as little as possible on the surrounding area (particularly the bladder and rectum).

EBRT can be used to treat a little bit of cancer, an intermediate level of cancer, or advanced local cancer. The area or "field" that the beams hit can be widened from just the prostate to include the surrounding area and even the lymph nodes in the pelvis or abdomen. Of course, when the radiation field is widened, the risk of complications is greater.

If a patient's prostate gland is large, hormone therapy may be used to shrink the size of the prostate gland prior to radiation treatments. If patients have high-risk cancer, hormone therapy is also given shortly before radiation therapy, during the course of the treatments, and then for a brief period of time after the treatments.

Best candidates for EBRT

If you have localized prostate cancer or if your cancer hasn't advanced too far beyond the protective prostate capsule, you may be a good candidate for EBRT. In general, to be considered a good candidate for EBRT, you have to be in fairly good health (other than having prostate cancer), but your health doesn't have to be as good as it does when choosing the prostatectomy or brachytherapy (the radioactive seeds discussed in the following section). Both a prostatectomy and brachytherapy are riskier than EBRT because you may encounter problems associated with anesthesia.

Before, during, and after EBRT

If you and your doctor agree that EBRT is the best treatment option for you, your doctor will do some preparation work, such as imaging your lower body with computerized tomography (CT) scans or magnetic resonance imaging (MRIs) to help target the radiation so that the beams are aimed just right. Just before the procedure, technicians will mark your body with special ink and will usually make certain arrangements so that with each radiation dose, you'll be in the same immovable position.

When it's time for the procedure, you'll be positioned on a special table. Then the machines will emit the radiation needed to destroy the cancer cells. The machines may sound noisy or even scary, but they won't cut you, and they won't penetrate your body with anything other than the radiation beams. You'll feel no pain.

EBRT isn't a one-time treatment — instead, you usually receive multiple doses of radiation. With EBRT, patients often get radiation treatments five days a week, for six or eight weeks in a row. Each therapy session only lasts for 15 minutes or so. EBRT treatments can be inconvenient, especially if you have to drive a considerable distance to get to the radiation center.

After you receive EBRT treatments, you may experience some side effects, such as fatigue and bowel or urinary problems. Many patients don't experience side effects during the first few weeks, but by the third or fourth week, the cumulative effects of EBRT may cause such problems.

Newer approaches to aiming radiation

Some newer forms of EBRT, which are becoming more widely used, involve aiming the beams better to try to make the radiation more effective or safer.

One new approach is *three-dimensional conformal therapy,* where computers aim extremely targeted beams of radiation at your prostate from different directions, all at the same time. Imagine Captain Kirk from the TV show "Star Trek" setting his phaser on "stun," while Mr. Spock and Dr. McCoy do the same with their phasers. Now imagine the three of them all concentrating their phasers on the same point at the same time, for major impact.

These combined beams can be aimed at the prostate more accurately than the beam used in regular EBRT, so the risk of damaging healthy tissues is lower, and additional radiation can be given more safely. In general, the more radiation you get, the better your chances for killing the cancer cells.

When you receive three-dimensional conformal therapy, a special plastic mold of your body is made ahead of time. Before you undergo the procedure, you're placed inside the body mold. The purpose of this body mold is to hold you as extremely still as possible so that you don't move at all during the treatments.

Intensity modulated radiotherapy (IMRT) is an even newer form of aiming beams in EBRT. With this approach, each beam is modified to produce a pattern of radiation intensities. (The other approaches use uniform intensities of radiation.) This aiming modification (which requires sophisticated computers) helps target higher doses of radiation to the prostate without damaging the surrounding organs.

Sowing brachytherapy seeds

Modern brachytherapy is a relatively new treatment for prostate cancer, although scientists have actually considered it a possibility for nearly a hundred years. Brachytherapy is more convenient than EBRT for most men, because brachytherapy only involves one procedure that takes about 45 to 60 minutes, whereas EBRT requires repeated treatments five days a week for six to eight weeks. Also, brachytherapy may enable your doctor to safely give your prostate a higher dose of radiation — although with EBRT, radiation can be given to areas farther removed from the prostate.

When you receive brachytherapy, you'll receive either a *general anesthesia,* where you're totally asleep, or a *spinal anesthetic,* where just the lower half of your body is numbed. The doctor will carefully position radioactive seeds into your prostate with the help of an ultrasound probe. More specifically, the doctor inserts hollow needles, which contain the radioactive seeds, through the skin behind the scrotum and into the prostate, under ultrasound guidance. Because the radioactivity in the implanted seeds only lasts for a few months at most, the seeds will be prepared elsewhere and then immediately sent to the hospital prior to your procedure. So those seeds will be ready and waiting for you.

Before the procedure, he maps out your prostate, often with the help of the CT scan image, and calculates the right seed dose for your prostate size, and the size and location of the cancer. The doctor then uses this information to create a very accurate gridlike pattern that will tell him where to insert the needles when you're under anesthesia.

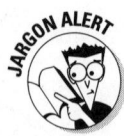

A few radiation oncologists use a device called an *endorectal coil* (a device that's inserted into the rectum and monitored with MRI) to implant the seeds. These doctors believe that endorectal coils help improve the precision of the seed placement. (The endorectal coil also is sometimes used to stage cancer. You can read about that use in Chapter 8.)

Sometime doctors use high-dose rate or *HDR brachytherapy* which involves radioactive seeds with iridium (rather than iodine or palladium). These seeds are inserted through needles and left in place for a short time, and then they are removed. (Other seeds can be left in the prostate indefinitely.) The process is repeated several times over the course of a day or so. External beam radiotherapy is always given in addition to HDR brachytherapy. Some doctors believe that HDR brachytherapy gives more radiation and fewer side effects. However, only a few radiation oncologists use this approach.

Best candidates for brachytherapy

For the most part, brachytherapy is given to men who are relatively healthy, because anesthesia is necessary with this procedure, and can be dangerous to the heart and lungs if patients are in poor health. The best candidates for brachytherapy are men who have localized cancer who are considered to be at low risk for developing advanced cancer — that is, patients with a PSA less than 11, a Gleason score less than 7, and a stage of cancer that's T1 or T2a. (Read about PSAs in Chapter 5, and read more about both the Gleason grading system and the TNM staging system in Chapter 8.)

With intermediate-risk cancers (PSA between 11 and 20, or Gleason score of 7, or stage T2b), many radiation oncologists give both EBRT and brachytherapy — although some give brachytherapy seeds alone. If the cancer is localized but high risk (PSA greater than 20, or Gleason score greater than 7, or stage T2c), or the cancer seems outside the prostate (stage T3), then EBRT (sometimes with or without brachytherapy) is given along with hormone therapy.

According to radiation therapy experts, brachytherapy seems to work best in patients who have prostates that are smaller than a volume of 60 cubic centimeters (cc), which is about the size of a tangerine. Prostate cancer size is measured by ultrasound, and most men have prostates that are less than 60 cc. When the prostate size is greater than 60 cc, it can be hard for the doctor to position the needles used to dispense the seeds. In this case, EBRT alone is a better option than brachytherapy. Sometimes a temporary course of hormone therapy (for three to six months) can shrink the gland sufficiently to make seed therapy feasible and desirable.

You may want to consider brachytherapy if

✔ You don't have severe urinary symptoms, such as frequency or urine blockage. Brachytherapy can worsen these symptoms even more than external beam radiotherapy.

✔ You haven't previously had a transurethral resection of the prostate, or TURP (because of benign prostatic hyperplasia of BPH, described in Chapter 4). If you've had a TURP, brachytherapy can cause many additional side effects.

Before, during, and after brachytherapy

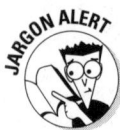

If your doctor is considering you for brachytherapy, he first needs to do a *transrectal urethral volume study* on you. This ultrasound test, which only takes about 15 minutes to perform, shows your doctor how large and how long your prostate is, giving him a map to base his treatment plan on. If the findings from the transrectal urethral volume study show him that you're a good candidate, and you're still interested in having the procedure, your doctor will schedule the procedure. *Note:* The transrectal urethral volume study is an outpatient procedure; the brachytherapy procedure requires you to enter the hospital, although most often, you can go home on the same day.

The doctor uses the information from the ultrasound study to create special templates that will actually be placed on your body during the procedure. These templates let your doctor know where to insert the needles that deposit the seeds in your prostate. Don't worry, you'll be sedated so that you don't squirm around while the doctor implants the seeds.

On the day of the procedure, the *anesthesiologist* (the medical doctor who administers the anesthesia to you prior to the procedure) will provide you with either a general anesthesia or a spinal anesthetic. Before the anesthesia is administered, the doctor may give you some Valium (generic name: diazepam) or another anti-anxiety drug to help you relax. After you're sufficiently anesthetized, the procedure will begin. (In most cases, your urologist will work together with a radiation oncologist to perform the brachytherapy.) The doctor will insert a transrectal ultrasound probe through your rectum so that he can position and inject the irradiated seeds right into your prostate.

Most of the radioactive seeds that doctors use today (which are made of either palladium or iodine) find a permanent home in your prostate. But don't worry: The radioactivity of both palladium and iodine decreases rapidly over time. For iodine, half the radioactivity is gone after two months; for palladium, half of it is gone after about 17 days. Thus, the seeds eventually lose their power and no longer pose any danger.

Your doctor will give you an antibiotic after the brachytherapy, to protect you against any infections that may crop up as a result of the procedure. He may also give you anti-inflammatory medications and painkillers. Some patients who have brachytherapy are sent home with a *catheter* (a tube inserted into your bladder to drain your urine) that's left in overnight. The catheter is removed by a doctor or nurse after a day or so. The catheter rarely needs to be left in for a longer period.

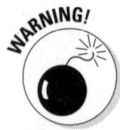

You may experience a little bleeding after the seeds are implanted, but you should be fine within a day or two. If you have any bleeding that begins 24 hours after the procedure, or if you have profuse bleeding at any time, contact your urologist to find out if you need to be checked out. You should also call the doctor if you pass any blood clots. If you can't reach your doctor, talk to the doctor who's filling in for him. If that doesn't work, go to the emergency room at the nearest hospital.

You may also have some problems with impotence right after the procedure. This problem should resolve itself in a few weeks or months (unless you were having impotence problems before you received the radiation treatments). However, some men lose their potency from the procedure either right away or months or years later, as the scarring from the radiation takes effect. Some of the other side effects of brachytherapy are urinary symptoms, rectal bleeding, and diarrhea.

Your prostate may be swollen and irritated after brachytherapy, and you may have problems with urinary frequency and urgency. Your urination is generally back to normal by six to eight months after the procedure. If you respond well to the anti-inflammatory and prostate-specific medications the doctor prescribes, as most men do, you shouldn't feel much pain. Your doctor may prescribe Flomax (generic name: tamsulosin) to help you urinate better or Ditropan (generic name: oxybutynin) to help slow down your bladder irritability.

In most cases, you'll be able to return to work within a few days of having brachytherapy, unless your job requires heavy lifting. If your job is physical in nature, wait another week or so before resuming your normal activities.

Some experts recommend using condoms for a while when you have sexual intercourse after undergoing the brachytherapy procedure. (You should be able to have sex within a week or so of the procedure.) The reason: to prevent the seeds from somehow escaping the prostate and entering the vagina during ejaculation. (This is highly unlikely, although it is theoretically possible.)

Following up

After your procedure, your doctor will follow up with periodic checks of your PSA levels. If the procedure is working, your PSA should fall to extremely low levels. Your PSA level will rarely drop to zero, as it does after surgery, because you still have a prostate and thus also have PSA-producing cells.

The exact level that your PSA should fall to is debatable. Some experts say 0.2 nanograms per milliliter (or ng/ml) is the right number, and others say 0.5 ng/ml, and still others say it's 1.0 ng/ml. After the PSA settles to its lowest level, the main thing doctors look for is a rise in PSA. A rise in the PSA level may indicate that treatment has failed you. However, in the first couple of years after radiation therapy, PSAs can rise temporarily because of a delayed inflammation effect. (This is true whether you have brachytherapy or EBRT.) If your doctor determines that brachytherapy has failed you, you'll need to work with him to devise a new plan.

When initial radiation isn't enough

If you have radiation treatments, you may never need any additional treatment for prostate cancer. Hopefully you'll be cured, and you'll live a long and prosperous life. Unfortunately, sometimes the cancer continues to advance, and additional treatments are necessary. Such treatments may come in the form of surgery, hormones, or newer options for managing advanced cases of cancer.

Looking at surgery

If you have radiation treatments, and your PSA scores and other indicators indicate that the cancer is still present, you may need to think about following your radiation treatments with surgery. Follow-up surgery does work, but it's not always the best choice, because the radiation often damages the prostate tissue, making it sticky and very hard to remove in a prostatectomy. If surgery is an option, it must be done by a very experienced surgeon.

Considering more radiation

Radiation didn't work for you, and you need more treatment, but sometimes more radiation may be what you need.

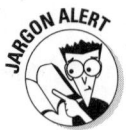

When brachytherapy is used to treat a recurrence of prostate cancer, it's referred to as *salvage brachytherapy*. Typically, salvage brachytherapy is performed on people who had EBRT for their initial treatment. Salvage brachytherapy is rarely performed if brachytherapy was used for the initial treatment. About 20 percent to 40 percent of patients who were initially treated with EBRT have a relapse of cancer and need further treatment, such as salvage brachytherapy. I believe salvage brachytherapy may result in a lot of complications, and currently I'm very cautious about recommending it. If you do decide to have it done, make sure it is performed by a very experienced radiation oncologist. (Some doctors also use salvage cryotherapy to freeze the cancer. You can read more about cryosurgery in Chapter 14.)

Hoping hormones help

If your cancer has advanced beyond the prostate gland, you and your doctor will need to discuss hormone therapy (also known as *endocrine therapy*,). Hormone therapy doesn't kill the cancer, but it can be effective at slowing down the cancer's wave of destruction (sometimes for years). See Chapter 13 for more information on hormone therapy.

Considering other options

Sometimes radiation therapy doesn't work. You may also find that hormone therapy isn't an effective treatment option for you. In these cases, *chemotherapy* (treating cancer with cancer-killing drugs) may be the best answer. (See Chapter 15 for a more in-depth discussion of chemotherapy.)

Other choices may also be warranted, such as joining a clinical study to try an experimental therapy or medication that's being investigated by medical researchers. (Read more about clinical studies in Chapters 15 and 21.)

Chapter 13

Slowing the Cancer with Hormones

*F*ew men like the idea of taking hormones. Of course, some athletes ingest male hormones to bulk up their muscles. (Which is illegal. It also has some awful side effects, such as shrinking testicles.) But the anabolic steroids that athletes sometimes take are *not* the same type of hormones that are used to treat men with prostate cancer.

The hormones that are used for treating prostate cancer are given to eliminate or block your own natural anabolic steroids, the most potent and important of which is testosterone. These hormones can slam the brakes on the continued growth of your cancer. Unfortunately, hormone therapy also may induce some annoying side effects, such as impotence, hot flashes, and mood swings.

Why do men put up with these aggravating side effects? Because studies have shown that hormone therapy often stops prostate cancer in its tracks for several years. Hormone therapy can't cure cancer but it can effectively extend many men's lives for many months or years. Hormone therapy is effective in about 85 percent to 90 percent of men. Hormone therapy can reduce the cancer or keep it from getting worse. Some physicians also recommend hormone therapy to patients who have curable cancers. With curable cancers, the hormones work to shrink the tumor before the patient undergoes radiation therapy or a prostatectomy.

In this chapter, I cover hormone therapy for men at all stages of prostate cancer. I talk about the specific drugs and the different categories of hormones that are usually used in hormone therapy, and I explain how they work to block prostate cancer (as far as is known). In addition, I discuss the pros and cons of using different types of hormones, and I cover the key side effects and what you can do about them if they occur.

Basic Info on Hormone Therapy

If you have prostate cancer, understanding the basics of hormone therapy is a very good idea for you and your family. (Hormone therapy is sometimes called *endocrine therapy,* because hormones are produced by endocrine glands in your body.) Even if your doctor isn't recommending hormone therapy for you now, you may need to take hormones at some point in the future, to prolong your life should your cancer become an advanced case.

Doctors use hormone therapy for men with different levels of cancer, so if your doctor is recommending that you start taking hormone medications, don't assume that you have a very advanced case of prostate cancer.

Understanding how hormone therapy works

With hormone therapy, the goal is to halt male hormone production and/or action to prevent further growth of prostate cancer. When hormone therapy (either medical or surgical) is administered to treat your prostate cancer, testosterone is decreased or blocked, temporarily delaying the spread of prostate cancer in many men. The testosterone and other natural anabolic steroids produced by the body make cancer cells grow. So, bringing testosterone to a screeching halt (or at least, slowing it down a whole lot) often significantly delays the spread of prostate cancer.

Comparing different forms of hormone therapy

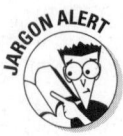

Doctors may use *monotherapy* (one therapy) or *combination therapy* (several different therapies at the same time) when treating patients with hormone therapy. Doctors may also consider *intermittent therapy* (treating patients with intermittent, or on and off, hormone therapy). For more on intermittent therapy, see the "Switching hormones on and off: Intermittent therapy" sidebar in this chapter.

In some cases, the *bilateral orchiectomy* (surgical removal of the testicles) is the best choice to shut down testosterone production, although it's a scary thought for most men. (Bilateral orchiectomy is a form of surgery, but it's considered a hormone therapy because it halts testosterone production.)

The first line of treatment: LH-RH agonist drugs

Most doctors who prescribe hormones rely upon *luteinizing hormone-releasing hormone agonist* (LH-RH agonist) drugs to do the job, at least initially. The LH-RH agonists cause two organs, the hypothalamus and the pituitary, to stop the testicles from making testosterone. Research indicates that as much as 95 percent of testosterone production can be shut down with LH-RH medications, which significantly delays any further spread of cancer.

LH-RH agonists are given as shots. They may be given in dosages that last one, three, or four months, or even longer. These shots must be administered by a doctor or a nurse under a doctor's direction.

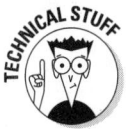

The key types of injectable LH-RH hormones that physicians may currently choose from are Lupron, Viadur, or Eligard (all of which have the generic name: leuprolide), Suprefact (generic name: buserelin), and Zoladex (generic name: goserelin).

Your doctor may decide that the LH-RH agonist medication isn't the best option for you, or she may want to add another hormone. Some doctors currently combine LH-RH agonist drugs with antiandrogens (I discuss antiandrogens shortly). Some doctors prescribe a hormone that was a popular treatment for prostate cancer 30 years ago — diethystilbestrol (DES), an estrogen.

Switching hormones on and off: Intermittent therapy

Some physicians are treating patients who have non-advanced prostate cancer with intermittent (on and off) hormone therapy. The hormones are given until the patient's PSA level drops to zero, and the tumor shrinks or at least is no longer spreading.

Generally, a patient takes the hormone therapy for at least 8 to 12 months and then stops. While he's off the hormones, his physician continues to carefully monitor his PSA level. When his PSA level goes up beyond a certain predetermined number, the hormone therapy is started up again.

While the preliminary evidence suggests that intermittent hormone therapy is safe, doctors still don't know for sure whether intermittent therapy provides equal or better survival rates than continuous hormone treatments. Clinical studies now underway may provide this information. Doctors do know, however, that men definitely prefer intermittent therapy over continuous therapy because intermittent therapy gives them a break from the side effects usually caused by hormone therapy (such as impotence and mood swings). When patients are off the drugs for a month or so, their libido usually returns, and they feel much better.

Hormonally speaking, who's the doc in charge?

You may wonder which type of specialist treats you with hormone therapy and monitors how well the medication is working to suppress your cancer. Often, the treating specialist is the urologist, because urologists frequently oversee cases of prostate cancer. Urologists sometimes prescribe hormone therapy because surgery has failed, or because they want to reduce the size of your tumor before surgery. Radiation oncologists may also treat you with hormones, because sometimes hormones are prescribed to reduce the size of your tumor before you have any radiation treatments. A medical oncologist

can also monitor your hormone therapy. (See Chapter 6 for more info about the different types of specialists who treat prostate cancer.)

When it comes to receiving hormone therapy, it really isn't important whether your particular specialist is a urologist, a radiation oncologist, or a medical oncologist. The important thing is that your doctor knows his stuff, answers your questions completely, provides you with excellent treatment, and carefully monitors your progress.

However, estrogen drugs are usually *not* the first line of defense for treating prostate cancer, because estrogens can cause very serious side effects that other medications (such as LH-RH agonists or antiandrogen medications) do not cause. Specifically, a large-scale study done for the Veterans Administration revealed that men who took a full dose of estrogens to treat their prostate cancer experienced an increased risk of cardiovascular problems, such as heart attacks and strokes. Consequently, estrogens are usually considered a sort of second-line form of hormone therapy for treating prostate cancer. (Read more about estrogen therapy in Chapter 15.)

Avoiding flares with antiandrogens

LH-RH agonists and estrogens stop the production of most testosterone, but they can't block *all* anabolic steroid production. About 5 percent or so of your total anabolic steroids are actually produced by your adrenal gland. Some experts believe that these steroids, even though they're much weaker than testosterone, can facilitate at least a little prostate cancer growth. Of course, this extra steroid production is a bad thing when you have prostate cancer, because you don't want any growth.

When you start hormone therapy with an LH-RH hormone, your body may react by creating a temporary surge of testosterone, which can last for several days. This surge in testosterone production is called a *flare*. After the flare ends, your testosterone levels plummet. Because the sudden flare of testosterone can theoretically temporarily fuel the growth of cancer cells, *antiandrogen drugs* are often used, temporarily, to prevent flares altogether along with LH-RH medicines. Antiandrogens work by blocking whatever testosterone-like substances may be around from interfering and working on the prostate cancer cells. This total shutdown therapy, blocking all androgen production, is called a *total androgen blockade.* With a total androgen block-ade, all testosterone and testosterone-like hormones are prevented from acting on the prostate cancer in your body. As a result, the invasive cancer can't penetrate the strong defense that's mounted by both the LH-RH antago-nist and the antiandrogen. However, the cancer will ultimately find a weak-ness somewhere and break through.

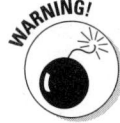

Testosterone flares can be a very serious problem for men who have advanced prostate cancer, because this extra surge of testosterone may be just enough to cause them to go from having no symptoms to experiencing pain. The extra testosterone from the flare may accelerate the cancer growth temporarily. In some extreme cases, the flare is enough to cause irreversible spinal paralysis. If you have advanced prostate cancer, and your doctor plans to use LH-RH therapy, he will probably also want to add an antiandrogen to the pharmaceutical mix to prevent testosterone flare. Your doctor may keep you on the antiandrogen for about a month or so. Flares usually aren't a prob-lem after the second and subsequent LH-RH shots.

Antiandrogen drugs are given as pills. Keep in mind that of the types of hor-mone therapies available, antiandrogens have the least number of side effects, although researchers don't know if taking antiandrogens alone can sufficiently block the spread of prostate cancer.

Casodex (generic name: bicalutamide) and Eulexin (generic name: flutamide) are two common antiandrogen drugs.

Comparing monotherapy to combination therapy

In the recent past, many experts believed that the best initial hormone therapy was the one that stopped all anabolic steroids (androgens) from working on prostate cancer. Therefore, they advocated long-term total androgen block-ade by combining an antiandrogen with an approach that stopped testosterone production (either an orchiectomy or LH-RH medication). Over the years, many clinical trials compared monotherapy (an LH-RH agonist or orchiectomy) with combination therapy.

The bottom line for all these studies was that, overall, long-term combination therapy didn't seem to be any better than monotherapy. Yet some experts still believe that combination ther-apy is better, especially for men who don't have very advanced cases of prostate cancer. However, experts do agree that giving an LH-RH medicine and temporarily given an antiandro-gen is the best strategy for preventing the flare, which usually is only a concern if you have very advanced prostate cancer. (Read Chapter 15 for more information on treating advanced cancer.)

The origins of the orchiectomy

The orchiectomy was based on a paper written in 1940 by Dr. Charles Huggins, a urologist who discovered that the removal of the testicles considerably slowed the rate of prostate cancer growth.

Dr. Huggins went on to make further discoveries. For example, he determined that taking female hormone medicine could achieve the same effect on men with prostate cancer as undergoing the orchiectomy. Both methods are considered hormone therapies, because they both stop the production of testosterone.

Dr. Huggins won the Nobel Prize in 1966 for his prostate cancer treatment research and discoveries.

Monotherapy with antiandrogens

In addition to prescribing antiandrogens with LH-RH agonists to prevent testosterone flare, some physicians are also using antiandrogens *alone* to treat patients who have prostate cancer that hasn't spread much beyond the prostate gland.

If your doctor uses monotherapy with antiandrogens, you won't suffer from many side effects caused by the other hormone drugs — you can skip the impotence, weight gain, hot flashes, and other side effects that are almost inevitably caused by LH-RH agonists and estrogens. On the negative side, common side effects of antiandrogens are diarrhea and swelling in the breasts.

The other downside of going solo with antiandrogens is that studies haven't shown whether antiandrogens alone provide men with as good an outcome, in terms of their survival, as combination therapy or LH-RH drugs. More studies are necessary.

Bilateral orchiectomy

Another way to shut down testosterone production is to surgically remove the testicles in a procedure called a bilateral (for both sides) orchiectomy (removal of the testicle) or orchiectomy for short. Understandably, this is not a popular choice among men needing hormone therapy, because the surgery causes instant and irreversible impotence, sterility, and other side effects. But you won't have to worry about testosterone making cancer grow, because testosterone production is permanently shut down. That factory is closed, and everyone went home.

The bilateral orchiectomy was the not-so-long-ago standard hormone therapy treatment for men with advanced prostate cancer. Although the side effects of the procedure (such as impotence, hot flashes, and decreased muscle mass and weight gain) are irreversible, doctors in many underdeveloped countries

today continue to use the orchiectomy, instead of hormone therapy in the form of drugs, to treat patients with advanced prostate cancer. This procedure is still used because it's relatively inexpensive and it's permanent — after the testicles are removed, no further shots or pills are necessary. But in the United States, Canada, and most other developed countries, physicians and patients usually choose hormone medicines over the orchiectomy to stop the testosterone action, because many men understandably have a major psychological hang-up with the thought of removing their testicles, even though the actual operation is short and relatively painless, with a quick recovery.

Figuring out if it's working

Doctors determine whether the hormone therapy is effective by monitoring your blood levels of prostate specific antigen (PSA). If your PSA is stabilized, your doctor should test your PSA levels every three months or so. But if your PSA is rising, it needs to be tested monthly. Your PSA level provides your doctor with an early warning system to help gauge if any cancer problems are starting again. Decreasing PSA blood levels are usually a good sign that the hormones are doing their job. Conversely, if your PSA levels are rising, your doctor will need to consider whether to change the dosage of the hormones, give you a different drug, or add even more drugs — sort of like calling in the National Guard to back up the regular troops.

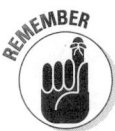

Even if your PSA level is low, you're feeling well, and hormone therapy is very effective for you, the downside is that the therapy will eventually fail. Figuring out how long hormone therapy will work for you is impossible, but for most men, it can effectively prevent any further spread of prostate cancer for at least one to four years, and sometimes for as long as ten years or more.

Understanding Your Doctor's Recommendation

Before your doctor recommends hormone therapy to treat your cancer, as well as which hormones may work the best for you, he first sizes you up as a possible candidate for hormone therapy, taking into account the following information:

✔ **Your life expectancy:** If your life expectancy is less than an additional five years, and your prostate cancer is confined to your prostate and isn't very high risk (see Chapter 8 on staging prostate cancer), you and your doctor may decide that it's not worth putting up with the expense or the annoying side effects of hormone therapy.

✔ **Your general health:** Your doctor may have considered you a candidate for a prostatectomy or radiation therapy because your cancer was localized, but your poor health made him decide against those choices, and to decide in favor of hormone therapy instead. Nearly all men can be given hormone therapy.

Even if your cancer is advanced, hormone therapy can be effective at lowering your PSA level and/or alleviating some symptoms for years. However, if you have localized cancer especially if you're without any symptoms, and have a life expectancy of less than five years, and you don't want to cope with the side effects that hormone therapy usually causes, you may wish to forego hormone therapy altogether.

Deciding If Hormone Therapy Is Right for You

Before you agree to launch your program of hormone therapy, be aware of side effects that may occur as well as the basic pros and cons of using hormones. This section covers these important topics.

Considering the risks you face

Hormone therapy can be tremendously beneficial and can effectively stave off your prostate cancer spread for years, but it shouldn't be taken lightly. When you take hormones (or have an orchiectomy), your body reacts to the orchestrated change in body chemistry. Some side effects of hormone medications may be annoying, aggravating, or really difficult, depending on the type of drug you take, the dose, whether you take one or more hormones, and your own physiology and general health. If you take hormones for a short period, you shouldn't have any problem tolerating their side effects.

When you take hormones, tell your physician about any side effects you experience. Don't be the strong and silent type who never complains. The downside of never complaining is that your doctor has no idea how much you're suffering, so he won't offer you any medications or other solutions to make you feel significantly better. Your family members will appreciate it too, because men who don't feel well can be very difficult people to be around.

The following sections describe common side effects you may experience when taking hormones.

It's getting warmer: Hot flashes — yes, in men

When most people think of *hot flashes* — which are momentary feelings of heat all over your body, like you were quickly thrown into a sauna and then tossed right out again — they think of older women going through menopause. But men can experience hot flashes, as well.

If you find that the hot flashes caused by your hormone therapy are really difficult for you to cope with, talk to your doctor. A variety of established medicines can help alleviate your hot flashes, such as a very low dose of estrogen or a hormone drug called Megace (generic name: megestrol acetate). Some alternative medicines may also help with hot flashes. (You can read about alternative medicines that may help you cope with the side effects of hormone therapy in Chapter 18.)

Coping with irritability and mood swings

Hormones can transform Mr. Nice into Mr. Extremely Irritable. If you're suffering from bouts of extreme irritability, don't worry: You're not having a total and permanent personality change. But the emotional impact of your irritable behavior can be tough for you (and your loved ones!) to take.

As much as possible, make a concerted effort to think first before snarling and lashing out. Count to ten when you find that your emotions are difficult to control. It really does help. You need to realize that, when you get used to the hormone therapy or it's done, Mr. Nice (or Mr. Average, or whoever you were before hormone therapy) will be back in the driver's seat of your mind again. If the hormone therapy is permanent, the mood swings will lessen with time. If the mood changes become too severe, ask your doctor about antidepressants or other mood-altering therapies. They usually work.

Lowered sex drive

When you take hormones to fight prostate cancer, your sex drive may be very low or even reduced to zero. With no sex drive, you'll likely become impotent.

Impotence may upset your partner, but it may not upset you a lot, because of your missing-in-action sex drive — except that you may feel bad that you really can't have intercourse with your partner while you're taking hormones. (But don't forget: Just because you can't have intercourse doesn't mean that you have to give up sex altogether. You can still pay attention to your partner sexually, even if you're not in the mood yourself.)

If you're on intermittent therapy, your doctor may eventually take you off hormones for awhile. In many cases, your sexual desire and potency will return after the drugs are out of your system and you begin producing testosterone again.

Looking at other side effects

In addition to hot flashes, irritability, and impotence, hormone therapy can also lead to a few other side effects. For example, some men experience very aggravating problems with *gynecomastia,* which is swelling and pain in the breast tissue (usually both breasts).

Gynecomastia can be lessened with a low dose of radiation therapy given before hormone therapy begins. Some men may also undergo surgery such as *liposuction* (suctioning of the fatty tissue in the breast) to help prevent gynecomastia, but this approach is rare.

Other side effects that may be caused by hormone therapy include:

- **Weight gain and redistribution:** You may gain about 10 to 20 pounds or so. (Some men experience more weight gain, while others don't have weight gain.) You may also find that you have weight redistribution, with your body fat gravitating to your thighs and arms rather than your belly. Vigorous weight control programs, with exercise and attention to your diet, usually help with this problem.

- **Loss of muscle mass:** Your body may become fleshier and looser while you're taking hormones, with less muscle definition than you had in the past. This side effect can be reversed with intermittent hormone therapy. Exercise also helps combat this problem.

- **Osteoporosis:** If hormone therapy continues for a very long time, you may develop *osteoporosis* (a condition characterized by the loss of bone density). If your doctor thinks that you're losing bone, and you're at risk for developing osteoporosis and bone fractures, he may prescribe calcium or vitamin D to help prevent any further bone loss. Some experts believe that bisphosphanase drugs, such as Aredia (generic name: pamidronate) and Zometa (generic name: zoledronic acid), may also help prevent osteoporosis. Exercise is another good prevention against osteoporosis.

- **Depression:** Having prostate cancer can induce depression, but taking hormones can sink you further into depression. However, this side effect isn't very common. If you think that you may be suffering from depression, talk to your doctor about it. You may need an antidepressant to help you recover from depression.

Focusing on the benefits

Hormone therapy has several benefits including the following:

- Hormone therapy can halt the growth of the cancer and extend your life for years.

✔ If hormone therapy is your first line of defense, you probably won't have to undergo surgery or radiation treatments.

✔ If you still have a prostate, hormone therapy can often improve any trouble you may have urinating.

Asking the tough questions

If your doctor suggests hormone therapy, find out why he thinks the treatment is appropriate for you, and then ask the following questions:

✔ "Are you suggesting hormone therapy as a first step before I try another treatment such as surgery or radiation, or are you suggesting that I only have hormone therapy?"

You want to know your doctor's overall plan.

✔ "What possible side effects can result from taking hormone therapies?"

Before you start taking hormones to quell the growth of prostate cancer in your body, you may think to yourself, "How bad can the side effects actually be?" After all, hormone therapy isn't as serious as having your prostate removed or as radical as having it irradiated. Your doctor should tell you about hot flashes, mood swings, and the loss of your sex drive — all are common side effects of hormone therapy.

✔ "How long will it take before you know if the hormones are delaying the spread of the cancer?"

Your doctor will likely tell you that your PSA level will show him if the therapy is working about three to four months after you start taking hormones.

✔ "Will I need more than one hormone?"

Some doctors believe that one drug is sufficient, while others prefer several medications. You may take two drugs for awhile and then taper down to one medication. Whichever way your doctor plans to go, be sure to ask her to explain her reasoning in simple terms.

✔ "Do you believe in giving hormone therapy early in treatment, or do you prefer to wait until I start experiencing symptoms such as pain?"

Many doctors believe in starting hormone therapy early on, and I'm one of them. Others prefer to wait until symptoms of advanced cancer appear. To be an aware patient, you need to know your doctor's philosophy on this issue. Ultimately, the decision to start hormone therapy early or late is really yours to make.

Preparing for Hormone Therapy

Most forms of hormone therapy require no preparation. For example, if you have an orchiectomy, you don't have to do anything — you just show up for the procedure.

When your doctor orders hormone therapy in the form of LH-RH medications, you receive the therapy in the form of injections. The shots are given at intervals of one month, three months, four months, or yearly, depending on the dosage your doctor orders. No preparation is necessary before getting the shots. You just make an appointment, go in, and get the injection.

If your doctor recommends hormone therapy in the form of antiandrogen pills (which are taken at least once a day), you need to get a blood test that checks your liver function before you start taking the drug. You'll then need get additional blood tests for the first three months after you begin taking the drug. (Your doctor will determine the frequency of blood tests.) These tests are important because antiandrogens in rare cases can cause minor liver damage, a problem that then subsides when you go off the drug.

Pondering Treatment for Patients with Initially Advanced or Resistant Cancer

If you've tried hormone therapy and it isn't working, either because it never worked or it worked awhile (maybe years) and now your PSA blood levels are rising, it's time to consider other options.

Dealing with advanced cancer

Sometimes the cancer is at an advanced stage when you're first diagnosed. This is not fun to hear, but if you work with your doctor, you can develop a good strategy for managing advanced prostate cancer. (Check out Chapter 15 for information on what to do about very advanced cases of prostate cancer.)

You may need to supplement your hormone therapy with other medications or treatments, particularly if your PSA level is on the rise. Your doctor may recommend experimental therapies or alternative remedies, which are not typical everyday treatments.

Listen carefully when your doctor tells you to think about such options, and ask why they may help you, how you'll know if they're working, what the pros and cons are, and what side effects they may cause. Your doctor may also recommend joining a clinical trial, which is often a very good idea.

Evaluating options for men who are hormone resistant

When your doctor recommends hormone therapy, he believes that it's your best choice for fighting back prostate cancer. But you can't always know for sure whether a therapy will work until you actually try it. When it comes to hormone therapy, some men are *hormone resistant.* If you're hormone resistant, the initial hormone therapy doesn't work for you (which is very rare), or it worked for awhile (sometimes for many years) but now it doesn't keep your PSA down and your cancer under control. When hormone resistance happens, you need to take a different course of action, such as undergoing chemotherapy or taking other types of medicine. (I cover these options in Chapter 15.)

When the initial hormone therapy doesn't work anymore, other hormone therapies, either alone or in combination with other drugs, may work to improve or stabilize your condition. For example, if you're on LH-RH injections and your testosterone level is not as low as it should be, your doctor may recommend an orchiectomy. Alternatively, if you haven't started taking antiandrogen pills, your doctor may recommend them, because they may help lower your PSA for awhile. Strangely, if you're already taking an antiandrogen, stopping it or changing to a different antiandrogen may make things temporarily better by lowering the PSA.

Other hormone pills, such as diethylstilbestrol (DES, which is an estrogen pill), may be added or substituted to give you a temporary benefit. Megace (generic name: megestrol acetate) is another supplemental hormone drug that may be effective. Because DES can cause problems with blood vessels, such as heart attacks, strokes, or blood clots, many physicians put patients taking DES on a small daily dose of aspirin or blood thinners.

The final hormone therapy that is sometimes prescribed late in the hormone-resistant phase is Nizoral (generic name: ketoconazole). This drug is normally used for fungal infections, but at high doses, it turns off certain parts of the adrenal gland, stopping production of testosterone-like hormones. Unfortunately, Nizoral has side effects, the most prominent of which is an upset stomach.

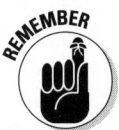

You have many options when it comes to second-line hormone therapy, but the juggling of hormones is an art that should be conducted by an expert (either a urologist or a medical oncologist).

Chapter 14

Considering Cutting-edge Treatments

*Y*ou and your doctor have seriously considered all the available choices for treating your prostate cancer, including surgery, radiation therapy, and hormone treatments — and maybe you also considered possible combinations of these different treatments. But now your doctor (or you) thinks that you need to also consider the new cutting-edge options for treating prostate cancer. You may be interested in a cutting-edge treatment because you have advanced cancer and/or you don't want to try hormone therapy. Or maybe you tried hormone therapy and it never worked, or it worked for awhile, and now your cancer is on the march again. Or maybe you have localized prostate cancer (cancer confined to the prostate), and you don't want to have a prostatectomy or radiation therapy because you're worried about developing impotence or incontinence.

In this chapter, I talk about cutting-edge therapies; I provide you with some basic information on how they work, and tell you their key pros and cons.

Icing the Cancer: Cryosurgery

Cryosurgery (which is also known as *cryotherapy* or *cryoablation*) refers to a relatively new procedure for treating localized prostate cancer in which the doctor uses very low temperatures to freeze the cancer cells. Cryosurgery may be a good treatment choice if you don't want to have surgery or radiation, but you still want to be treated. Cryosurgery is sometimes also used as a *salvage therapy* (an additional local therapy that's used to treat the cancer when the initial treatment is not successful) after radiation treatments, when your doctor feels that more radiation treatments won't help you. Unfortunately, so far, cryosurgery after radiation produces serious side effects, such as urethral burning, incontinence, and rectal injury. But the good news is that doctors are working on lowering the risks of developing these side effects.

Cryosurgery has been used by some doctors since the 1970s, but it didn't gain prominence until the early 1990s (with the development of new probes and more advanced ultrasound technology). However, many doctors are still uncertain and highly skeptical about cryosurgery, so don't assume that your doctor will be thrilled about the idea if you mention it to him.

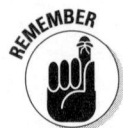

Cryosurgery has been a Medicare-approved procedure for treating prostate cancer since 1999. Most other health insurance companies cover this procedure, as well. Cryosurgery is the only specifically Medicare-approved nonsurgical procedure for treating localized cancer after radiation has failed.

Looking at the tip of the iceberg: How cryosurgery works

Cryosurgery is usually performed in the hospital, so if you decide to have the procedure, you'll need to plan on a one- or two-day hospital stay. Before the procedure, your doctor performs a *transrectal ultrasound* (a test that I cover in Chapter 6) to determine where the cancer is, how large it is, and how much space it takes up inside your prostate. You may also have a computerized tomography (CT) scan and/or a bone scan (also covered in Chapter 6) to make sure that the cancer hasn't spread to your lymph nodes or bones. (If it has spread, cryosurgery won't be performed.)

Right before the procedure, you're sedated with anesthesia. You receive either a *general anesthesia* (which makes you unconscious for the procedure) or a *spinal anesthesia* (which numbs you from the waist down). In most cases, cryosurgery takes about an hour or two.

Urologists are the doctors who generally perform the cryosurgery procedure. During the procedure, the doctor uses liquid nitrogen to put your prostate cancer cells into a deep freeze that they'll never recover from. (Some doctors prefer to use argon gas rather than liquid nitrogen.)

First a saline solution is inserted into the area to separate the rectum from the prostate and protect it from the deep freeze. Before physicians began using saline solutions, cryosurgery caused a lot more rectal damage. Then the urologist inserts the cryoprobes through your skin, between your scrotum and rectum, and into your prostate. When the probes are situated just right to cover the entire prostate, the doctor injects the liquid nitrogen (or argon gas) and freezes the prostate. Doctors use anywhere from five to eight probes to obtain uniform freezing throughout the prostate.

When the liquid nitrogen or argon gas is injected, it forms a ball of ice in the prostate. When the ball of ice melts, the cancer cells rupture and die. Doctors usually do at least two freezing and melting cycles over the course of one procedure, just to make sure they get all the cancer. Sort of like tying your shoelaces with a double knot to make sure they don't come undone.

During the procedure, the doctor uses a *transrectal ultrasound probe* (a special device, inserted through your rectum, that enables the doctor to view your prostate) to carefully monitor what he's doing. With the probe, the doctor can see exactly where the gland is freezing. He can then make the adjustments necessary for freezing the entire prostate, which theoretically destroys the prostate but also the prostate cancer.

The doctor will usually also insert a special warming catheter into your *urethra* (the canal that carries urine from your bladder to the outside; it travels right through the prostate gland) to keep it from freezing during the procedure.

Pros and cons of cryosurgery

Cryosurgery has advantages and disadvantages. The following list covers some of the primary advantages:

- ✔ If the procedure works, it kills the cancer by putting it into a deep freeze. So far, results have shown that when the prostate is biopsied again after cryosurgery, most of the time, no further cancer is present, and the prostate specific antigen (PSA) blood test usually goes down to low values and stays there.

- ✔ The procedure requires no incisions, and it doesn't result in any blood loss.

- ✔ The procedure can be repeated, if necessary. (Some treatments, such as brachytherapy, can only be performed once.)

- ✔ Doctors can tell right away how well the prostate has been covered by the liquid nitrogen (or argon gas), because they can see the ball of ice that forms. When the prostate is completely covered with the ball of ice, the doctors know that the entire prostate (and all the cancer) is being treated.

Here are some of the primary disadvantages of cryosurgery:

- ✔ If the cryoprobes aren't targeted very carefully by an experienced physician, the healthy tissue surrounding the prostate can be damaged — despite the use of a warming catheter to protect the urethra and saline solution to protect the rectum. If healthy tissue is damaged, significant side effects such as urethral burning, incontinence, and rectal problems can occur.

- ✔ Very few urologists perform this procedure. Some doctors (including me) believe that the information available on cryosurgery is just too preliminary to consider favoring it over a prostatectomy or radiation treatments.

- ✔ The nerve bundles that control erections often unavoidably get frozen during the procedure. Consequently, this freezing of the nerve bundles leads to impotence. Some doctors have successfully performed nerve-sparing cryosurgery, enabling their patients to avoid the impotence problem; but until nerve-sparing cryosurgery becomes more prevalent, impotence will continue to be a substantial risk with cryosurgery.

Turning Up the Heat: Microwave Therapy

Some researchers believe that prostate cancer can be eradicated with *microwave therapy,* a new treatment that uses very high temperatures to destroy prostate cancer cells. This therapy has also been used to successfully treat benign prostatic hyperplasia (BPH). See Chapter 4 for more on BPH.

Microwave therapy, like radiation and cryosurgery, seeks to destroy the prostate, and therefore the prostate cancer, without actually removing it surgically.

Men who have localized prostate cancer and don't want surgery or radiation therapy are the best candidates for microwave therapy. Microwave therapy may also be a good treatment for patients whose radiation therapy has failed. Microwave therapy can be administered more than once.

How microwaving works

Microwave therapy (which is also known as *thermal ablation therapy*) is currently being clinically tested on patients with localized prostate cancer.

A variety of machines can be used to deliver microwave therapy to the prostate. For example, the doctor may use a rectal probe or a heating probe inserted into the urethra to deliver the microwave heat. Basically, these instruments focus microwaves into the prostate to heat it up and systematically destroy it, along with the localized prostate cancer. The microwave devices are engineered to try to preserve the urethra and cut down on side effects.

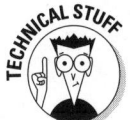

Doctors are also testing the heat generated from high-intensity focused ultrasound (HIFU) as a treatment for destroying localized cancer. This approach is more noninvasive than the other heat approaches, and small preliminary trials that are being conducted in Europe seem to be promising.

Pros and cons of microwave therapy

The main benefit of microwave therapy is that, if it works, the cancer cells are destroyed, and the problem is solved without radioactive seeds inserted in your prostate or exposure to high doses of external beam radiation therapy. In addition, doctors can treat you again with microwave therapy if they feel that additional treatment is needed. With some of the heating systems, little or no anesthesia is needed; yet another advantage.

The primary disadvantage of microwave therapy is that healthy tissue may accidentally be destroyed along with the bad tissue. Also, if you decide to undergo microwave therapy, you need to find a doctor who's very experienced at performing the procedure and is conducting a clinical trial, because this form of therapy isn't yet approved in the United States.

Not enough evidence is available to determine whether microwave therapy is as effective at treating prostate cancer as surgery and radiation. However, the technology behind the procedure is continuing to improve, and more and more doctors are gaining valuable experience. Someday it may become a popular method for treating local prostate cancer. Unfortunately, if the cancer spreads beyond the prostate but is still in the general area, it is harder to treat with microwave therapy than it is with radiation or a non-nerve-sparing prostatectomy.

Looking at Gene Therapy and Immune Therapy

Researchers are currently performing clinical trials to test the effectiveness of *gene therapy* (inserting genes into the cancer in order to kill or change it) and *immune therapy* (using viruses to stimulate the immune system) on prostate cancer.

Gene therapy and immune therapy are both in the infancy stage. To date, the results have been promising, but neither has provided a cure for prostate cancer. So don't expect your doctor to be enthusiastic about signing you up for a clinical trial unless you've exhausted all other options, such as surgery, radiation therapy, or hormone therapy.

Considering gene therapy

With gene therapy, certain genes are inserted into the DNA of the cancer cells to either correct the defect of the cancer cells and turn them into normal cells, kill the cancer cells, or get the cancer cells to produce substances that help the body's immune system fight off the cancer.

Genes can be inserted into the cancer cells in a variety of ways.

- ✔ The most popular way to administer gene therapy is to use special viruses to carry the gene into the cancer cells. These viruses are specially modified to make them harmless to the patient. After the genes are inserted into viruses, the viruses are put into the prostate where they proceed to transfer the genes to the prostate cells (including the cancer cells). This type of gene therapy is usually used to destroy cancer cells.

- ✔ Another way that gene therapy can be administered is to put the viruses into the prostate cancer cells *ex vivo*. With this procedure, the viruses are inserted into cancer cells that have been taken out of the body. After the gene is transferred to the cancer cells, via the viruses, the cancer cells are then reintroduced into the patient. When the patient's own immune cells get close to these infected cancer cells, they recognize the cancer cells as foreign cells and destroy them. The ex vivo procedure is also a type of immune therapy.

Analyzing immune therapy

Immune therapy is used to increase your immunity to your prostate cancer. In addition to immune therapy that is performed with genes, which are inserted into the cancer cells to stimulate the immune system, immune therapy can also be performed by using other approaches:

- ✔ **Cellular immune therapy:** This therapy involves taking the immune cells from a patient's own blood and mixing them with prostate cancer cells or substances from the cell outside the body to increase the blood cells' immunity to prostate cancer. After the immune cells are mixed with the substances, they are injected right back into the patient and theoretically help fight off the cancer.

✔ **Antigen therapy:** With this form of immune therapy, substances that are present in either the prostate cell or the prostate cancer cell are injected into the patient (sometimes along with other immune booster drugs) in the hopes that the body will develop an immunity to the substances in the prostate or the prostate cancer cell and then destroy the cancer. In a sense, this therapy is similar to vaccinations.

The pros and cons

The pros and cons of gene and/or immune therapy are largely theoretical. They may offer great benefits, but that's not yet known. A great many researchers are betting that some form of gene and/or immune therapy will eventually make great headway toward some cancer cures including prostate cancer. Currently, virtually all approaches that have gotten far enough to be tried on patients are strictly controlled and studied in clinical trials. These trials are usually conducted at major academic medical centers (I talk more about clinical trials in Chapters 15 and 21).

If you're told about a gene or immune therapy for your prostate cancer, and especially if there are claims that it works great, be careful. In my opinion there are a lot of questionable doctors and/or organizations, especially outside academia, promoting these newer approaches (especially immune approaches) when in fact they are worthless or even harmful.

Evaluating Experimental Drug Therapy

Drug therapies are a different form of treatment for prostate cancer. Chemotherapy is one common form of drug therapy. When you receive *chemotherapy,* you're given drugs that poison your cells — the cancer cells, but it may also kill healthy cells.

Chemotherapy has been amazingly successful at treating some forms of cancer, such as some forms of leukemia and testicular cancer, but so far it hasn't been as miraculous at treating prostate cancer. I should also add that chemotherapy hasn't been tested as extensively with prostate cancer as it has with other forms of cancer. On the other hand, chemotherapy (especially combinations of different chemotherapy drugs) is beginning to show some success at significantly increasing the quality and quantity of the lives of prostate cancer patients.

Chemotherapy drugs are now being routinely used by medical oncologists to treat patients with advanced prostate cancer when other therapies have all failed. They are also sometimes given to high-risk patients with local disease (patients with PSAs over 20, a TNM classification of T2c or higher, or a Gleason score between 8 and 10 — see Chapter 8) before and after initial therapies such as surgery are used. Sometimes chemotherapy is used with hormone therapy, and sometimes it's used instead of hormone therapy. (See Chapter 15 for more info on treating advanced prostate cancer with chemotherapy.)

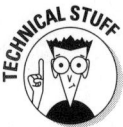

Designer small molecule drug therapy is a new cutting-edge type of chemotherapy treatment. With this form of therapy, the important abnormal processes in the genes and proteins of the cancer cells are discovered, and then a very specific drug is actually developed to halt that particular abnormality in its tracks. This therapy has had some startling success with other forms of cancer, such as leukemia. Doctors hope that this therapy will one day be used to successfully treat prostate cancer. I'm convinced that this approach will be tried in prostate cancer in the near future, once researchers better understand the molecular abnormalities that occur with prostate cancer.

Joining Clinical Studies

Clinical studies are specialized research experiments that are performed to test medications or other treatments. Clinical studies for prostate cancer often (but not always) test drugs or other therapies on subjects with advanced cancer, for whom other therapies have failed. Some men already have a very advanced case of prostate cancer when they're first diagnosed. (This doesn't happen a lot, but it does happen.) In such cases, the man may want to join a clinical study to have a chance at trying a cutting-edge medication or treatment.

Some of the therapies that I describe in this chapter are currently being tested in clinical studies, such as gene therapy, immune therapy, and the newer drug therapies. If you fit the criteria that the researchers are looking for, you may be able to join one of these studies.

Clinical studies are important to consider, because not only can they benefit mankind and medical science but they can also benefit you. (For more on clinical studies, see Chapters 15 and 21.)

Chapter 15

Treating Very Advanced Cancer

In This Chapter

▶ Evaluating the different treatments for advanced cancer

▶ Coping with difficult symptoms and side effects

Sometimes men receive effective treatments for their prostate cancer and then never have to worry about it again because they're cured. Other times, the cancer isn't totally eradicated, and secondary treatments are necessary.

But if these secondary treatments don't work, and the PSA starts rising again, then initial hormone therapy is necessary to further control the cancer. Eventually, however, (and it may take as long as ten years) almost always the PSA (and symptoms) increase, and the patient is considered *hormone resistant*. At this point, the physician must tell the patient that his cancer is a very advanced case.

In other circumstances, the patient may be initially diagnosed with an advanced case of cancer that's spread beyond the prostate gland, and maybe to the lymph nodes and/or the bone. The patient is put on hormone therapy and the PSA declines, and symptoms, if any, decline or even disappear. But eventually, the PSA increases, and the patient is considered to be hormone resistant.

This chapter discusses the treatments to consider when you're facing hormone-resistant (advanced) cancer, including secondary hormone therapy (which is described in more detail in Chapter 13), chemotherapy, experimental options, and therapies offered in numerous clinical studies you may be eligible to participate in. I also discuss the potential side effects of advanced cancer and how to manage them.

Looking at Your Treatment Options

If you have an advanced case of prostate cancer, the most important thing to know is that you still have hope for prolonging your life, because many treatments and options are available to help stave off the growth of the cancer. If you have a conscientious doctor and you follow her instructions carefully, you can often limit the cancer growth for years.

Trying hormone therapy . . . again

Maybe you tried hormone therapy, and the hormones you used didn't work well for you — they either failed to slow down the cancer, or stopped working after awhile. Thus, you have hormone-resistant prostate cancer. That doesn't mean that all the hormones your doctor may consider trying are inevitably useless against prostate cancer — instead, you and your doctor have a large array of hormones to choose from, and one of them may help you fight back those advanced cancer cells. Maybe the hormone you need is in the form of an antiandrogen, an estrogen, or a steroid. I cover secondary hormone therapy extensively in Chapter 13.

Considering chemotherapy

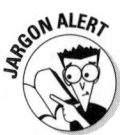

Chemotherapy refers to anti-cancer drugs that are given (either orally, intravenously, or by injection) to attack the cancer cells. A variety of different types of chemotherapy drugs are available for treating prostate cancer. If your treatment plan includes chemotherapy, your urologist and oncologist will decide which drugs are the best ones for you to take.

Medical experts disagree on how well chemotherapy works against prostate cancer and on when chemotherapy should be tried to help treat the disease; however, chemotherapy may be your best option for extending and improving the quality of your life when you have advanced prostate cancer. Chemotherapy isn't generally regarded as the front-line defense for treating prostate cancer, but sometimes it's the last best hope.

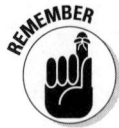

When physicians use chemotherapy to treat advanced cancer, they usually continue to administer hormone therapy, as well.

Discussing the drugs

With chemotherapy, you basically take a special kind of controlled poison to kill cancer cells. The drugs are designed to go after the cancer cells, but they also harm healthy cells, especially those that are fast-growing (like cells in the intestine or blood). Because the cancer cells are weaker, they are often the first cells to die. Medical oncologists have become very skilled at delivering just the right amount of poison to kill the cancer cells without doing undue harm to you.

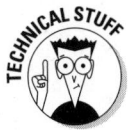

Some key drugs that are used in chemotherapy for prostate cancer are Novantrone (generic name: mitozantrone), Navelbine (generic name: vinorelbine), Taxotere (generic name: docetaxel), Emcyt or Estracyt (generic name for both: estramustine), Adriamycin (generic name: doxorubicin), and Paclitaxel (generic name: taxol). Sometimes these drugs are combined. For example, estramustine can be combined with Paclitaxel, Taxotere, or other chemotherapy drugs.

Radioactive elements, such as Strontium-89 or Samarium-153, are sometimes used with (or instead of) chemotherapy to treat patients with advanced prostate cancer. These drugs sometimes help to reduce the pain from spread of the cancer to bone, especially when it's in more than one or two locations.

Researchers are constantly testing new drugs, or established drugs in new combinations, in clinical trials. They also test drugs that were previously used for something else. One such drug, thalidomide, is under clinical study as a potential chemotherapy treatment for men with prostate cancer. Yes, this is the very same drug that caused pregnant women to have very deformed babies long ago. However, because men can't get pregnant, that problem is not a concern when treating prostate cancer. Preliminary studies indicate that thalidomide combined with docetaxel may help treat men with advanced prostate cancer.

Weighing the pros and cons of chemotherapy

The primary advantage of chemotherapy is that it can be an effective way to prevent cancer cells from advancing any further. However, it doesn't provide a cure; instead, it provides you with a temporary stopgap measure to help extend your life. Chemotherapy is like a policeman, standing in the street directing traffic, who holds up his hand to (hopefully) stop any further growth of cancer cells. Unfortunately, the cancer cop will eventually have to put his hand down, and the cells will start growing again.

Some of the stronger cancer cells eventually develop a resistance to chemotherapy. So, even if chemotherapy works well for you now, the sad truth is that it just won't work forever. However, the "when" of how long chemotherapy can extend your life may often be in terms of many months, so chemotherapy can be extremely effective at extending your life.

The primary disadvantage of chemotherapy is the side effects, which may be severe. Side effects can include

- Nausea and vomiting
- Loss of appetite
- Weight loss

> ✔ Hair loss
>
> ✔ Extreme fatigue

Some chemotherapy symptoms are worse than others, but they may be worth putting up with if the treatment improves your situation. Some men don't experience any side effects. For example, Jake, who has advanced prostate cancer, takes his wife out for a nice long lunch immediately after his chemotherapy. Jake has had no problems with nausea and vomiting — or any of the other side effects that may result from chemotherapy.

You may be like Jake and have no side effects (and I hope that's the case), but you really don't know for sure how you're going to react to chemotherapy until you actually have a few sessions under your belt.

Evaluating experimental options

When treatments such as surgery and/or radiation, and hormone therapies (both primary and secondary) just don't work anymore, and the cancer cells are proliferating anyway, you've moved from being considered hormone resistant to hormone refractory. At that time, you need to consider not only standard chemotherapy options but also experimental options to help you cope with your advanced cancer.

One option is to join a clinical study. Clinical studies (which are also known as a clinical trials) refer to research that's performed by doctors and others to test medications and treatments. With clinical studies for prostate cancer, researchers are looking for medications and other treatments that can cure prostate cancer, prolong life, or perform other positive goals.

One major upside to participating in a clinical study is that because clinical trials are usually performed at major medical centers and because many types of doctors are involved, the care is usually outstanding. Also you may have access to drugs and treatments that just aren't available to the average man with prostate cancer. One downside to joining a clinical study is that some studies give all participants the new therapy being tested, but other studies don't. So if you're in a *randomized study,* which divides the participants into two groups, you may not be in the test group that receives the therapy being tested. Instead, you may be in the test group that receives a different medication or even a *placebo* (a pill that doesn't contain any medication at all). If the study is randomized and blinded, the patients' doctors don't know which patients are getting which drug (or placebo). Researchers perform these studies so that they can determine how the people who received the new medication fared when compared to those who didn't receive it.

Another downside of clinical studies is the fact that the studies may not be finished in time to help treat your advanced cancer. (But your participation helps other men who may be in the same predicament in the future.)

Generally, experimental drugs can only be given to patients who join clinical studies. But very occasionally, the U.S. Food and Drug Administration (FDA) allows some patients, particularly patients with advanced cancer or other very serious diseases, to use medications that are currently being tested but aren't yet approved for treatment. This special permission is called *compassionate use*. You can ask your oncologist for more information about this subject, but you should know that the compassionate use mechanism is rarely used in prostate cancer.

Managing Difficult Symptoms and Side Effects

Many men with advanced prostate cancer share several common medical problems that they need to discuss with their physicians and work on managing. These symptoms or side effects may stem from the prostate cancer itself, or they may develop as a result of the treatments.

Prostate cancer is prostate cancer, even if it moves beyond the prostate

Some people don't realize that if the cancer advances to your bones or other organs, even though you may no longer have a prostate gland (because you had a radical prostatectomy), you're still having a problem with prostate cancer. You don't have bone cancer (a rare form of cancer that starts in the bones) or another form of cancer. Instead, you have prostate cancer that started in your prostate and then spread to your bones. This spread is called *metastasis*. Because the particular makeup of prostate cancer is unique, even when it has spread to the bones (or anywhere else), a pathologist would be able to view the cancer cells in the bones under a microscope and recognize them as being prostate cancer cells.

Removing cells from your bones to see if they are cancerous would be difficult and painful. So doctors use the prostate specific antigen (PSA) blood test to determine if your prostate cancer is spreading. Because only prostate cancer cells generate PSA, your physician should order regular PSA tests to monitor your levels of PSA. If your PSA levels are still rising after treatment, your doctor will know that the prostate cancer cells are growing, and that more action needs to be taken to prevent them from spreading any further. If your PSA levels are going down, that's great news. If they're continuing to stay at the same level, that's not as good as having them go down, but the fact that they're staying the same is fairly good news.

Some of the more common medical problems that men with very advanced prostate cancer may experience include:

✔ **Pain:** If the cancer has spread to your bones or spine, pain may emanate from those areas of your body. Possible treatments include

- Prescribed medications: Nonsteroidal anti-inflammatory drugs (NSAIDs) such as ibuprofen and Celebrex (generic name: celecoxib), steroid medications such as prednisone or hydrocortisone, or narcotics such as oxycodone or morphine can help you cope with the pain.

  Don't worry that you'll become a drug addict if you take narcotics to manage your pain. Researchers have demonstrated that people who use narcotics to alleviate pain are much less likely to become addicted than people who take narcotics to attain a state of euphoria. Of course, people in severe pain may become physically dependent on narcotics if they take them day after day in increasing dosages. But if you're under the care of a good physician whom you can trust, you really shouldn't worry or even think about becoming a drug addict. Doctors are monitored by the Drug Enforcement Administration (DEA), a federal policing organization, so they have to follow very strict guidelines when prescribing controlled drugs such as narcotics.

- Radiation: You may be able to gain very significant pain relief with radiation therapy. Ask your doctor for more info about radiation therapy for pain, especially if you're suffering from bone pain that is coming from only one or two specific areas of the bone.

All doctors are trained to manage some pain. In general, medical oncologists are better than other doctors in treating patients with pain as a result of cancer. Also, some doctors specialize in managing pain. If pain is still a problem for you after receiving treatment from your doctor, ask for a referral to a pain specialist. Dealing with cancer pain is never ideal, but when you're in expert hands, your cancer pain can usually be controlled.

✔ **Anemia:** Your cancer may cause you to develop *anemia* (a low red blood cell count), which is one of the causes of weakness and fatigue from cancer. Under normal circumstances, when the body doesn't have enough red blood cells, a hormone called erythropoietin kicks in and stimulates the bone marrow to produce more. When the patient has advanced cancer, this extra red blood cell production isn't enough. However, genetic engineering has produced a medicine, called Epogen or Procrit (both with the generic name epoetin alpha), that boosts the red blood cell production in cancer patients even further. Injections of this medicine can often make your anemia better. But in some cases, you may require a blood transfusion to build up your blood cell count. In other cases, oral iron supplements can help take care of the problem. Your doctor can tell you which treatment is best for managing your anemia.

✔ **Bladder problems:** If you're having difficulty urinating, tell your doctor. You may have a bladder infection or bladder irritability, both of which can be treated with medications. If you have a blockage, you need to be treated right away. If you still have your prostate, and the blockage is being caused by tissue, you may need to undergo surgery to have the cancer tissue removed.

✔ **Kidney blockage:** With advanced cancer, the local cancer sometimes starts to grow into the bladder and block off the *ureters* (narrow tubes that carry the urine from your kidneys to your bladder). This blockage can cause a swelling of the kidney, resulting in pain and infection. If both kidneys are blocked, the result can be kidney failure. Doctors can temporarily alleviate this problem by putting permanent tubes, called *double J catheters,* up through the ureters from the bladder to the kidney. These tubes, which are inside your body, allow the urine to come down from the kidneys into your bladder. Doctors can also alleviate the blockage by inserting a permanent tube through your back and directly into one or both kidneys. This procedure is called a *percutaneous nephrostomy.*

✔ **Osteoporosis:** Men with advanced cancer sometimes suffer from *osteoporosis,* a condition characterized by bone substance loss. Hormone therapy often accelerates this condition. Osteoporosis can lead to an increased risk of bone fractures and delays in the healing process. When you have osteoporosis, minor falls can cause a broken arm or leg, or, at worst, a fractured hip. (Bone fractures are also more common in men whose prostate cancer has spread to the bones, because the cancer weakens the bone, allowing it to be fractured more easily.)

If you're diagnosed with osteoporosis, your doctor may recommend prescribed doses of calcitriol (vitamin D) or other medications. In fact, some preliminary studies indicate that calcitriol may be effective at fighting back prostate cancer cells. (You can read more about this possibility in Chapter 18.) Some doctors may prescribe calcium or vitamin D to keep you from ever developing osteoporosis in the first place.

The bisphosphanates are another type of drug that is often used to help stabilize or improve osteoporosis. Some experts believe that these drugs can also stabilize or reduce the bony lesions that may result from advanced prostate cancer. Two bisphosphanate drugs that are currently being used are Zometa (generic name: zoledronic acid) and Aredia (generic name: pamidronate disodium). Many more potent bisphosphanates are currently under development.

✔ **Severe fatigue:** Some treatments, such as hormone therapy or chemotherapy, and even the prostate cancer itself can have a significant effect on your energy level. As a result, you may need to take frequent breaks or naps.

✔ **Muscle weakness:** Prostate cancer can really sap your strength, making you feel weaker than you used to be. Avoid heavy lifting or performing any difficult tasks.

- ✔ **Depression:** If you experience depression, see a psychiatrist or therapist who's knowledgeable about treating people with severe illnesses such as cancer as well as treating people who have depression.

- ✔ **Decreased mental function:** Some men report difficulties with their memory or overall cognitive abilities. To help with this problem, make sure you get at least seven hours of sleep at night and you rest when fatigued.

- ✔ **Chronic constipation or diarrhea:** These problems may stem from your illness or the medications or treatments you're receiving. Whatever the cause, make sure that you tell your doctor about your symptoms.

- ✔ **Edema:** This condition, which is characterized by water buildup in the body, especially in the legs and the scrotum, sometimes is seen in men with advanced prostate cancer. Ask your doctor for help with this problem.

- ✔ **Weight loss:** If you experience a weight loss of more than ten pounds, be sure to tell your doctor. Your treatment may need to be changed, or you may need a new medication. You may also have to learn to live with this weight change as part of the price of your therapy.

I realize that this is a long list, and you may feel like just giving up hope. Don't do it. Ask your doctor and others who know about treating advanced prostate cancer and its side effects to help you formulate the best possible treatment plan. Ignore the naysayers — just go around them, like the blocks to progress that they are. At some point, you may exhaust all your treatment options, but until you follow every possible path, you're not done looking.

Part IV
Changing Your Lifestyle to Combat Prostate Cancer

The 5th Wave
By Rich Tennant

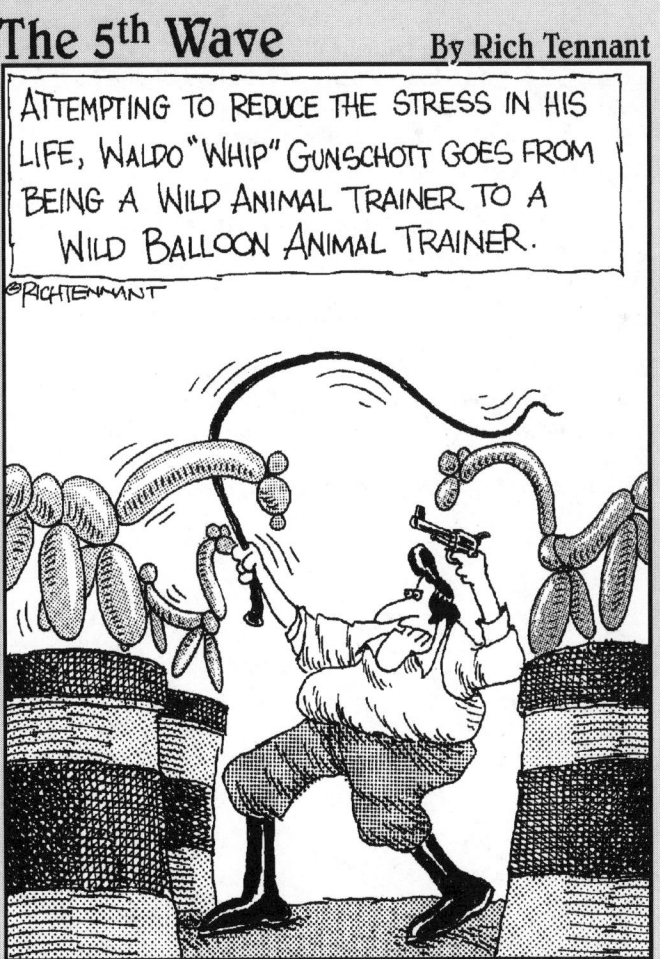

ATTEMPTING TO REDUCE THE STRESS IN HIS LIFE, WALDO "WHIP" GUNSCHOTT GOES FROM BEING A WILD ANIMAL TRAINER TO A WILD BALLOON ANIMAL TRAINER.

In this part . . .

This part concentrates on the lifestyle changes you can make to improve your health when you have prostate cancer. (Yes, you *can* feel better even though you have cancer.) For example, prostate cancer can bring plenty of extra stress into your life; I discuss good tactics for dealing with this stress in Chapter 16.

Exercising offers plenty of health benefits. Dumping bad habits that can keep you sick, such as smoking and drinking, can help you feel better, as well. I cover both of these topics in Chapter 17.

Alternative options are important to many people. Even if you've never tried before, alternative remedies can be very appealing when you have prostate cancer. In Chapter 18, I talk about the pros and cons of some key alternative options (such as taking selenium and vitamin E).

Chapter 16

Stress-busting When You Need It Most

*P*eople react in different ways when they find out that they have prostate cancer. Fear is the most common reaction. Other common reactions are anger, depression, and distress. The combination of these reactions, as well as the continuing burden of coping with the cancer diagnosis itself — figuring out with your doctor how best to treat and beat the disease, and then actually getting the treatment — can create an enormous burden of stress. You may have thought that, on a scale of 1 to 10, your stress levels were already at 10 before you found out that you have cancer, but after you receive the cancer diagnosis, you move into a whole new realm of personal stress.

When you recover from the initial reeling shock, it's important to take charge of the stress monster so that you can continue to manage your everyday life as well as cope with the prostate cancer. Some studies indicate that stress may play a role in causing the occurrence or recurrence of prostate cancer. If these studies are correct, they offer yet another reason for getting a handle on your stress.

This chapter shows you how to cope with your stress burden and the depression that may come along with it.

Easing Stress with Relaxation Therapy

You're never going to be happy about having prostate cancer. You'll have ups and downs as you deal with your diagnosis and eventual treatment. However, you have options for helping you reduce the severe stress. Relaxation therapy is one common method of relieving stress that's effective for many people with a variety of ailments.

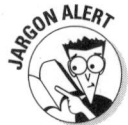

Relaxation therapy is a self-help tactic where you use your mind to calm your body and bring your stress levels down from a very high and painfully intense place to a more tolerable and calmer state. Using relaxation therapy, you voluntarily and consciously concentrate on relaxing one part of your body at a time until you succeed at relaxing your whole body.

I know, I know, when you're struggling to figure out what the heck to do about this cancer problem, the last thing you want to think about is relaxation. It probably doesn't even seem remotely possible to relax. Instead, you want to go kill that cancer, somehow, some way, without destroying your body and your life in the process. Or maybe you'd really like to calm down, but your body is in a very tense state (and understandably so), and you feel like you're ready to pounce on someone or jump out of your skin. Both of these feelings are very normal for a person in the midst of an emotional crisis caused by a diagnosis of prostate cancer. Eventually, you need to master your stress so that it doesn't control you and derail you from acting against the cancer.

Looking at the key benefits (and one possible drawback)

Your problems won't evaporate when you relax, but they may seem more tolerable. When you feel calmer, you can work on a better and more reasoned plan for dealing with your prostate cancer. You can also make your current life much more tolerable. And, you can make living with you a better experience for those you care about, because you won't be freaking out about your cancer diagnosis.

The only drawback to relaxation therapy (if you can call it a drawback) is that you have to take some time — at least 15 to 20 minutes — out of your busy schedule to lie down and actually do the therapy. But most people consider the benefits of relaxation therapy to be well worth the brief time that needs to be spent on it. As you get better at relaxation therapy, you can achieve relaxation in a shorter period, but that shouldn't be your primary goal.

Mastering basic relaxation therapy techniques

Relaxation therapy is easy for most people. Of course, when you're totally stressed-out because of your cancer (as well as whatever else life is throwing at you now), calming down may take a little more time than when your biggest problem is, for example, deciding how to spend extra money or where to go on vacation.

Relaxation therapy requires a little concentration and a lot of quiet. The following steps provide some basic how-to info. If you'd like to explore relaxation therapy more, you can purchase books or audiotapes on the subject.

1. **Lie down.**

   No, relaxation therapy isn't about taking a nap, although you may actually fall asleep if you become relaxed enough.

   You may want to close the blinds or turn off the lights before you start your relaxation therapy session, unless darkness makes you more tense. You may also want to make sure that you're wearing loose clothes. It can be hard to relax when your belt is too tight, or your tie is driving you crazy. Loosen your cinched-in belt and take off that tie.

2. **Choose a starting point on your body and begin mentally relaxing each part of your body.**

   Some people start at their feet and mentally work their way up to their heads, while others start the exercise at their head and end up at their toes. You decide where to start and where to finish. (I assume that you're a foot person, so I gauge my instructions to start at the feet. If you prefer to start at the head, follow the same suggestions in reverse order.) So, as you lie there, imagine that your feet are becoming increasingly relaxed, loose, and tension-free. Take deep, slow breaths, and tell yourself (in your mind or aloud) that your feet are becoming heavy and warm.

   Tell yourself that you can no longer move your feet with your own free will. You willingly give up control of your feet because they're so heavy. Continue to imagine this relaxed feeling as you mentally tell yourself that you're more and more relaxed, more and more peaceful, and you mentally move throughout your body, up to your knees and then to your upper legs. Let go of your tension, everywhere that you find it, until you are resting effortlessly. Let your body be supported by the surface you're lying on and feel the gentle pull of gravity. End the exercise at your neck, mouth, and eyes.

3. **Use** *mental imagery* **(using your mind to picture a place that's relaxing to you) to accompany the slow relaxation of your body.**

   Maybe your idea of a calm spot is the ocean, the mountains, or the desert. Think about a place where you feel safe and happy. Imagine how it looks, sounds, and smells. Feel the temperature and imagine the colors of your calm spot. Make it as real as you can in your mind. As you think about a pleasant place, your muscles unconsciously relax, and your body begins to release tension.

Take your time when performing relaxation therapy techniques: Don't rush through it. Don't move to another part of your body until the one you're concentrating on is completely relaxed.

When you master the simple relaxation therapy technique described here, you can use it in other settings. You can perform the technique in ten minutes behind the closed door of your office or bedroom (if you leave the door open, people may interrupt), or even in the waiting room before a hormone therapy shot or a radiation treatment.

Some people do well with relaxation therapy, while for others, vigorous physical exercise is more effective for reducing stress. If you decide to use exercise to help you de-stress, choose an exercise you like (or hate the least), such as bicycling, swimming, running, or walking. Maybe you can also get some quality time with a family member by exercising together. (You can read more about the value of exercise in Chapter 17.)

High stress and PSA levels

Some studies indicate that high stress levels may be linked to abnormal levels of *PSA* (prostate specific antigen, a tumor marker for prostate cancer). A study led by Arthur A. Stone, PhD, of State University of New York at Stony Brook, and reported in *Health Psychology* in 1999, found significantly higher PSA levels among men who reported high stress. The study looked at 318 men. After controlling for the impact of age, the researchers found that men with high stress levels, based on psychological tests for anger, nervousness, and their ability to cope with their daily lives, were three times as likely to have abnormal PSA scores than the men who weren't so stressed-out. (Sixteen percent of high-stress men had high PSA scores, versus 4.8 percent of low-stress men.)

The researchers didn't follow up with the men to determine which of them developed prostate cancer, so it can't be determined from this study that high stress causes an elevated PSA level. But the results do seem to suggest that if you've been diagnosed with prostate cancer, you should keep your stress levels down. And if you haven't been diagnosed with prostate cancer, you should also work to keep your stress down to a tolerable level.

Pulsing Down with Biofeedback

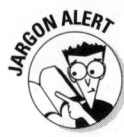

Biofeedback is a stress-reducing technique in which you use computerized data about your body to help you purposely slow down your blood pressure, your pulse, your breathing, and other body functions. Changing the levels of these bodily functions can help you feel better and less stressed-out. Interestingly, with some responses such as body temperature, your goal is to very slightly *raise* your temperature, because your body temperature drops a little when you're stressed-out. Before you begin any sessions, your biofeedback therapist will explain the goals you need to achieve. (And if he doesn't, ask him to do so.)

During biofeedback sessions, the therapist hooks you up to a computer and some sensors. (If this makes you think of Frankenstein being strapped down to a table while a scientist darts about pressing levers, think again — it really isn't that bad.) For example, the therapist may slip a sensor around your finger to take your pulse. Other sensors may be attached to your body to measure your external body temperature and muscle activity. The sensors take periodic readings of your body reactions, and the computer converts this information into a representation (such as a line graph) that you can see on a monitor. As you relax, you see changes on the computer screen, so you can tell if the biofeedback is working. If you tense up, you see this reaction displayed on the computer monitor, as well. You're taught to use the information on the monitor to help change your body reactions on your own. Your goal is to bring down the stress measures and keep them down, well below the high-stress level.

You may find that any first-time success you have with biofeedback can have the surprising effect of briefly propelling your body reactions back up into Stressland. For example, the indicators start to drop, so you get excited, which then raises your pulse back up again, causing the indicators to go back up. Don't worry — many people can master biofeedback (although it's not for everyone, especially Type A over-achievers who equate success with doing something rather than with relaxing). Even if you think that you're an over-achiever, consider giving biofeedback a shot, anyway. It may work very well for you.

Some studies have demonstrated that people who master biofeedback don't need to be connected to the computer to use the skills acquired during biofeedback sessions. They're able to generalize the same techniques that calm them down during biofeedback to other environments. They (and hopefully you, too) can relax whenever they want, without the help of the biofeedback equipment and therapist. (Of course, you shouldn't select your daily commute as one of your favorite relaxation times. You need to be fully alert when driving! Instead, choose a time when you're home, a slow time at the office, or somewhere where you can relax without any problem.)

> ## Petting therapy
>
> Studies have shown that petting a cat, dog, or other pet can actually lower your blood pressure and make you feel much calmer and happier. If you have a pet that can be petted (a pet lizard is a little rough on the hands, so Lizzie the lizard may not work well for this particular exercise), sit down next to Fido or Fluffy and gently stroke her for at least a few minutes. You'll both benefit from this very simple low-tech activity.

Analyzing the pros and cons of biofeedback

The primary advantage of biofeedback is that, if it works, it can help calm you down considerably.

The main disadvantage of biofeedback is that you have to find a therapist who uses this form of therapy — not everyone does. In addition, your insurance company may not pay for biofeedback sessions. Another negative is that biofeedback therapy is not a quick-fix solution; it takes at least a few sessions for you to know if it's working (which may be more time than you're willing to invest). Biofeedback doesn't work for everyone.

Finding biofeedback therapists

Psychologists and other therapists are more likely than psychiatrists to perform biofeedback therapy. Ask your doctor if she can recommend a biofeedback expert. You can also call your county medical society for recommendations of medical doctors who use biofeedback. If you live near a university or a large hospital, call the public relations staff to find out if they can recommend anyone on staff who offers biofeedback sessions.

Looking Into Your Eyes: Understanding Hypnotherapy

If you're like most people, when you hear the word "hypnotist," you probably think of an exotic-looking man wearing a turban and standing on a stage. He chooses a volunteer from the audience and proceeds to put him into a trance.

He then gets the poor guy to perform ridiculous acts, making him cluck like a chicken or act in other totally stupid ways. But this carnival image of hypnosis doesn't do justice to what hypnotherapy can actually achieve in helping you alleviate the stress in your life. *Hypnotherapy* can't cure your cancer, but it may assist you in limiting panic and fear so that you can work with your doctor to create an effective treatment plan. Hypnosis can also help you resolve other problems, such as quitting smoking or losing weight.

With hypnotherapy, the therapist first talks to you about the goals you hope to achieve with the therapy (for example, attaining a calmer, more relaxed state), and the problem you hope to resolve (such as reducing your stress so that you can better cope with your prostate cancer).

When you're ready to undergo hypnosis, the therapist may ask you to relax and imagine a place where you feel safe and calm. She may play soft music or use visual imagery to help you achieve a hypnotic state. The hypnotic trance is akin to when you first start to fall asleep. (The state where others tell you that you're nodding off, but you deny it.) When you're in a light hypnotic state, the therapist makes suggestions to you based on your goals.

Don't worry — you can't be induced to rob the local bank or perform a hit on someone. After experiencing hypnotherapy, your moral values remain intact and in good working order.

Hypnotherapy is somewhat similar to relaxation therapy — or at least it starts out that way — because both use basic calming techniques. But the end-goal with hypnotherapy is not to make you relax or fall asleep but instead to actually help open up your unconscious mind so that you can actively listen to important ideas or thoughts that may help you.

You may also be able to master *self-hypnosis.* With this type of hypnosis, you give yourself hypnotic suggestions to help you calm down, stop smoking, lose weight, or change other behaviors.

Most hypnosis practitioners are psychologists or medical doctors, but some practitioners don't have an a medical or doctoral degree. Ask your physician if she can recommend a competent hypnotherapist.

Pondering Meditation and Prayer

If relaxation therapy, biofeedback, or hypnotherapy doesn't really suit you, or if you're looking for something to supplement these therapies and help you reduce the tremendous stress that a diagnosis of prostate cancer can trigger, consider meditation or prayer. Meditation or prayer (or both) can help you achieve the positive goal of relaxing your body to meet the tough challenges you face.

Meditation may sound like some sort of exotic Eastern (and I don't mean Connecticut) exercise, but you can master the basics to enable you to relax your body and brain.

Meditation is a focused state in which you block out all outside distractions and instead concentrate on achieving a state of internal calmness and peace. (Of course, if the fire alarm goes off, you'll hear it.) When you meditate, your breathing slows down, and the many concerns of the day fade into the background. When you're calm and focused, you can make much better and more reasoned decisions about how to deal with the challenges that prostate cancer can bring, such as making treatment decisions and dealing with the side effects that may occur with your treatment. Meditation may also help you cope with the emotional demands of prostate cancer (such as the fear and distress).

Meditation takes practice, so don't expect to feel like a new man after just one meditative session. You can pick up meditative skills from psychologists and other experts, or you can take a class. Check with your local community college to see if it offers such a course.

For more info on meditation, check out *Meditation For Dummies,* by Stephan Bodian (Wiley Publishing).

If you're an atheist, prayer probably won't work well for you. But if you're religious or you think that there *may* be a supreme being out there, prayer is one way to consciously reach out and communicate your concerns and fears to a higher power than you, relinquishing control of your emotional or physical pain. Telling your higher power about your problem and asking for help can often provide you with tremendous relief. For me, prayer was an important part of the way I handled my prostate cancer. You may find that receiving some help from someone in your religious faith group can also be very useful. You can ask the members of the faith group to pray for you, as well. Some groups call this a *prayer circle.*

Battling Depression

You may feel stressed-out as you struggle to cope with your cancer, figure out what treatment to choose, and fathom how the disease is affecting you now as well as how it may affect you later on. But sometimes the key problem isn't stress. Instead, it may be depression.

Depression is a severe form of sadness, and it's a very common and highly treatable problem. It can be easy to lapse into a depressive state when you encounter a tough problem like prostate cancer. But you can overcome depression, and you don't have to get any parts of your body irradiated or removed in order to treat it. The main problem is in recognizing possible depression in yourself so that you know when it's a good idea to talk to your doctor about it. Here are some indicators of possible depression:

✔ You frequently (once or twice a week) wish that you were dead, or you develop a plan to commit suicide. Thinking about death is actually normal when you're diagnosed with cancer. Hoping for death, however, is not normal — it's a sign that you need help.

✔ You gain or lose ten pounds or more. Weight loss or gain is a possible sign of depression.

✔ You rarely sleep through the night (and it's not because of urinary problems), and you wake up early in the morning to worry about your problems. Finding out that you have prostate cancer is enough to impair the sleep of the most stable man on the planet. But if you're having trouble sleeping night after night, you may be lapsing into a depressive state.

✔ You feel like you're worthless and that everything is hopeless in your life. A diagnosis of prostate cancer is a shock to any man, and it can throw you completely off your stride. But if you start blaming yourself or assuming that the prostate cancer is your fault because you think that you're a worthless human being, you may be suffering from depression, and you may need help climbing out of the hole.

If you exhibit any of the behaviors or feelings listed here, you're either severely depressed or you're at risk for developing depression. Tell your primary care doctor about your depressive symptoms or see a psychiatrist who is knowledgeable about the latest medications for depression.

Benefiting from Counseling

You don't have to be a drug addict, mentally ill, or have some other dire psychological problem in order to benefit from counseling. Real men see psychiatrists, psychologists, and other therapists when they're facing a crisis (and being diagnosed with prostate cancer definitely qualifies as a crisis). Some therapists specialize in treating people with chronic disease or cancer:

Discovering how therapists can help

A therapist can help you identify how you feel, help you accept that your emotions are normal, and work with you so that you can concentrate on making a plan to fight the cancer rather than endlessly and uselessly wonder "what if?"

Sorting out therapists

Differentiating psychiatrists from psychologists, social workers, and other therapists can be confusing. Here's a basic primer for you:

✔ Psychiatrists are medical doctors who treat people with a wide variety of mild, moderate, or severe emotional problems. They can also prescribe medications, such as antidepressants for depression and antianxiety drugs for patients in a panic mode. Psychiatrists are often excellent at diagnosing emotional problems. Because psychiatrists are doctors, they can also understand your prostate cancer and how it may be affecting you emotionally.

✔ Psychologists aren't medical doctors. They are therapists who have a doctorate (PhD), or an advanced degree, in psychology. Psychologists can't prescribe medicine, but they can teach you coping skills to help you deal with the stress you're facing.

✔ Social workers, who are also often therapists, usually have a master's degree in social work. They concentrate on helping people find practical solutions to their problems.

✔ Therapists may have a master's degree in psychology or counseling. They can't prescribe medication, but they may be effective at teaching you methods of stress reduction, such as hypnotherapy or relaxation therapy.

Make sure that any therapist you see has a professional license issued by your state. Most therapists proudly display their license in their office. You can also check out their license at the state professional licensing board, which is usually located in a department of professional regulation at the state capital.

Therapists also can help you by challenging irrational ideas and replacing them with common-sense ideas. This form of therapy is called *cognitive behavioral therapy,* or CBT. Imagining that you somehow deserve prostate cancer, and that it's probably a punishment for something you did (or didn't do) in the past, is one example of an irrational idea. Assuming that whatever happens, happens, and that there's nothing you can do to treat the cancer is another example of an irrational idea. The rational counterpart to these ideas is that no one knows for sure what causes prostate cancer, but it may have to do with your age, race, medical history, or other factors that are beyond your control. No evidence exists to indicate that getting cancer is some sort of involuntary atonement for your past bad behavior.

Tracking down a good therapist

You can use many different ways to find a good therapist, but the best way involves networking with others, including professionals (such as your urologist or oncologist or even other therapists) and your friends, relatives, and co-workers. Ask them the names of therapists who understand serious illness. You can also ask members of the clergy for their recommendations of therapists. Asking for referrals from many different people gives you a wide variety of therapists to choose from.

The downside of this process is that when you tell people you're looking for a therapist, they'll know that you need help. If having people know about your prostate cancer worries you, you need to think about whether networking is worth pursuing.

Chapter 17

Working on a Healthy Lifestyle

*W*hen you're diagnosed with prostate cancer, you may think that there's no longer any point to working on good health habits, like exercising, losing weight, eating a better diet, or doing any of the other healthy things that your doctor urges you to do, such as giving up smoking or drinking. When you already *have* cancer, the thing that most people are trying to avoid in the first place, what's the point of practicing healthy habits? Many men who are newly diagnosed with cancer often think, "Bring on the nicotine, the alcohol, and the fatty goods galore, and the heck with my fitness routine!"

But they're wrong. Studies indicate that incorporating healthy habits into your life may help you avoid cancer. The studies also show that healthy habits may help prevent recurrences or the progression of prostate cancer.

In this chapter, I talk about the benefits of exercise, weight loss, and eating a healthy diet. I also tell you about getting rid of bad habits, such as smoking and drinking, that harm your health and may increase your risk of developing, or suffering a recurrence of, prostate cancer.

Benefiting from Exercise

A sedentary couch-potato lifestyle probably didn't cause your cancer to develop in the first place, but constant physical inactivity isn't good for what ails you. Exercise can cause a psychological rush, making you less likely to feel depressed, stressed-out, or upset. Exercising generates *endorphins,* which are brain chemicals that act as mood boosters. Rather than guzzle down a few beers or slump in front of the TV, how about swimming a few laps or walking around the block a few times to help you feel better? It works!

Of course, if you're receiving anti-cancer treatments or you're recovering from surgery, radiation, or hormone shots, you're not ready to run any races, and you should take it very easy. But when your doctor says that you're ready to start moving again, getting healthier by getting physical is a smart anti-cancer strategy.

Taking it slow at first

Men with prostate cancer can have very different overall levels of health. Some men who are diagnosed with cancer are otherwise physically strong and fit, while others haven't exercised in years, spending most of their time behind a desk or maybe riding around on a golf cart.

How much you exercise depends on how active you are. Active men can generally exercise far more vigorously, and for longer periods of time, than sedentary men can.

So, if you've been leading a pretty low-key and inactive life, you shouldn't jump right into your new exercise program by running the Boston Marathon or climbing Mount Everest. You need to build up slowly with exercise, as your own doctor can tell you. In fact, it's very important to check your exercise plan with your doctor first.

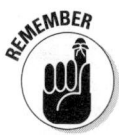

No matter what your physical fitness level, your doctor may recommend a stress test before giving you the all-clear to exercise. *Stress tests* determine the effect of exercise on your body. When you take a stress test, you perform a simple exercise, like walking on a treadmill, while machines measure your heart rate and blood pressure. On the other hand, if your doctor knows that you're in good physical condition (other than having prostate cancer), he may give you an immediate thumbs up to start exercising.

Stretching and walking can help

Stretching and walking are excellent exercises for most men, with or without cancer. Imagine yourself walking all over the cancer, killing it dead. Other good exercises are bicycling, swimming, and jogging.

The federal government devised a walking plan that's easy to follow (see Table 17-1) and allows you to build up slowly. You can use the program just as it is or adapt it to your needs.

During the warm-up portion of the walking program, walk at a comfortable pace and then work up to a brisker pace for the exercise portion. When you're ready for the cool-down phase, start walking slower so that you can get your heart rate down.

Table 17-1		A Very Simple Walking Program		
Week	Warm-up	Exercise (Walking)	Cool-down	Total Time
1	5 min.	5 min.	5 min.	15 min.
2	5 min.	7 min.	5 min.	17 min.
3	5 min.	9 min.	5 min.	19 min.
4	5 min.	11 min.	5 min.	21 min.
5	5 min.	13 min.	5 min.	23 min.
6	5 min.	15 min.	5 min.	25 min.
7	5 min.	18 min.	5 min.	28 min.
8	5 min.	20 min.	5 min.	30 min.
9	5 min.	23 min.	5 min.	33 min.
10	5 min.	26 min.	5 min.	36 min.
11	5 min.	28 min.	5 min.	38 min.
12	5 min.	30 min.	5 min.	40 min.

After you complete Week 12, gradually increase your brisk walking time (the exercise portion of the program) to 60 minutes, three or four times a week.

Don't have very much time to exercise? Walking doesn't take a lot of time; almost everyone can budget a short period of time for walking on most days. Eliminate a few mindless TV programs, and there you have it — enough time. Take your partner or child with you on your walk for some quality time together.

Dropping a Few Pounds

Whether obesity can cause prostate cancer is unknown, although some researchers believe that it can — they point to a higher prevalence of prostate cancer among overweight men. (Studies also suggest that obese men with prostate cancer have a higher death rate than their leaner counterparts.) What is known is that obesity can contribute to health problems, because it puts an extra strain on your body.

Weighing in on simple, quick, and safe weight-loss tips

In addition to exercising more and eating a healthy diet (and fewer overall calories), you may want to consider adopting other simple weight-loss strategies:

- ✔ If you need to go two or three floors up or down in a building, take the stairs.

- ✔ Don't pile your plate up with food — no matter how good it looks. If you do, you may feel like you have to eat it all. Instead, take modest portions of food. Then, if you're still hungry five minutes later, you can take another modest portion.

- ✔ Fill up on veggies rather than on sweets or breads. Consider a variation of what your mom may have told you: A tomato (or broccoli) a day keeps the oncologist away.

Chewing on necessary nutritional tips

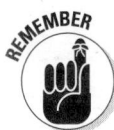

If you remember just one thing about nutrition, remember this: Fruits and vegetables are good, especially tomatoes — it's practically impossible to eat too many fruits and vegetables. If you simply keep this one statement in mind, adopting it as your sort of mantra or motto, you're going to be less likely to pile on the cake, cookies, and calorie-laden carbohydrates that can make you fat and unhealthy.

Many vegetables and fruits have built-in *antioxidants,* or cancer-fighting ingredients, such as vitamin C. (You can read more about antioxidants in Chapter 18.) Fruits such as apples, oranges, and tomatoes are especially good for you because they're high in vitamin C. Fruits and vegetables that are bright in color are often high in antioxidants.

Tomatoes are especially good because not only do they contain antioxidants and fiber, but they're also naturally high in *lycopene* (a substance that also can be taken as a supplement). Some small preliminary studies have shown a drop in the prostate specific antigen (PSA) levels of men with prostate cancer who have taken lycopene supplements. Because rising PSA is the last thing a man with prostate cancer wants, these results are promising, but research is ongoing. (You can read more about lycopene and other supplements in Chapter 18.)

In addition to eating more fruits and vegetables, cut back on red meat and high-fat foods like whole milk or cheese. If you drink alcohol, do so in moderation or consider avoiding it altogether. (See "Stopping or cutting back on heavy drinking," later in this chapter, for more about alcohol.)

According to the research . . .

Preliminary research performed at the UCLA Jonsson Center in Los Angeles, California, indicates that prostate cancer cell growth may be slowed when patients combine daily walking with a low-fat, high-fiber diet. Other studies also have supported the benefits of eating foods high in fiber (such as tomatoes).

In another study of more than 47,000 men who were followed from 1986 to 1998 (reported in a 2002 issue of the *Journal of the National Cancer Institute*), researchers found that eating foods with tomato sauce twice or more per week was associated with a significantly lower incidence of prostate cancer. Bring on the low-fat pasta!

Doing Away with Unhealthy Habits

When you're under extreme stress, as you are when you're fighting prostate cancer, giving up habits that serve as an emotional crutch can be even harder. When you have prostate cancer, you may feel drawn to problem health habits more than ever before, as you attempt to alleviate stress by self-medicating with nicotine, alcohol, or food. Maybe you feel like smoking calms you down, or perhaps you believe that alcohol helps you tolerate the stresses and strains you're under.

Here are some key reasons why resisting your bad health habits can be so hard when you're diagnosed with prostate cancer (or any other form of cancer):

- **You feel sorry for yourself.** Having prostate cancer really is a bum deal, but smoking or drinking up a storm won't help you.

- **You're depressed.** You may be unconsciously self-medicating your depression and anxiety with nicotine, alcohol, or fatty comfort foods.

- **You think that staying healthy is pointless.** "Live for today, for tomorrow you may die" seems like a motto with real relevance to you now, but you can hasten your own death by overdoing bad health habits.

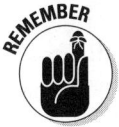

This isn't *Star Trek,* and resistance is *not* futile. With the diagnosis of prostate cancer, you've been given a jolt to your body and soul. You need to stand up and make an action plan for fighting back. New, healthy habits should be a part of your action plan.

Quitting smoking

For years, people have known that smoking causes lung cancer and *emphysema,* a potentially fatal respiratory ailment. Recent studies have also indicated that smoking may cause other forms of cancer as well, including bladder cancer and prostate cancer. Tobacco is extremely addictive — if you don't already know this, you'll find it out when you stop smoking and start experiencing physical and psychological withdrawal symptoms. But kicking the habit is doable!

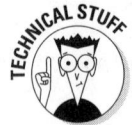

When you draw on a cigarette, the nicotine goes from the "cancer stick" to your brain in ten seconds flat. If you smoke two packs of cigarettes a day (40 cigarettes), you receive 400 daily nicotine hits to your brain. Every time your brain is hit with a nicotine jolt, it releases *adrenalin* (a hormone), which in turn makes your blood pressure and heart rate go up. Nicotine also triggers your brain to release a chemical called *dopamine,* which enhances pleasure. When you're hooked, it's hard to stop smoking. But you can quit, and the health benefits you receive when you stop smoking are well worth it!

Ending your habit with medication

Some people stop smoking cold turkey, while others rely on over-the-counter or prescribed medications to end their addiction.

The popular medications known as *nicotine replacement therapy drugs* actually contain a dose of nicotine. These medications are available in gum form, skin patches, nasal sprays, and inhalers. With nicotine replacement therapy, you take one dose of non-smoked nicotine and gradually cut down your intake of nicotine until you quit altogether. Instructions are provided for each form of nicotine therapy: Make sure you read them. Researchers disagree on how effective nicotine replacement therapy is.

If you use nicotine replacement therapy drugs, *you should not smoke.* You can become very ill from the excessive nicotine you receive from both smoking and nicotine replacement therapy.

Clinical studies have shown that a non-nicotine drug called *Zyban* (generic name: bupropion) may also be effective in helping you quit smoking. This prescription drug is also used as an antidepressant (sold under the name Wellbutrin), usually in higher doses than those given for quitting smoking.

Trying smoking cessation therapies

You may be able to end your smoking habit with hypnotherapy (which I discuss in Chapter 16) or individual or group counseling sessions. These therapies really can't be ignored when attempting to overcome a smoking habit. Some studies indicate that a combination of medication (either nicotine replacement therapy medications or Zyban) and therapy provides the best long-term results. Ask your doctor for more information on smoking cessation therapies.

Stopping or cutting back on heavy drinking

If you have a drinking problem, you need to face up to it and conquer it. This is very easy to say and very hard to do, especially when you're under the extreme stress of coping with prostate cancer. But drinking doesn't empower you. Instead, it further impairs your ability to deal with your cancer.

Some researchers believe that regular alcohol abuse can cause or contribute to the development of prostate cancer. The evidence is insufficient to either back up or refute this theory, but I can tell you with certainty that regular excessive drinking (more than three or four glasses of beer or wine per day, or more than two shots of gin, vodka, whiskey, or other forms of hard alcohol) is a very bad idea for anyone, with or without cancer.

Excessive drinking harms virtually every system in your body. It can cause your pancreas and liver to become inflamed. It can cause anemia and increase your risk of infection. If your immune system is struggling to combat the illnesses that result from heavy drinking, it'll be less able to work on effectively fighting your cancer.

Knowing if you have a problem

Many heavy drinkers and alcoholics aren't aware that they're problem drinkers. They may deny the problem, they may think that their troubles justify their drinking, or they may rationalize the problem in some other way, such as by blaming others who are supposedly driving them to drink. The reality: Unless you're strapped down and the alcohol is being poured down your protesting throat, no one's forcing you to drink.

Some people are alcohol abusers, while others are alcoholics. *Alcohol abusers* have a psychological dependency on alcohol. With alcohol abuse, the degree of dependency may not be as severe as it is for alcoholics, but it can easily lead to alcoholism. *Alcoholics* are both physically and psychologically dependent on alcohol. Because of their physical addiction, alcoholics not only want to drink but they *need* to drink. They may try to give up drinking for short periods (usually days), but almost invariably, unless they have medical or therapeutic assistance, they become so physically and psychologically uncomfortable that they soon resume their drinking.

Whether you're an alcohol abuser or an alcoholic, you know that you have a problem if you meet at least one of the following criteria:

✔ You fail to fulfill your responsibilities to your family or employer as a result of your excessive drinking.

> ✔ You've been arrested for a problem that's related to alcohol, such as driving under the influence or attacking someone after you drink too much.
>
> ✔ You drink despite the serious family and relationship problems that are either caused or worsened by your excessive drinking.

According to the Substance Abuse and Mental Health Services Administration (SAMSA), about 6 million people in the United States have an alcohol abuse problem. In addition to the 6 million alcohol abusers in the United States, another 8 million people (or about 10 percent of all drinkers) are alcoholics.

Getting help from a support group

Some organizations, such as Alcoholics Anonymous (AA), provide assistance and support to people who are addicted to alcohol. These organizations meet regularly. They don't require dues, but they do require a sincere commitment to giving up drinking. Just cutting back isn't good enough. You can also visit the Web site of Alcoholics Anonymous at www.alcoholics-anonymous.org.

Alcoholics Anonymous is the most famous of these support groups, but you can find others. If you need help overcoming a drinking problem, ask your doctor to recommend such a group.

Enrolling in a rehab program

You may need to get your drinking under control by entering a rehab program. The most famous rehab clinic is the Betty Ford Clinic, which was named after the wife of former president Gerald Ford. You can find thousands of other rehab programs and facilities throughout the United States and Canada. *Residential programs,* where you live at the treatment center for weeks or months, are the best rehab programs, but if you're undergoing treatment for cancer, you may need to go to a facility that offers outpatient treatment. If you do enter a residential program, the medical director needs to be fully aware of your prostate cancer.

Getting depression under control

If you have a drinking problem, you may also be dealing with depression. In fact, many researchers believe that depression may actually be a possible cause of alcohol abuse. If depression is causing your alcoholism, you may unwittingly be using alcohol in an attempt to self-medicate, even though drinking is a pretty inefficient method for improving your mood, because alcohol is a depressant. It may initially make you feel happy and less inhibited, but when the alcohol's effect kicks in, so does the depressed mood.

Depression often improves when you take antidepressants. When they work, these medications can stabilize your mood and enable you to overcome your depression and think more clearly. There are many different antidepressants for doctors to choose from. Work with your doctor to determine which antidepressant is right for you.

Therapy can help you handle your depression and your drinking problem. Seek a therapist who understands both chronic alcoholism and other serious medical problems, such as cancer or chronic illness. Ask your doctor to recommend a good therapist, or ask your partner to help you find one. You may find that your partner is thrilled to help you overcome your problem any way possible. (See Chapter 16 for more about depression and the different types of therapists who can treat it.)

Chapter 18

Alternative Remedies

*V*itamin or mineral supplements, when used to help cure a medical problem (such as prostate cancer) or to relieve its symptoms, fall into the realm of *alternative remedies,* as do special diets or other nontraditional treatments. Researchers are currently studying whether alternative remedies may be useful as supplemental prostate cancer treatments, and whether they offer some additional value for preventing prostate cancer from developing in the first place. In addition, alternative remedies may sometimes help men cope with some of the side effects of traditional treatments such as hormone therapy. Finally, anecdotal evidence suggests that some alternative remedies may add some additional benefit to existing established therapies such as surgery and radiation.

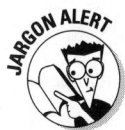

Your doctor may refer to some alternative remedies as *alternative medicines, complementary medicines,* or *alternative therapies.* All of these terms refer to nontraditional treatments and medications.

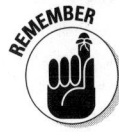

But don't get swept off your feet by the potential benefits of alternative remedies — scientific evidence has not yet adequately proven their effectiveness. In general, alternative remedies are best considered as preventive measures against cancer rather than as remedies for cancers that need treatment now. Alternative remedies should *never* be used as a substitute for treating cancer that's already been diagnosed.

In this chapter, I provide information on what is currently known about how alternative remedies can help men with prostate cancer. I also talk about how you need to be careful and use common sense when trying alternative remedies.

Weighing the Pros and Cons

Many men — even those who've never tried alternative remedies before — become fascinated by the idea that some special plant or vitamin (or yet-to-be-discovered elixir) may be able to cure prostate cancer or even prevent it from developing in the first place. While no magic cure for prostate cancer is available, current studies are being performed to determine if alternative remedies can help prevent or halt a recurrence of the disease. Major breakthroughs may occur, and when that happens, I'll be standing up and cheering loudly. But for now, you need to understand that a note of caution is in order when using alternative remedies. You need to keep in mind both the basic pros and cons.

The benefits of alternative remedies

Some preliminary studies indicate that some alternative remedies, especially lycopene, vitamins E and D, and selenium, may be effective at preventing prostate cancer from developing or recurring. (You may hear your doctor refer to these treatments that are used to prevent cancer from occurring in the first place as *chemoprevention medications.*) Alternative remedies may also give you some hope when traditional medicines don't seem to be working that well. Alternative remedies also may provide men with some relief from the side effects of treatments for prostate cancer (see "Easing Treatment Side Effects with Alternative Remedies," later in this chapter).

Danger! Don't rely solely on alternative medicine

Don't be like Frank, who relied solely on alternative treatments and diet. Frank went on a strict *macrobiotic diet* (a vegetarian diet in which you consume mostly fresh vegetables and whole grains like brown rice, corn, and oats), which he says others told him would cure his prostate cancer. They urged him to forego surgery or radiation treatments, and he agreed. Frank rigidly followed the strict diet. He also adhered to the other recommendations associated with the diet, such as singing and dancing every day and taking lots of vitamins. Unfortunately, the special diet and the other advice Frank rigorously followed didn't work. Frank's prostate specific antigen (PSA) blood levels kept going up steadily, indicating that his prostate cancer was advancing. By the time Frank finally returned to his doctor for conventional treatment, the cancer had spread and wasn't curable anymore, although it was still treatable.

The macrobiotic diet wasn't necessarily bad, but Frank should have continued to see his physician and had the treatments he recommended.

The downside of alternative remedies

Men sometimes put too much hope in studies that may be performed on only a handful of men or based on some slickly written ad copy on a product that hasn't been tested at all. Even worse, some men may decide to take unproven alternative medicines and forego traditional treatments that can save or at least extend their lives. I'm not saying that all alternative remedies are bad, but setting aside your doctor's judgment and reasoned medical opinions for something a newspaper ad touts or some pitchman tries to sell you on the Internet is a very foolish and even life-threatening way to go.

I urge you to very carefully weigh the possible benefits along with the very real risks of alternative remedies and share your decision with your physician. Be sure to tell your doctor if you're taking *any* form of alternative medicine, no matter how confident you are that the drug is natural and, therefore, can't hurt you. Some alternative remedies may interfere with medications your doctor prescribes to treat your prostate cancer, and some alternative drugs may impede the effectiveness of chemotherapy medications. You certainly don't want to inadvertently decrease or neutralize the cancer-killing properties of the medications your doctor orders. To be safe, tell your doctor about your alternative remedies. He will let you know if the remedies present a risk. (In most cases, you won't have any risk, but you don't want to choose the one drug that's problematic.)

Another disadvantage to alternative remedies is the troubling lack of uniformity from one product to the next. Studies show that manufacturers of supplements are sometimes weak in the area of quality control. As a result, supplements may not always have as much vitamin E (or whatever supplement they're selling) as the package indicates. Some products that are imported from other countries and sold as supplements have been found upon random inspection to include low levels of vitamins or herbs, or none at all; some have also included dangerous drugs (such as Coumadin, a blood thinner), as well as other harmful or useless substances.

If you decide to take vitamin E supplements (or any other alternative remedies), find a brand that's made in the United States or Canada, where controls and inspections are the most stringent. Stick with that brand, and ignore any big sales that other sellers may offer.

Considering Vitamin E and Selenium

If your doctor agrees, you may wish to consider using an alternative remedy — such as the most popular options today: vitamin E and selenium — as a preventive measure after having treatment for prostate cancer.

Surprising findings on vitamin E and beta carotene

Few cancer physicians thought much about vitamin E before the Alpha-Tocopheral Beta Carotene Cancer Prevention Study (ATBC) results were released in 1998. This study was performed to determine whether taking vitamin E or beta carotene reduces the risk of lung cancer among smokers. The findings were not at all what the researchers had expected.

Sadly, the study showed that neither vitamin E nor beta carotene helped to prevent lung cancer. But researchers found something else quite fascinating: The researchers were surprised to discover that the study subjects who were taking vitamin E experienced a 32 percent reduction from the norm in the development of prostate cancer. And the men who already had prostate cancer experienced a 41 percent drop in the disease's death rate.

The researchers also found that taking high doses of beta carotene was associated with a 23 percent *increased* risk of developing prostate cancer and a 15 percent *increased* risk in the death rate. In addition, they found out that subjects who smoked and took beta carotene were *more* likely to develop lung cancer and die from it, than smokers who avoided the supplement. Further studies are needed, because researchers still don't know whether the negative effect from beta carotene is limited only to smokers. At this point, it appears that vitamin E may be beneficial, but you should avoid taking beta carotene supplements.

I know what you're thinking: "These statistics look pretty good, and I should start taking that vitamin E." The problem is that when researchers discover something that the study wasn't intended to test (such as testing for lung cancer, and then finding out something about prostate cancer), those results often aren't reliable, and they may even be false. The National Cancer Institute is spending a lot of time and money on the large SELECT trial that I describe in the "Considering Vitamin E and Selenium" section in this chapter to determine whether vitamin E and selenium really are effective at preventing prostate cancer.

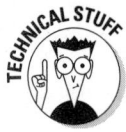

The federal government of the United States is currently sponsoring the Selenium and Vitamin E Cancer Trial (SELECT). This massive clinical study follows 32,000 men who've never been diagnosed with prostate cancer. The subjects, located at 400 different sites, will be studied for 7 to 12 years. The study subjects are mostly older than age 55; however, the minimum age requirement for black study subjects is 50 years, because black men have a significantly higher risk for developing aggressive prostate cancer at a younger age. When the study is complete and the results are in, SELECT will ultimately demonstrate if and how well both selenium and vitamin E work as preventive drugs against prostate cancer. Unfortunately, the results from this study won't be available for at least several years. Until then, I can't tell you whether selenium and vitamin E will help you. However, I can provide you with some basic info that you can present to your doctor if you decide to try an alternative approach.

Vitamin E: A potential lifesaver?

Researchers won't know for sure whether vitamin E is good or bad for you until the clinical trials are finished, although the current information regarding vitamin E and the prevention or recurrence of prostate cancer is cause for cautious optimism. (See the "Surprising findings on vitamin E and beta carotene" sidebar in this chapter for more information.) Some physicians are already recommending supplemental vitamin E to their patients, either to prevent prostate cancer or to keep PSA levels down after treatments for cancer. These doctors aren't waiting for the long-term study results.

The primary benefit of taking vitamin E is that it may help prevent the development or recurrence of prostate cancer. Of course, if you stay cancer-free, you won't actually be able to tell if you're still healthy because of the vitamin E or because of another reason. But does it really matter?

The primary disadvantage of taking vitamin E is that you have to pay for this over-the-counter supplement yourself, and studies may eventually show that it doesn't help prevent cancer. Also, if you take very large doses of vitamin E supplements, you could have a problem with blood thinning. Follow the instructions!

If you want to obtain vitamin E from the foods you eat, or if you want to supplement your vitamin E pills with foods rich in vitamin E, consider the following foods (some are cooking oils used to prepare food):

The popularity of nontraditional remedies

Whether doctors like the idea of alternative remedies for treating prostate cancer or not, many patients use them. In a study of 84 patients with prostate cancer (reported in a 2002 issue of *Urology*), 37 percent said that they used unconventional treatments. About half were taking megadoses of vitamins A, E, and C, and about 12 percent were taking selenium. Other studies have shown that many prostate cancer patients are taking herbal remedies such as saw palmetto or lycopene. (There is no evidence that saw palmetto offers any benefits to patients with prostate cancer.)

Unfortunately, many patients don't tell their doctors about the vitamins, herbs, or other remedies they're taking unless directly asked. Keeping this information from their doctors presents a problem, because these supplements may interact with the medicines their doctors order. Some physicians also worry that high doses of vitamins may interfere with the results of radiation therapy and chemotherapy.

✔ Wheat germ oil

✔ Almonds

✔ Soybean oil

✔ Lettuce

✔ Watercress

✔ Sunflower oil

✔ Nonfat milk

✔ Peas

Selenium: Can it reduce your risk?

Selenium is a nonmetallic trace element that's normally present in your food and water. Some researchers believe that taking selenium daily may help prevent the development of prostate cancer. Some researchers also believe that selenium may help prevent a resurgence of prostate cancer among men who've already been treated for the disease. Whether men with prostate cancer may be deficient in selenium is not clear, but selenium may provide some protection against the development of prostate cancer. The SELECT study (discussed earlier in this section) should reveal whether selenium helps prevent prostate cancer. Unfortunately, you have to make decisions now; you can't wait 3 to 12 years for the SELECT results.

Even if your doctor doesn't see any value to taking selenium, he probably agrees that selenium isn't harmful to men with prostate cancer. Of course, you shouldn't take doses that are higher than those recommended on the label of the bottle. More is not always better: Often, more is worse, because high doses of just about anything can make you sicker.

Promising results on the effects of selenium

One of the first studies for determining the effects of selenium was actually performed to find out if taking selenium protects against the development of skin cancer — the researchers weren't interested in prostate cancer. In this study, which was released in 1996, researchers concluded that selenium provides no protection against skin cancer. However, the men who took selenium during the study had a 60 percent reduced incidence of prostate cancer. (As with the vitamin E study, the researchers were looking for something else; their unexpected findings, however, are still very valuable for doctors and patients.) The results of the study are promising, but they don't provide definitive proof that selenium can help prevent prostate cancer — that would require a more focused study.

Toeing the line with selenium

In one rather weird-sounding study from Finland (reported in 1998), researchers analyzed the collected toenail clippings (no kidding) of 33,000 men for selenium. (Selenium collects in the toenails.) After careful analysis of all the toenail clippings, researchers found that high levels of selenium in the toenails was associated with a significantly reduced rate of advanced prostate cancer. (And you probably thought that toenail clippings were trash.) Whether these findings mean that selenium is somehow associated with a lower rate of prostate cancer, or whether it causes a lower rate of prostate cancer, is not yet known.

A disadvantage of taking selenium is that it's not usually covered by health insurance, so you have to pay for it yourself. Make sure that you buy selenium that's made and packaged in the United States or Canada, and then stick with that brand to avoid potential problems with the lower levels of vitamins you may find in brands made in other countries.

If you prefer to obtain your daily dose of selenium from food rather than from pills, you'll be happy to discover that some foods are very high in selenium. Of course, you can also take a selenium supplement *and* eat foods that are high in selenium. Keep in mind that it can be hard to eat enough food to obtain the same level of selenium found in a capsule of selenium. The following foods are high in selenium:

- ✔ Whole wheat bread
- ✔ Bran
- ✔ Oats
- ✔ Brown rice
- ✔ Barley
- ✔ Fish
- ✔ Meat
- ✔ Turnips
- ✔ Garlic

Fighting Prostate Cancer with Your Diet

Diets have always been a major consideration with prostate cancer. Most of the research on the connection between diet and prostate cancer suggests that diets low in fat (especially saturated fats from red meats) may reduce the risk of prostate cancer. Not all fats are bad, however; fats from fish and some vegetables may actually be beneficial in preventing or fighting prostate cancer. This fact may explain why the rate of clinical prostate cancer is much lower among Japanese men, who eat a diet high in fish and fiber, than it is among U.S. men, who eat a diet high in red meat and fatty foods. Consider this: If a Japanese man moves to the United States, in two generations his family rate of prostate cancer will increase to the same rate found in American men, possibly because of adopting an American diet. However, until further studies are done, the impact of diet can't be known for sure.

Avoiding quack therapies on the Internet

When you have prostate cancer, especially an advanced case, you can feel pretty desperate. Unfortunately, plenty of people in cyberland are eager to prey on your fears and anxieties, and they'd love for you to shell out your hard-earned bucks on their useless products. Sure, some extreme solutions may work, and you may even think, "What can it hurt to try?" Well, you can lose a lot of money, and such remedies can be useless at best and harmful at worst.

When evaluating alternative therapies promoted on the Internet to treat prostate cancer (in addition to talking to your doctor about it, which you should always do), consider whether the sellers of the product or treatment make any of the following types of statements:

- **The product will cure your prostate cancer.** The fact is, after the cancer has started, the only known cures are surgery or radiation. Other treatments, such as hormone therapy or cryosurgery, can delay the spread of cancer, but no drugs, including "natural" supplements, can cure your cancer. Anyone who says differently is lying.

- **You shouldn't (or don't need to) tell your doctor about the product.** You absolutely *should* tell your doctor about any alternative remedies before you take them. Maybe she won't approve, or maybe she'll give you the thumbs up. If your doctor doesn't like an alternative therapy, she'll tell you why.

- **The product is a good substitute for surgery, radiation treatments, hormone therapy, or any other treatments your doctor is recommending.** This is terrible advice that can lead to cancer spread and death. Don't gamble with your life.

- **This remedy has cured other patients — check out all the testimonials.** There are many ways to get testimonials from people: One way is to pay them. Another is to obtain statements from true believers. Even if the testimonials are authentic, you don't know if a testimonial given by John Doe in 1999 is still valid. You don't even know if John Doe is still alive.

The bottom line is, be a skeptical consumer. You can also check on a broad array of remedies on the searchable Quackwatch Web site run by physician Stephen Barrett at www.quackwatch.com.

To find out more about the specifics of diets, check out some the many diet books on the market. (You may want to check out *The ABC's of Nutrition & Supplements for Prostate Cancer,* by Mark A. Moyad, M.P.H., from Sleeping Bear Press.) Some formally programmed diets that may be useful include the Mediterranean diet, the macrobiotic diet, the Dean Ornish diet, and the Pritikin diet. However, don't rely on diet alone to treat your cancer unless your doctor specifically recommends that you do.

Checking Out Other Alternative Remedies

Selenium and vitamin E aren't the only alternative medicines for men hoping to prevent prostate cancer from developing or recurring. Many researchers are also looking into whether nonsteroidal anti-inflammatory medications (NSAIDs), such as aspirin or Motrin, can reduce the risk of prostate cancer. So far, the findings are conflicting and unclear. In addition, naturally occurring substances (or supplements) such as lycopene and fructose may also be beneficial to men with prostate cancer, both during and after treatment.

However, keep in mind new fads are always coming out, and when this book goes to press, some people may well be saying, for example, that eating dehydrated sea turtle eggs cures prostate cancer. This is just one outrageous example of what someone may come up with as a hot new "cure."

PC-SPES

Although it may sound like some government formulation, the PC-SPES name is actually based on *PC,* for prostate cancer, and *SPES,* for the Latin word for hope. Some of the purported ingredients in PC-SPES were chrysanthemum, licorice, saw palmetto, and other herbs.

In 2002, the U.S. Food and Drug Administration (FDA) banned PC-SPES as a prostate cancer treatment, based on the fact that some formulations of the herbs also contained substances that are dangerous for some patients, such as Coumadin (generic name: warfarin), a drug that thins the blood and can cause a bleeding problem, Xanax (generic name: alprazolam), a strong anti-anxiety medication, and other drugs. These substances were not listed on the bottle label.

Some doctors think that unadulterated forms of PC-SPES (one that is pure, without the extra drugs/ingredients that caused the FDA to pull it off the market) may still merit further study. At this point, however, PC-SPES is not an option for men in the United States.

Naturally occurring alternative remedies

Lycopene, a substance found naturally in tomatoes, may prevent prostate cancer as well as stop it from recurring. Lycopene can also be taken as a dietary supplement, but few studies have been done on lycopene supplements. Some small clinical trials performed on men with prostate cancer have indicated that lycopene supplements may cause a drop in PSA levels, although larger studies are needed to confirm that the supplements can help prevent cancer. In the meantime, I advise against taking lycopene supplements, because there just isn't enough evidence showing whether they're okay or not. Instead, go natural and adopt this motto: "Eating a tomato a day may help keep the oncologist away."

Some preliminary evidence suggests that other substances found in certain foods may help prevent prostate cancer from occurring or recurring, as well. These substances include fructose (found in many fruits), soy, flaxseed, vitamin D, calcium, and green tea. Some of these substances can be found in more purified forms as supplements, but check with your doctor before buying and using them.

Easing Treatment Side Effects with Alternative Remedies

Alternative remedies, such as vitamins, herbs, and supplements, may also help with the side effects you may experience when receiving traditional treatments for prostate cancer (particularly hormone therapy, which I discuss in Chapter 13).

Cooling hot flashes

In addition to the regular hormone medications that are often prescribed for alleviating hot flashes, you can also find a variety of alternative remedies that some experts claim are beneficial if you ingest them in some form, such as a supplement. These remedies include

- ✔ Soy
- ✔ Flaxseed
- ✔ Vitamin E
- ✔ Green tea
- ✔ Chamomile
- ✔ Licorice
- ✔ Black cohosh
- ✔ Chastberry

Boning up with vitamin D

Some reputable physicians indicate that an increased intake of vitamin D (cal-citriol) may help ease *osteoporosis* (a bone disorder that results in a loss of bone density) induced by hormone therapy. Some evidence suggests that vitamin D is useful for prostate cancer prevention or recurrence. You can obtain vitamin D preparations over the counter, but I think having your doctor prescribe it for you is better, because vitamin D can be harmful.

Here's another vitamin D tidbit: Vitamin D is actually produced in the body by sunlight when sunlight comes in contact with skin cells. So getting some sun (but not too much!) may actually be good for prostate cancer prevention.

Settling your stomach with ginger

Some forms of therapy, such as chemotherapy and hormone therapy, may cause nausea and heartburn. If you don't want to take a standard remedy for these stomach problems, consider a low dose of ginger. (When you were a small child, your mother may have given you ginger ale to help settle a sick stomach. Unfortunately, most of today's ginger ales don't have any ginger in them.) You can also ask someone to buy or make you ginger cookies or ginger snaps. Ginger is also available as a tea.

Part V
Coping with the Aftermath Effects of Prostate Cancer

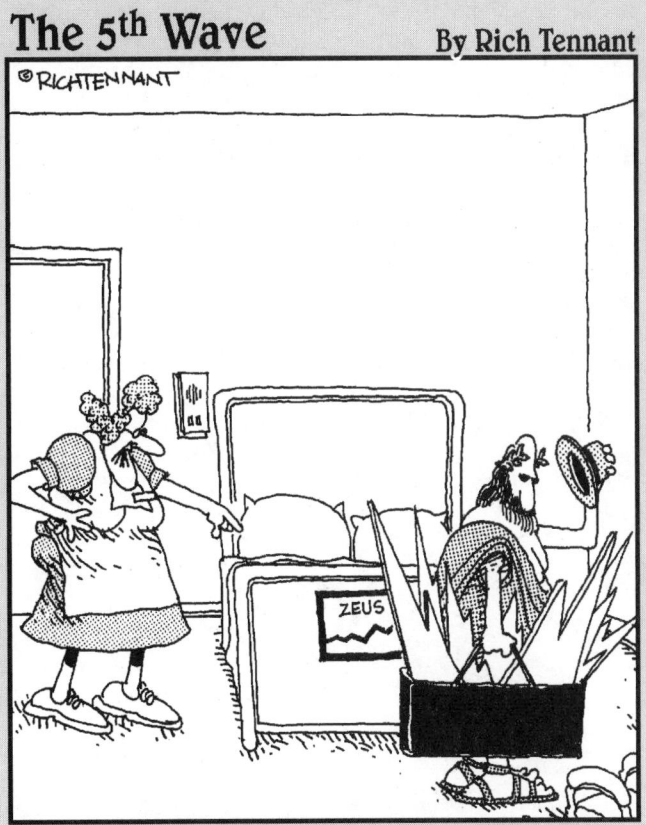

The 5th Wave
By Rich Tennant

"Mr. Zeus! What are you doing out of bed? After your operation, the doctor said you shouldn't even be shorting out lamps yet, let alone hurling thunderbolts ...!"

In this part . . .

This part discusses the common concerns many men have when coping with the aftermath effects of prostate cancer. For example, many men worry about becoming impotent, although for many men with prostate cancer, it's only a temporary problem, if it's a problem at all. Impotence may not become a problem for you, but if you do have trouble getting or keeping erections, I discuss many good ways to deal with the problem in Chapter 19.

A lot of men also worry that prostate cancer will cause permanent incontinence. In reality, incontinence is usually only a temporary problem for men with prostate cancer, or it just doesn't happen at all. In Chapter 20, I cover the different types of incontinence and what you can do if you suffer from it.

Here's another troubling thought for men with prostate cancer: "What if the cancer comes back even after treatment?" Chapter 21 discusses the signs that may signal a recurrence of the cancer (such as a rising PSA level).

Chapter 19

Resolving Erectile Problems

*W*hen an enraged Lorena Bobbitt cut off her husband's penis in 1993, the story hit the news big. Men everywhere cringed at this extreme disfigurement and the severe pain it must have caused the victim. Fortunately, Mr. Bobbitt's severed penis was miraculously reattached, and, according to reports, it's fully functional. What does this groan-inducing story have to do with prostate cancer and the erection problems it may cause? Well, if doctors can actually reattach and repair a man's severed penis, there certainly must be hope for men whose penises are still connected to their bodies but aren't working at maximum capability.

I'm not saying that *impotence* (the inability to get or maintain an erection) is a thing of the past, nor am I saying that any man can achieve full sexual potency after treatment for prostate cancer. But if prostate cancer has affected your ability to have erections, you still have plenty of hope and plenty of options to choose from. Even when the entire prostate gland must be removed to cure the cancer, sexual potency can often be preserved through prostate surgery that spares the nerves that control erections.

In this chapter, I explain how and why prostate cancer sometimes affects sexual potency. I also discuss the options for overcoming erection difficulties, which include mechanical devices, oral and injectable medications, and penile implants.

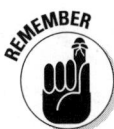

Be sure to talk to your partner candidly before you choose an injectable drug or any of the other remedies described in this chapter. Your partner may have a different opinion about which remedy is best. You may find that your partner wants to take an active part in your decision-making process.

Considering Causes of Erectile Dysfunction

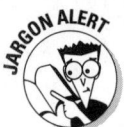

Erectile dysfunction (ED) is the term used by most physicians to describe any trouble with starting or keeping erections to the point where you can't successfully have sexual intercourse. (Doctors often use the initials ED because they believe that the term erectile dysfunction sounds too negative.) ED encompasses a broad range of difficulties with erections: It refers to the man who can't get an erection at all, to the man whose erection is a little soft and easily lost, and also to the man who has some relatively minor and occasional trouble maintaining an erection.

Some medical conditions, such as diabetes or other diseases that cause circulation or nerve problems, can cause erectile dysfunction before any cancer treatments ever start. Problems with erectile performance also can be temporarily caused by psychological problems (such as worrying about your prostate cancer). In fact, prostate cancer and other prostatic diseases are rarely the actual cause of the impotence. Treatments, on the other hand, can affect the quantity and quality of erections.

Surgery

When doctors perform a radical prostatectomy, they completely remove the prostate gland. (You can read more about prostatectomies in Chapter 11.) When the prostate gland is removed, ejaculation is no longer possible; only dry orgasms can occur (which is just fine for many men and their partners). But the nerves that control erections are located very close to the back of the prostate, on both sides. If the cancer is bad, the doctor may have to remove the nerves (on one or both sides) along with the prostate. Removing both nerves during surgery causes permanent erectile dysfunction.

However, these nerves can often be spared. When *nerve-sparing surgery* is performed, the erections are often unaffected or only temporarily impaired. It can sometimes take awhile (3 to 12 months or longer) for the natural ability to have an erection to come back after you undergo nerve-sparing surgery.

Radiation therapy

You may have heard that radiation treatments don't impair your potency at all. The reality is that radiation therapy may cause temporary or long-term problems with erectile dysfunction because of inflammation or scarring that can occur around the nerves.

The odds for developing a potency problem are about the same with radiation as they are with a nerve-sparing prostatectomy done in expert hands; however, radiation gives much better results than the prostatectomy when the nerve-sparing surgery is not performed. (See Chapter 12 for more on radiation therapy.)

Hormone therapy

Hormone therapy lowers your sex drive and sometimes (but not always) impairs your ability to have erections. When the hormone therapy is over, your ability to get an erection usually returns.

During hormone therapy, hormones are used to decrease or block your testosterone, because testosterone makes cancer grow faster. But because testosterone is the main hormone responsible for your sex drive, when you decrease the effect of testosterone, you also block your ability to have erections as well as your urge to merge with your significant other.

Take Tom and Linda, for example. They had no sex life while Tom underwent hormone therapy for 15 months, because Tom lost his sex drive altogether. He also had problems with fatigue, joint pain, depression, hot flashes, and sleeplessness, none of which made him feel sexy either. He had his last hormone shot in December. By June, according to Linda, they were "back in the saddle again." Tom just felt better one day, so he decided that it was time for what he called "a test drive." Linda was fine with that, and she says that everything worked very well, just like before he was diagnosed with prostate cancer.

Getting older doesn't always cause impotence

Some men (and even some doctors) may mistakenly attribute their erection problems solely to aging, especially if they're age 65 or older. This is one of the quandaries of ageism that men sometimes face. However, when a man older than 65 suddenly begins to have problems with his erections, it isn't the result of a simple aging problem. Instead, the problem may be a result of diabetes or another illnesses that needs to be treated. Most urologists are very familiar with the diagnosis and treatment of erectile dysfunction. But if your urologist insists that your erectile dysfunction is just a consequence of aging alone, and that nothing can be done about the problem, get another medical opinion.

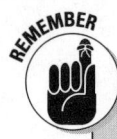

Orgasms without erections

Men can actually have an orgasm without having an erection and without ejaculating. The nerves that control and produce orgasms aren't located in or around the prostate gland, so even if your prostate gland is surgically removed — and even if you can't have an erection anymore — you can still have an orgasm.

Men who have orgasms without erections sometimes say that they feel a little weird at first, probably because they're used to the kind of orgasm that includes an erection and ejaculation, and they perceive that their former experience represented the normal way of doing things. But men who have orgasms without erections also say that their orgasms are highly erotic, very satisfying experiences.

The ability to have orgasms without an erection means that men can continue to enjoy an active sex life with their partners, even if penile penetration isn't a part of that sex life. Generally, the non-erect penis must be manually or orally stimulated for the orgasm to occur. In addition, it usually takes longer to achieve orgasm with a non-erect penis than it does with an erection. It may take at least several minutes of direct stimulation before the orgasm occurs.

Sometimes, orgasms don't happen, no matter how diligently your partner (or you) keeps trying. It just works out that way sometimes — it isn't anybody's fault. However, if you're one of the many men who thought that you'd never have an orgasm again because of your problem with erections, this information may be very welcomed by you.

Finding Natural Ways to Improve Your Love Life

If your erections are either unsatisfactory or completely nonexistent, you can still rev up your sexual experiences in many different and natural ways. For example, if you smoke, you should stop. Smoking can impede your ability to have or keep erections. You can give up smoking by using nicotine replacement medications or trying one of the other smoking cessation ideas I offer in Chapter 17.

You may also want to give up drinking. Alcohol is a depressant, and one thing it depresses is your love life and your ability to have erections. So lay off the booze! See Chapter 17 for more reasons why minimizing your alcohol consumption is important.

You should also keep in mind that you can express your love for your partner with more forms of sex than just sexual intercourse (which requires an erection). You can try oral sex or mutual masturbation, for example.

It may help to think back to the days of your youth, when sex meant whatever you could achieve in the back seat of your father's car. These sexual escapades didn't include penetration, and yet you were still often able to attain sexual gratification.

Another important point to keep in mind is that you can have orgasms without having any erections at all. (See the "Orgasms without erections" sidebar in this chapter.)

But if intercourse is your preference (and it is for most couples), you can almost always achieve it with one of the methods I describe in the sections that follow.

Uplifting Experiences: Devices That May Help

To understand the devices that can help you achieve erections, you need to know a little about how normal erections work. Two narrow cylinders of spongy tissue (called the *corpus cavernosa*) run along the inside length of your penis. During sexual excitement, inflow valves in your penis open to increase the blood flow into the cylinders. After the cylinders fill with blood, the outflow valves in your penis close, trapping the blood inside the cylinders. The blood causes the cylinders, and therefore the penis, to swell and get hard. After the orgasm has occurred, the outflow valves open again and let the blood drain out, causing the penis to return to its flaccid state.

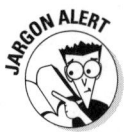

The *vacuum constriction device* is one type of mechanical device that can help you achieve erections. These devices are pumped up either manually or electronically.

Vacuum constriction devices rely on the basic principles of a vacuum. To use such a device, you place a chamber over your penis and then pump the air out, creating a vacuum. This partial vacuum causes increased blood flow inside your penis. As your penis becomes engorged with blood, you achieve an erection. When the vacuum device causes your penis to swell sufficiently (or as erect as you can get it), you remove the chamber and place a small, thick rubber-band–like device around the base of your penis. This band helps the blood stay in your penis so that you can maintain your erection for at least a brief period of time. You have to keep the band on, otherwise you'll quickly lose your erection. However, when intercourse is over, the band *must* come off — if you leave it on, you can do yourself harm. Take a look at Figure 19-1 to see how the vacuum device is used.

Use it or lose it?

Many doctors tell men that they shouldn't worry about having erections after undergoing surgery or radiation treatments that can impede or prevent erections. They tell these men that if it's going to happen, nature will simply take its course, and the ability to have erections will gradually come back again. However, many doctors who specialize in treating erectile dysfunction disagree: They encourage sexual activity as soon as possible after treatment. They believe that the nerves and muscles that control erection can actually *atrophy* (shrink up and die) if they aren't used for a long period of time, and if you make no attempt to have an erection, you may ultimately lose your ability to have an erection.

Who's right? No one knows for sure. However, if your doctor believes that it won't harm anything to resume sexual activity within weeks or months after your treatment for prostate cancer, follow his advice, even if you have to use artificial means (like a vacuum device or one of the other options I describe in this chapter) for awhile.

Some vacuum devices are available with a prescription, while others are available over the counter at your local pharmacy or medical supply store. These devices cost anywhere from $150 to $500, depending on how fancy they are and where you buy them. In general, the vacuum devices that require a prescription work better than the units you can buy over the counter at your local pharmacy, but they also cost more.

The primary advantage of the vacuum device is that it can help you get an erection. Men who are able to get at least some erections on their own may benefit the most from this type of device.

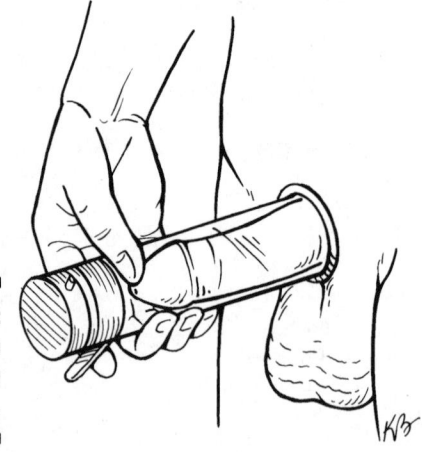

Figure 19-1:
A vacuum
pump
device.

The disadvantage is that your penis may feel cold or "funny" to you and your partner. In addition, you may experience a slight feeling of pain from the constriction band that helps you maintain the erection. Some men say that they just can't manage to have an orgasm after achieving an erection with these devices. Many couples complain that this approach is not very romantic; for some, it can be a deal breaker. Alternatively, some couples think that the device is okay, and they're happy that it helps them achieve erections.

Happily Ever After with Viagra and Other Medications

If you have minor difficulty obtaining or keeping erections, medications can often help resolve the problem.

Revving things up with Viagra

Viagra (generic name: sildenafil citrate) is the most well-known and commonly used drug for treating impotence. A few years ago, former Congressional representative Bob Dole touted Viagra in high-profile TV commercials while recovering from prostate cancer.

Viagra was first approved as a medication to treat erectile dysfunction by the U.S. Food and Drug Administration (FDA) in 1998. (Some men with normal sexual potency are also taking the drug, but it's only recommended for men who're having erectile difficulties.) This prescribed drug costs about $10 a pill.

Unlike the medications that are taken for such problems as chronic hypertension, thyroid disease, or diabetes, you don't take Viagra daily. Instead, you take it about an hour or two before you have intercourse. Doctors recommend actively thinking about sex and performing manual stimulation after taking the drug, to help encourage the erection along. Viagra works best if you take it on an empty stomach. The effects of the drug should take hold within an hour of taking it.

Viagra helps many men achieve erections, and it may work for you, as well. As with all drugs, however, it does have pros and cons. The primary benefits are:

✔ Most men tolerate Viagra well, with no or only a few minor side effects. (I discuss these side effects shortly.)

✔ Viagra can help you sustain an erection for up to four hours, so you can set your own sexual pace.

The primary drawbacks of Viagra are:

✔ It may cause minor side effects such as headaches, flushing (reddening) of the body, mild stomachaches, and temporary blurred vision. (Only rarely are these side effects so uncomfortable that the man stops taking the drug.)

✔ It often only works after prostate cancer surgery if one or both of the nerve bundles that control erections are spared.

If you're taking nitroglycerin (which is often used to treat heart pain) or other drugs like nitroglycerin, you can't take Viagra, because the combination of the two drugs can lead to a sudden and sometimes fatal drop in blood pressure. Talk to your doctor to find out if you're currently taking any heart medications or any other drugs that may react with Viagra.

Some men consider Viagra to be a godsend that fully restores their sex lives; other men consider the drug to be a major disappointment, because, for them, it only helps to achieve a sort of mushy erection that's insufficient for actual penetration, and its effects wear off very quickly. If Viagra doesn't work for you, consider the other options that I describe in this chapter. You should also know that several other drugs similar to Viagra are close to getting approved in the United States. It appears that one of these other drugs may work when Viagra doesn't, so stay tuned.

Viagra worked for them

Tad was impotent for several months after his nerve-sparing prostatectomy, but he and his wife Emma were determined to continue an active sex life. They found that Viagra helped Tad have erections, although Emma points out that a lot of touching and cuddling and some mutual masturbation was still necessary. (Which was fine with them, because they enjoyed this kind of lovemaking before they ever heard of prostate cancer.)

Emma and Tad figure that the penis is a muscle that needs to be stimulated, and that the Viagra worked with them to make it happen. After about eight months, they realized that they no longer needed Viagra, because Tad's potency was back to normal again.

Shooting for improved potency: Injectable drugs

If Viagra doesn't work for you, you can try a self-injected medication. When I say self-injected, I mean that you inject the medication directly into your penis (actually, directly into one of the two *corpus cavernosa,* the narrow cylinders of spongy tissue in your penis). The injection can hurt a little (most men say that the injection feels a little like a mosquito bite), but if the medication brings back your erections, you may decide that the gain is worth the minor pain. Your doctor will show you how to properly perform the self-injection.

If you're queasy around needles, and you don't like the idea of injecting your-self with medication, you may want to try a *self-injecting device.* This device includes a hidden, spring-loaded needle that contains the medication. When you're ready to use the self-injector, you simply press a button, and the needle injects the medicine into your penis.

The two most common self-injectable drugs for treating erectile dysfunction are Caverject (generic name: alprostadil) and Genabid (generic name: papaver-ine). Some men also have success with Trimix, which is a combination of alprostadil, Vasomax (generic name: phentolamine), and Genabid.

Injectable drugs are prescribed medications. They can cost anywhere from $5 to $25 (or more) per injection.

Self-injected medications, like other ED treatments, come with pros and cons. The primary benefits of self-injected medications are:

- ✔ The erections you achieve with the medication are often as firm and feel as normal as the erections you experienced before you had prostate problems.
- ✔ The effects of the medication usually last about an hour or so.

The disadvantages of the self-injected medications are:

- ✔ You're limited in the amount of injections you can give yourself. Some doctors recommend no more than 12 shots a month, while others rec-ommend no more than one a day. Taking more shots than your doctor recommends can cause dangerous scarring.
- ✔ You need to see your doctor about every three months for a checkup when using self-injected medications. Your physician will inspect your penis to make sure that you don't have any damage or scar tissue buildup.

✔ You have to plan ahead before using injectable drugs, because they need to be injected about 15 minutes before you have sex. Some men believe that these drugs spoil sex, because the rushing around takes away the spontaneity and the romance.

✔ Self-injected medications can cause *priapism,* or an abnormally long-lasting erection. This condition may sound pretty good when you're having so much trouble getting an erection in the first place, but having an erection that lasts for four hours or more can actually be a painful and scary experience. This side effect isn't common, but it can happen. If it happens to you, call your doctor or go to the emergency room right away. The doctor can administer an injection to reverse the priapism. Priapism that continues untreated for longer than four to six hours can cause permanent damage. That thought alone should help you overcome any embarrassment you may have about reporting your extended erection.

Musing about MUSE: The implantable pellet

If self-injections aren't right for you, you may want to consider the *Medicated Urethral System for Erection,* or *MUSE* (generic name: alsprostadil). MUSE is a medicated pellet, roughly the size of a grain of rice, that you insert into the urethra of your penis. MUSE is the same drug that's in Caverject, the injectable form of the drug. When you place the MUSE in your urethra, it gradually dissolves and finds its way into the corpus cavernosum, where it does its job just like the direct penile injections.

MUSE is a relatively new entry in the world of erectile dysfunction medications. It was first approved by the U.S. FDA in 1996. The pellets cost about $20 each, and you insert them yourself.

They did their homework

Carol, whose husband Jake was diagnosed with prostate cancer when he was 55, says that much of their success with coping with impotence stemmed from the fact that they discussed the possibility of it happening before Jake's surgery. They read up on the various aids that were available and agreed that they'd be willing to experiment if necessary. When Viagra and a vacuum device didn't work, Jake tried a self-injected medication. The injections worked, and they've been using them for two years.

As with all medications and therapies, MUSE has some benefits and draw-backs. The primary advantages of MUSE are:

- ✔ The preparation is easy. You urinate to help lubricate the area, and then you insert the pellet.
- ✔ Inserting the pellet is generally painless.
- ✔ MUSE is often effective at inducing an erection when Viagra fails.

The primary disadvantages of MUSE are:

- ✔ The effects of the drug are sometimes erratic.
- ✔ Some men complain that MUSE doesn't produce firm enough erections.
- ✔ You need to plan ahead carefully, because it only takes about five to ten minutes for the medication to kick in.
- ✔ Side effects may include minor leg swelling and a feeling of burning or warmth in your urethra. In some rare cases, your sexual partner may complain of a burning feeling during intercourse, as well. However, this burning sensation will not cause any permanent harm to your partner.

Considering Penile Implant Surgery

You tried Viagra, the vacuum constriction device, the self-injected medica-tions, and MUSE, and none of them worked for you. Or maybe they worked, but they just required way too much effort. Perhaps your doctor told you that penile implant surgery is your one remaining choice for restoring sexual potency. If this is the case, don't be discouraged or afraid. You may find that the penile implant is actually the best and most effective choice for your situation.

Looking at your choices

Penile implants are comprised of one or several rods that are permanently inserted (under anesthesia) in the two cylinders of spongy tissue (corpus cavernosa) inside your penis. These cylinders normally fill up with blood and become hard when you're sexually aroused. The implant fills this same role when your own cylinders aren't working. All penile implants are contained inside the body, so they can't be detected. In addition, they are measured to fit into your penis in such a way that the size of your erection is the same or very close to your erections in the past.

You have several different types of penile implants to choose from:

- **Semi-rigid or malleable implants:** These implants are semi-rigid, so you can manipulate your penis into either an up or down position. If you keep your penis in the erect (or up) position, it may appear as though you have a permanent erection, so no wearing tiny bathing suits — unless you're really into showing off! In the down position, your penis can generally be concealed fairly easily — unless you insist on wearing very tight clothing. With this implant option, you're always ready. This choice is the simplest and most popular penile implant. See Figure 19-2 for an example of this type of implant.

- **Inflatable implants:** With this type of implant, a pump is attached to an artificial cylinder that fits in the penis. To achieve an erection, you just press on the appropriate part of the penis to activate the pump. This option is depicted in Figure 19-3.

- **Three-piece prosthesis:** This implant is made up of a fluid reservoir and inflatable cylinders that fit inside the natural cylinders of spongy tissue in your penis. When the pump is activated by gently pressing on a certain part of the scrotum, the penis becomes erect. Pressing another part of the pump makes the penis become flaccid (or limp) again. This implant is the most complicated and expensive option, as well as the most functional. See Figure 19-4.

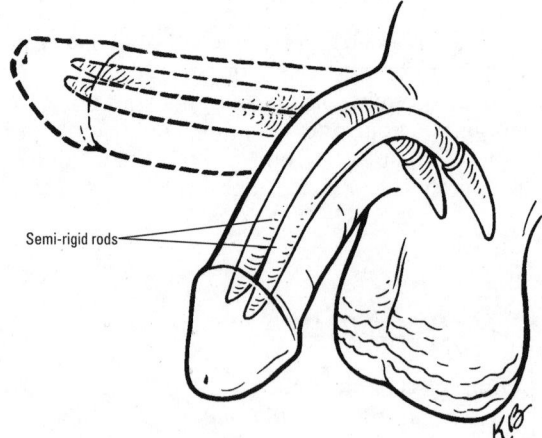

Semi-rigid rods

Figure 19-2:
Semi-rigid
implant.

Overcoming your fear of surgery

If your doctor is telling you (or if you feel, for reasons of preference) that a penile implant is your last best hope for satisfactorily regaining your sexual potency, you're probably not jumping with joy at the prospect. For one thing, you may be nervous about having surgery, especially if you've already had a prostatectomy. But even if you've never had surgery before, it can still be a nail-biting decision.

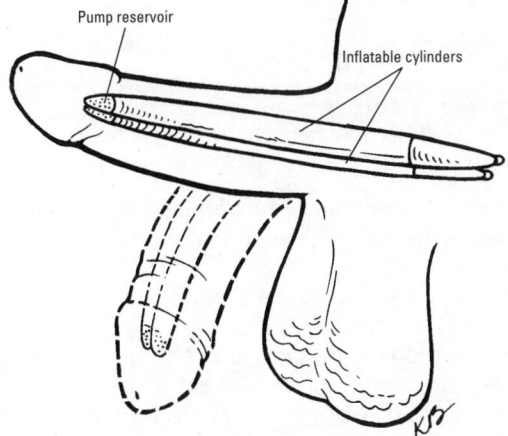

Figure 19-3:
Inflatable
implant.

You may worry that the surgery, which is performed in the same general area as the prostatectomy, will somehow shake up any leftover cancer cells. You may fear that these aroused cancer cells will then multiply wildly throughout your entire body. You may conclude that you're better off letting things be.

The fact is, penile implant surgery doesn't cause cancer to recur, nor does it cause new cancers to develop. So you don't need to worry about the surgery triggering another case of cancer.

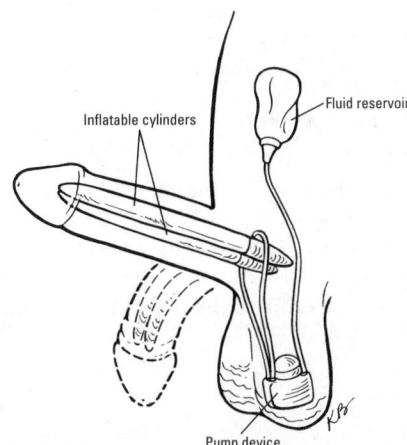

Figure 19-4:
Three-piece
prosthesis.

Weighing the pros and cons

Before you decide to undergo surgery for a penile implant, you need to understand the benefits and drawbacks of the procedure.

The primary benefits of the penile implant are:

- You don't have to mess with external devices.

- You don't have to take any drugs to achieve an erection. (The drugs that help you obtain an erection may negatively interact with other medications you take.)

- You don't have to do any complicated planning when you want to have sex. You're much more in charge of your own sex life.

The primary drawbacks of the penile implant are:

- **Risk of infection:** Infections may occur after the surgery, despite careful infection control by the doctor and the operating room staff. When infections develop in the genital area, they can be very hard to treat because of their location in the body. If an infection does occur, all or part of the penile implant will likely have to be removed, and implanting another one then becomes more difficult.

- **No turning back:** The other approaches (such as vacuum devices or injections) will likely be ineffective should the implant ever be removed.

- **Mechanical breakdowns:** If the implant breaks down (and it eventually will if given enough time), all or part of it will need to be replaced, and it can only be replaced with surgery. Fortunately, mechanical breakdowns are not common, and most implants last at least five to ten years.

- **High cost:** Penile implant surgery can cost $10,000 and up. Don't assume that your health insurance will cover the procedure. Always check before scheduling the procedure.

Knowing what to expect

Your doctor will tell you ahead of time what he plans to achieve with your penile implant surgery. When you clearly understand what your doctor is recommending, you can decide whether or not you want to go along with his plan. You don't have to understand exactly how the procedure is done, but you do need to know whether the procedure is likely to be successful, and about any of the problems that may occur.

Here are some questions to ask your doctor before you decide to go ahead with the penile implant surgery:

- ✔ "How long will it take me to recover from the surgery?"
- ✔ "How long should I wait before having sex?"
- ✔ "Are there any potential problems that I should watch out for after surgery, such as bleeding, pain, or other problems?"
- ✔ "Are there any limits to how often I can use my implant, or is the sky the limit?"
- ✔ "About how many times have you performed this surgery?"

  You don't want a doctor who's just learning the procedure. Make sure the doctor has performed the procedure at least 25 times.

- ✔ "About how many years can I reasonably expect the prosthesis to be good for, and how will I know if a replacement is needed?"

Comparing methods for inducing erections

It can be hard to decide which method for inducing an erection is best for you. You have to take into account such key factors as how much the method costs, how long the method takes to induce an erection, and how long your erection is going to last when using it. For example, maybe implant surgery costs thousands of dollars, but you don't have to pay any additional expenses (you won't need Viagra or any of the other options I describe in this chapter), and you can have sex whenever you and your partner feel like it. On the other hand, maybe the thought of surgery scares you, and you'd rather try one of the other options. The following chart enables you to discover the basic facts about each method at a glance.

Method	Estimated Cost	Time It Takes to Induce an Erection	How Long the Erection Lasts
Viagra	$10/pill	About an hour	Up to 4 hours
Injectable drugs	$5–$25 each	About 15 minutes	About an hour
MUSE	$20 each	About 5–10 minutes	About an hour
Vacuum devices	$150–$500	A few minutes	No more than half an hour
Surgery	Thousands of dollars	Anytime	As long as you want it to

If you decide that penile implant surgery is right for you, ask your doctor what you should do (or must do) before and after the surgery. For example, he may not want you to eat or drink anything after midnight the day of the surgery. (This is a common precaution used with most types of surgery. By not eating, you're less likely to throw up or choke on your anesthesia.) The doctor will also warn you not to take blood thinner medications, such as Coumadin or the herb ginkgo biloba, because they can cause you to bleed excessively during surgery. The excessive bleeding can make the surgery harder to perform or impair the healing process.

Chapter 20

Dealing with Urinary Incontinence

*U*rinary incontinence refers to the loss of control over the release of your urine. It can be a temporary problem that occurs after surgery or radiation, or it can be a longer-lasting problem.

For many men, incontinence is annoying and embarrassing. However, many highly effective treatments can be used to manage the incontinence problem, no matter how minor or severe. In this chapter, I talk about the different types of incontinence and the importance of considering whether you have a short- or long-term problem. I also cover techniques (such as bladder retraining, Kegel exercises, medications, and lifestyle changes) that can help you recover from or lessen your incontinence. You may benefit from an injection of collagen, so I explain how this treatment works. In severe cases, surgery may be the best answer for you, so I also provide information on incontinence surgery.

Identifying Incontinence

Prostate cancer can directly or indirectly create incontinence problems, at least temporarily. Rarely, the disease itself can affect the control you have over your urination and cause you to have some minor "accidents" before you're ever treated. Even more rarely, major incontinence can occur if the prostate cancer is advanced. But most of the time, incontinence is a side effect of the treatment you have for prostate cancer.

Incontinence usually improves: One study's highlights

Doctors March and Lepor of New York University Medical Center studied incontinence in 145 of their patients three months after having a radical prostatectomy, and then a year after surgery. Their findings were reported in a 2001 issue of *Current Urology Reports*.

The doctors found considerable improvement among most of the men in the study. For example, three months after their surgery, 56 percent of all the men used no pads (which means that they had no problem at all with incontinence). One year after their surgery, 81 percent of the men weren't using any pads. In looking at the other extreme, 12 percent of the men had to use large pads all day three months after their surgery. But at the one-year point, less than 1 percent of these men were using large pads.

Time may or may not heal all wounds, but it certainly works quite well when it comes to resolving many of the problems associated with incontinence. In my experience, the return of complete continence is even better now than when Doctors March and Lepor analyzed their patients. This is especially true among surgeons at major medical centers, such as myself, who perform this surgery frequently. Up to 50 percent of my patients either never wear pads or stop wearing pads after one month. That number increases to 95 percent to 98 percent after one year.

Your body and bladder often need time to adjust to the treatments for prostate cancer. How well you're doing, incontinence-wise, immediately after an anti-cancer procedure, is not always indicative of how you're going to do for the rest of your life. However, if you have no control at all over your bladder right after treatment, you can probably expect that you'll continue to have some problem with incontinence for at least awhile. And if you have a minor problem with dribbling urine after treatment — one that requires you to wear just one pad a day inside your jockey shorts — you may find that the problem quickly resolves completely.

In general, permanent incontinence is rare with any prostate cancer therapy. But temporary incontinence is more likely to be a problem after a prostatectomy than after radiation treatments, because to remove the prostate, the surgeon has to get very close to the major valve (or sphincter) controlling urine flow, and consequently, risks damaging the sphincter. Also, once the prostate is removed, the surgeon has to reconnect the bladder to the urethra, which is very close to the sphincter. Radiation can sometimes cause temporary incontinence, too. Thankfully, the situation usually improves, by quite a lot. How long it takes for incontinence to improve or go away altogether varies, but it may be about a year or so before it gets as good as it's going to get.

Checking out the key symptoms

You may think that figuring out whether you have urinary incontinence is easy. If you can control your bladder, you don't have it, and if you can't control your bladder, you do. But many other urinary symptoms are often associated with incontinence. These symptoms include:

✔ Difficulty emptying your bladder completely

✔ Feeling like you need to urinate often, even though you just went

✔ Dribbling or leaking urine

If you experience any of these symptoms, tell your doctor. He can determine what type of incontinence you're experiencing and recommend the best treatment option.

Determining your incontinence type

Incontinence comes in several different forms. You can have a mixed form of incontinence, but most problems with incontinence fall into one of these categories:

✔ **Stress incontinence:** This is the most common form of urinary incontinence resulting from surgery for prostate cancer. The main problem with stress incontinence is a weak *sphincter* (the muscle that opens and closes to let urine out). Stress incontinence is characterized by a leaking or dripping of urine when you laugh or sneeze — sort of like when people say that they laughed so hard, they wet their pants, except with stress incontinence, it doesn't take a rolling-on-the-floor kind of laughing to make you lose your urine — just a mild chuckle can be sufficient enough to induce this response. (Laughter is a great way to beat the blues, so instead of giving it up, make sure that you plan ahead, with pads or special jockey shorts that have built-in padding.) A person suffering from severe stress incontinence may drip out urine most of the time while standing, but rarely while sleeping in bed.

✔ **Overflow incontinence:** This type of incontinence is characterized by a constant loss of urine throughout the day. Overflow incontinence is sort of like a maddening drip from your kitchen sink faucet, which can seem like Chinese water torture to your brain when you pay attention to it, making it hard to distinguish from severe stress incontinence. Pads can take care of this steady flow, but you also need to contact your urologist, because the main problem here is not a weak sphincter, as with stress incontinence, but is that your bladder, which is always full, isn't getting emptied properly. Retention may be caused by a blockage of the bladder (a problem that occurs with benign prostatic hyperplasia, or BPH; see Chapter 4) or by scar tissue that forms after surgery or radiation.

✔ **Urge incontinence:** Urge incontinence, which is rare and often temporary, is the most common type of incontinence that may be felt after radiation therapy. This type of incontinence is characterized by the feeling that you constantly have to go the bathroom right away, or the dams are going to burst. This is the most torturous form of urinary incontinence. Most of the time, even though you feel like you have to urinate a huge amount — because the pressure is so bad — when you actually do urinate, only a little bit comes out. The problem is that your bladder is hypersensitive, and even a small amount of urine causes an extreme feeling of bladder urgency.

Evaluating your incontinence: A dribble or a flood?

Incontinence problems can vary a lot from man to man. Maybe the problem is just a little trickle every now and then. Or maybe the problem requires a few pads a day to absorb leaked urine. For a few men, the problem is more like a flood than a few drops. The severity of the incontinence depends on the individual, the type of anti-cancer treatment he had, and other factors. You need to keep in mind that most men get better over time.

Your doctor may ask you several questions to help evaluate the severity of your condition. Here are a few examples of the types of questions she may ask:

✔ "Are there situations in which you're more likely to lose control of your urine, such as when you laugh or cough? Or is your incontinence pretty much a constant and steady problem?"

✔ "What kinds of pads are you using, and how many do you go through in a day?"

✔ "Are you having problems with incontinence during the night, when you're asleep? If so, about how much urine are you losing while you're asleep?"

✔ "Have you tried to resolve the problem on your own? If so, what did you try? Did it help?"

Be honest when you tell your doctor about any herbal remedies, supplements, or other methods you tried in an attempt to improve your condition. And be sure to tell her what happened when you used them.

Wishing you were dry

Some men believe that incontinence is worse than impotence. (Although men with potency problems may not agree.) You don't have to have sex to function in society, but you do have to empty your bladder several times a day. If you're struggling with bladder control, you may be agonizing over whether you may have an accident. You may also be worrying about smelling bad.

Pads and disposable undergarments often include deodorizing substances, so the smell factor shouldn't be a key concern. If you're using enough pads, as well as pads that are large enough, you should also be safe from embarrassing accidents. So the main problem for most men, understandably, is that they just don't *like* wearing pads or disposable undergarments. These items make them feel like they're old and incompetent, or like they're not in charge. Or they may make them feel like babies. The experience of incontinence may be more emotionally distressing than physically upsetting. Sometimes it helps to know that many men face this problem and it should also help to know that incontinence is usually a temporary problem that improves over time.

Tell your doctor how you feel about your incontinence, and be candid. After getting over the initial dismay, many men find that they don't mind minor incontinence; if you don't speak up, your doctor may think that you fall into this category of men. She may also be unaware of the severity of your problem, thinking that you're only losing a few drops of urine every once in awhile rather than losing daily bucketfuls. So make sure you tell her how your incontinence is affecting you.

Padding the Problem

You may need to buy some padding to help you cope with your incontinence. Wishing it away just doesn't work!

There are many different types of incontinence products available today. You can buy disposable undergarments or pads that fit inside your underwear, or you can purchase washable underwear with a built-in absorbent lining. Tim, a man who was treated for prostate cancer, joked with his daughter Tiffany that they could both use maxi-pads. (Of course, he bought his own pads.) But, in fact, some men do buy sanitary napkins, pretending that they're purchasing them for their wives or girlfriends. Sanitary napkins can be effective if your incontinence is minor.

If you're too embarrassed to buy pads at the local supermarket or pharmacy — because you're afraid you may end up behind someone you know at the check-out counter — you can purchase the items you need at a local medical supply store. Nearly every city has such a store, where people can buy crutches, supplies to treat diabetes, special bandages, and packing for wounds. And, oh yes, incontinence supplies. You can also buy incontinence products on many different Web sites online. Find such sites using a search engine such as www.google.com or www.yahoo.com.

Drying Out: Working on Solutions

You don't have to just accept your incontinence, even if you have a severe case. And you shouldn't be embarrassed or afraid to talk to your doctor about it: Urologists hear about cases of incontinence all the time. Your doctor won't think any less of you if you tell him about your problem. The incontinence isn't you or your doctor's fault, but if you work together, you can often come up with one or more solutions to help improve the situation.

Giving medication a try

One TV ad for an incontinence medication depicts men and wome who are frantic to go to the bathroom, and who leave their golf game or their board meeting in a rush to find a toilet. In the background, someone sings, "Gotta go, gotta go, gotta go." Then the tormented people start taking the drug that's advertised — the problem is apparently solved, and they live happily ever after. Medications *can* help many men, but they don't help everyone.

Several prescribed drugs are available to help you regain some control over your incontinence, as well as lose the feeling that you must urinate right now or you'll burst. Medications such as Detrol (generic name: tolterodine tartrate), Ditropan (generic name: oxybutynin chloride), or Urispas (generic name: flavoxate hydrochloride) may help improve your incontinence situation considerably. ***Note:*** Urispas is not recommended in men with any cardiac problems, because it can cause or worsen heart rhythm problems.

The key benefit of these drugs is that, if they work, they can give you some control back. The key disadvantage is that they may cause some (usually minor) side effects, such as dry mouth, constipation, headache, and drowsiness.

Sometimes over-the-counter cold medications with epinephrine and antihistamines can help improve your incontinence problem. In addition, the antidepressant imipramine may provide relief. You don't have to be clinically depressed to benefit from imipramine, which is also used to treat chronic pain syndromes. These medications work by slowing down the bladder and, to some extent, making the sphincter stronger.

If your urge incontinence is severe, Pyridium (generic name: phenazopyridine), a special bladder anesthetic, may help control the pain. This drug is available over the counter or in a prescribed dose from your doctor. It only works for a little while, and it doesn't work for everybody. Pyridium turns your urine bright yellow, so don't be alarmed if your urine becomes an interesting new color after you take it.

For more information on incontinence treatments and medications, contact the National Association for Continence (NAFC) at P.O. Box 8310, Spartanburg, SC 29305; phone 800-BLADDER (800-252-3337); Web site www.nafc.org/site.

Working on bladder retraining

Bladder retraining, or training yourself to urinate on a particular schedule (like once every hour) whether you have to go or not, may help you avoid accidents and overflows. These exercises can sometimes lessen bladder urgency and also help empty bladders that retain too much urine. Ask your urologist to recommend a bladder-retraining regimen.

Keying in on Kegels

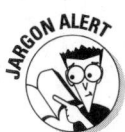

You may also benefit from *Kegel exercises,* which are special exercises for the bladder sphincter that help you practice starting and stopping the flow of urine. These exercises can help you retain your urine better and longer. They are especially beneficial if you have stress incontinence.

Kegel exercises are recommended to both men and women with incontinence problems. They were initially developed for women who developed incontinence after childbirth by Dr. Arnold Kegel in 1948. The exercises have since been adapted for men.

Here's how the exercises work: When you urinate, pay attention to how the sphincter muscles feel during this process (which isn't something you normally pay attention to) — gain a good sense of where these muscles are located and how they feel when they're contracted and relaxed. After you identify how it feels to stop and start urinating voluntarily, tighten and loosen your sphincter muscles without urinating. (At first, you may wish to try this in the privacy of your own bathroom.) When you tighten your urinary sphincter, hold it contracted for the count of ten, and then release it for the count of ten. Do these exercises several times a day. After you become more comfortable and confident with the exercises (after a few days, or a week or so), work your way up to ten sets each day.

You should discuss the details of your Kegel exercise program with your doctor, because too many sets can make your sphincter unduly fatigued. Also, be sure that you *don't* hold your breath when you contract your sphincter muscle. Holding your breath during the contraction is a natural reaction, but you want to keep on breathing for best results.

You can practice Kegel exercises in your car, at work, or anywhere else. For more details on how to perform Kegel exercises, check out this Web site: www.phoenix5.org/Basics/treatsides/incontinence/kegelOSU.html.

The collagen connection

If stress incontinence is still a problem for you after a year or so, you may want to get a collagen injection. This relatively minor procedure involves injecting collagen directly into the *urethra,* the canal in the penis through which urine flows to the outside of your body. The collagen creates a snugger passageway in the urethra, giving you less of a chance to leak a large amount of urine. The collagen is similar to the substance that some movie stars have injected into their lower lips (although the incontinence application seems far more sensible to most doctors — especially urologists like me!). Collagen injections usually only last for several months to a year, and then they have to be repeated. They are best for minor degrees of stress incontinence.

The collagen injection is an outpatient procedure that requires a little special preparation. First, you need to be tested to make sure that you're not allergic to collagen. The doctor or nurse gives you a small injection into the skin. If you don't have a reaction to the injection, you're not allergic. If you're good to go, the doctor then uses a *cystoscope* (a device that allows the doctor to see inside your urethra) to determine where (and if) he can inject the collagen for the best results.

Sometimes your anatomy is such that the doctor can predict ahead of time that collagen won't work for you. (So he won't go ahead with the procedure.) If he thinks that collagen may help you, and you decide to undergo the procedure, you'll receive anesthesia to make you unconscious while he injects the collagen.

A drawback to using collagen is that it may wear off or become absorbed by your body after a short while. Also, if the doctor uses too much collagen, you can develop a blockage (which is also bad). Some people may have an allergic reaction to the collagen or develop an infection after the procedure. In extremely rare cases, the collagen can make patients even more incontinent.

Make sure that your doctor has experience with this procedure. Ask him how many collagen injections he's performed on men with incontinence. If the answer is at least 20, your doctor is likely skilled at performing the procedure.

Making some lifestyle changes

You can also make some simple lifestyle changes to help control your incontinence.

- ✔ Drink plenty of fluids during the day, but ease off fluids after dinner and/or three to five hours before bedtime. Remember, whatever fluid goes in must also eventually come out!

- ✔ If you have an incontinence problem, don't cut back on fluids during the day to make yourself urinate less. Cutting back on fluids can lead to dehydration. It can also increase your risk for bladder infection — because germs won't be getting flushed out of your bladder as often as they should. Try to drink about eight to ten glasses of water (or more) each day.

- ✔ If your bladder is feeling very irritated, you may want to eliminate such bladder irritants as caffeinated drinks (coffee, tea, and soda), chocolate, and highly spiced or acidic foods and drinks. Caffeinated drinks also can be dehydrating, as can alcohol.

- ✔ You also may find some relief with an over-the-counter drug called Prelief (generic ingredients: calcium glycerophosphate and magnesium stearate). Prelief minimizes the acidity in caffeine, spicy foods, and chocolate, and can make your irritable bladder feel better. Check with your doctor before taking Prelief.

- ✔ If you smoke, it's a very good idea to stop smoking, not only for general health reasons, but also to help your bladder. Nicotine can cause painful bladder spasms and also may worsen your incontinence problem. Coughing from smoking obviously can make stress incontinence worse. Read about smoking cessation in Chapter 17.

- ✔ If you're overweight, weight loss can help your incontinence problem, because, very simply, less weight means less pressure on your bladder. Eat more vegetables — they'll help you lose weight and they're better for you anyway!

Considering surgery

Sometimes the best efforts of you and your doctor don't work, and the incontinence is just much too severe of a problem. (In most experienced surgeons' hands, less than 5 percent of men with prostate cancer have severe incontinence a year or more after their surgery.) Even if your incontinence isn't severe, you may still find it to be far too aggravating for you. In these cases, you may find that surgery is the best way to resolve your incontinence so that you can return to your normal life again. In the following sections, I give you the basics on urinary sphincter prosthesis surgery, the gold standard, and sling surgery, a newer option.

Urinary sphincter prosthesis surgery

The most common type of surgery for incontinence is the insertion of an artificial sphincter around the urethra near the bladder. If you have no control or almost no control over your bladder, your incontinence problem may have been caused by damage to the sphincter muscle during surgery or radiation treatments. Aging can sometimes make the sphincter muscle work less efficiently, as well.

With this procedure, the artificial sphincter is implanted around the part of the urethra that connects to your bladder, and a control unit is implanted in your scrotum. This prosthesis is totally inside your body, so it can't be seen externally. To urinate, you press on the device inside the scrotum. The artificial sphincter then opens for a short time, allowing urine to flow. Then the sphincter gradually shuts automatically. The device works sort of like the automatic door at your local grocery: You press a button (or step on the pad), and the door opens. After a period of time, it closes automatically.

Before you agree to have urinary sphincter prosthesis surgery, consider all the pros and cons. The key advantage to having urinary sphincter prosthesis surgery for your incontinence is that it can help end the leaks. The key disadvantage for any surgery is that the procedure can have complications, and sometimes it may not give you the effect you're hoping for. For example, the artificial sphincter device may become infected and need to be replaced. The device may also develop mechanical problems. Another disadvantage is that the artificial sphincter may squeeze on the urethra too much, causing a hole to form. In these rare cases, the device needs to be removed, and the hole allowed to heal. After the wound heals, another device can usually be inserted. A final disadvantage you should consider before agreeing to urinary sphincter prosthesis surgery is your insurance may not cover this procedure, so be sure to check with your insurance company before you agree to the surgery.

The urinary sphincter procedure can be a complex surgery, so you need to make sure that you find a very skillful and experienced urologist to perform the procedure. If you opt for this surgery, make sure that your doctor has at least 25 urinary sphincter procedures under his belt. Before you undergo urinary sphincter surgery, ask your doctor the following questions (as well as any other questions that you can think of):

✔ "What kind of improvement can I expect right after — or soon after — this procedure?" (Total continence, some improvement, or something else?)

✔ "How long will it take before I notice if the procedure is working for me?" (Days, weeks, or months?)

✔ "Are there any serious symptoms that I should watch out for right after the procedure?" (Such as blood in the urine, pain with urinating, or something else?)

✔ "What's the approximate probability that this particular procedure will work for me?" (Ten percent? Fifty percent?)

After you receive your doctor's answer, evaluate whether the odds are worth undergoing the procedure. Also, keep in mind that even if the odds of success are good, the procedure still may not work. (Nothing is 100 percent.)

Sling surgery

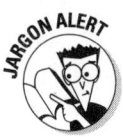

Recently, some surgeons have tried *sling surgery,* a surgery that was previously reserved for women who had stress incontinence after childbirth. With sling surgery, a strip of tissue taken from the patient is wrapped around the urethra like a sling (sometimes an artificial material such as Gortex is used instead), elevating it and thereby (hopefully) providing just enough resistance to impede urine leakage — but not enough to stop urination completely.

Although the results from this type of stress incontinence surgery seem promising, I'm still not convinced that sling surgery works in enough men and/or for a long enough period of time to replace urinary sphincter prosthesis surgery as the leading method to resolve your incontinence, but it's an option worthy of your consideration. If the sling surgery doesn't work, urinary sphincter prosthesis surgery can still be done.

Chapter 21

What to Do When Treatment Doesn't Wipe Out Cancer

*T*he treatments you had to fight prostate cancer may have been very effective, but they apparently didn't wipe out the cancer completely. Technically, the cancer isn't *back* again, because it never really went away. You (and probably your doctor, too) thought and hoped that it was gone for good. But instead, the cancer was still there, somewhere underneath it all, and you and your doctor just didn't realize it. Cancer can be very sneaky like that. If your doctor told you that you were cured, it doesn't mean that he's incompetent or that he was fibbing. Many men are cured of prostate cancer through surgery or radiation treatments, but some men have recurrences of the cancer.

In this chapter, I talk about the signs that may suggest that prostate cancer is growing in your body again. I also tell you what to do if you find that the cancer is growing again.

Sometimes you notice signs that your prostate cancer may be a problem again, and sometimes your doctor flags a possible problem with the cancer, based on your test results or on his own past experience. For example, a rising prostate specific antigen (PSA) blood level is one indicator of prostate cancer (see Chapter 5 for more on PSA); back pain may be another indicator of the disease. You shouldn't become obsessive, but you do need to stay vigilant so that you and your doctor can react to any burgeoning problems. You also may want to consider joining a clinical study, in which you may receive experimental drugs or treatments that wouldn't otherwise be available to you. I cover both of these options in this chapter.

Recognizing the Signs of a Recurrence

In the past (before you were actually diagnosed with prostate cancer), you may have ignored some of the symptoms that can indicate a possible problemwith your prostate, such as back pain. (Although many men don't have any symptoms before they're diagnosed.) But now that you've been diagnosed and treated for prostate cancer, you know that the bury-your-head-in-the-sand approach isn't going to work well for you. If you notice any indicators that your prostate cancer may be on the move again, you need to contact your doctor as soon as possible. Working together with your physician, you can formulate your war plans to fight back the cancer monster.

Your doctor can flag a recurring problem with cancer through regular checkups. Some men fail to see their doctor as frequently as recommended, because they assume that they're just fine. Even physicians who've had cancer themselves sometimes make this mistake. But seeing your doctor on the schedule he recommends after treatment is really important. When you have regular checkups, your doctor can detect rising PSA levels and ask you about symptoms. He can also look you over in person and examine you for any problem areas. If you don't have regular checkups, you may require radical therapies (which you otherwise may not have needed) by the time you finally do go to see your doctor.

Rising PSA levels

If your PSA levels are starting to go up, your cancer may be growing again. You shouldn't panic if your PSA level goes from .1 to .2 after surgery — this level of change is minor, and it may be the result of laboratory error. (Technically, you should have a zero PSA level after surgery because you no longer have a prostate gland. But labs usually report some low levels of PSA in men who have had surgery.) However, if your PSA level starts to exceed .4 or .5 after surgery, the cancer may be making a comeback, and this is one comeback you must fight.

Maybe you didn't have surgery. Instead, you had radiation treatments to wipe out your cancer. But now your PSA levels, which had been pretty stable and low, are starting to rise. If you had radiation therapy, and your PSA level is above 1.0, you may have cause for concern, so consult with your doctor about what to do next.

After you have radiation therapy, especially in the first couple of years afterwards, your PSA level may be elevated slightly from prostatic inflammation caused by a delayed reaction to radiation treatment. So if your PSA starts going up abruptly after radiation therapy, don't panic. The rise may not be from cancer. Talk to your doctor.

If the cancer is recurring after surgery or radiation therapy, your PSA level will almost always rise before you experience any symptoms. So if you're having back pain and your PSA is low and stable, cancer is not the likely cause of your pain. This is also true for patients on hormone therapy (see Chapter 13), although rarely, patients on hormones may have symptoms or signs of a recurrence of cancer without experiencing changes in their PSA level.

If you had hormone therapy to stem the tide of the cancer, and it worked for a little while, but now your PSA level is going up again steadily, the hormones are no longer working to prevent the growth of the cancer cells. This is very advanced cancer, also called *hormone-resistant prostate cancer,* which I discuss in depth in Chapter 15. With hormone-resistant prostate cancer, PSA values may not be such an outstanding warning test as it is in other less serious stages of prostate cancer. So keep in touch with your doctor, and don't assume that merely getting regular PSA tests is sufficient. For more info on PSA levels, see Chapter 5.

Developing symptoms

Although you shouldn't rely on PSA tests alone, I can't emphasize enough that your PSA level can almost always tell you if the cancer is coming back long before you notice any symptoms. However, patients whose PSA levels are rising are often super-sensitive to any symptoms they may have, and they often think that their symptoms are due to cancer, which is usually not the case.

The following symptoms may indicate that your cancer is starting to spread again:

✔ A loss of appetite combined with a weight loss of ten or more pounds.

✔ Pain in your back or legs (which can indicate bone pain).

   Remember that such pain doesn't always indicate cancer. Back and leg pain can be caused by a number of different things — however, you should still see your doctor to rule out a recurrence of cancer.

✔ Tiredness and some shortness of breath with mild exercise.

   This symptom, when caused by cancer, is usually the result of a low red blood cell count.

If you experience any of these symptoms, see your doctor right away. These symptoms don't necessarily mean that your cancer's back; you could have another problem altogether. But it's always best to see your doctor, just to be on the safe side.

Don't Panic, Work with Your Doctor

When you think that prostate cancer is a problem for you again, your first reaction may be sheer panic followed by anger — a common reaction among many men. The panic comes from a feeling of "Oh, no! What can I do now? I'm going to die!" Then you may feel angry and aggrieved, especially when you did every single thing the doctor told you to do. Whatever therapy you had, it now looks like it didn't work, because the cancer may be a problem for you again.

Don't panic and keep the symptoms of a possible recurrence to yourself, thinking that telling your doctor about the symptoms will somehow make the problem real. Don't imagine that you can make the problem go away if you don't think about it. This line of thinking is childish, but sadly, many people who have cancer recurrences actually think this way. Don't make the same mistake. Instead, share your symptoms with your physician. Very often I find that patients' fears aren't justified at all, and they worry themselves sick waiting to see me at their next clinic visit. Because stress can make you feel worse, finding out that you're fine can help take a great load off your mind. If your fears are justified, you and your doctor can work out a new treatment plan.

After you tell your doctor about your suspicions, he'll examine you and order a PSA test and possibly a bone scan to determine if the cancer has spread to your bones. If you were initially treated with radiation (and not a prostatectomy), your doctor may want to biopsy your prostate again. (See Chapter 7 for more on biopsies.) Cooperate fully with your doctor so that he can help you come up with a good plan for treating your cancer.

Some people complain that their doctor seems to lose all interest in them when they return with fears that their cancer has returned. This reaction may be the result of a perception of failure on the part of the doctor. Nobody likes to fail, including hard-driving physicians. But doctors are still supposed to soldier on, even with the tough cases. If you tried several times to communicate with your doctor about your fears of a recurrence, and you don't seem to be getting anywhere, you may need to find a new doctor. And don't waste time worrying and wondering about your doctor's feelings or motivations. Focus on your own problem.

After your doctor offers his expert medical opinion on what may be wrong with you and what you should do about it, you can seek a second opinion from another doctor if you feel that you need one. In fact, many physicians encourage you to seek a second opinion.

If you decide that you want to get a second opinion, ask your doctor for the name of a physician who subspecializes in urologic oncology. Seeing a doctor at an academic medical center may be a good bet, because urologic oncologists (urologists who specialize in treating cancers of the genitourinary system) are more likely to be aware of the latest therapies, and many of them also perform clinical trials. Very often, the urologic oncologist will reassure you that your doctor knows his stuff, and will send you back to him. If you feel that your doctor doesn't want you to seek a second opinion, ask other doctors who aren't directly treating you for recommendations. You can also call medical centers, check the Internet, and ask your friends or relatives for the names of good cancer specialists. (See Chapter 5 for advice on finding a doctor.)

Evaluating Your Treatment Choices

If you experience a recurrence of cancer, your doctor will help you determine how advanced it is and whether it has spread beyond the prostate. If the cancer is reappearing and confined to the prostate, you generally have more choices than you do if the cancer has spread to other parts of the body. Depending on the type of treatment you had initially, you need to work with your doctor to select the best treatment for dealing with your cancer as it currently stands. For example, if you had a prostatectomy initially, you can't have surgery again — your prostate is gone. However, you may be able to have radiation treatments (Chapter 12), hormone therapy (Chapter 13). Alternatively, if you've had radiation therapy, you may be able to cure or at least suppress that cancer with surgery (Chapter 11), cryosurgery or microwave therapy (both covered in Chapter 14), or hormone therapy.

If the cancer has advanced a great deal, you may want to join a clinical study (see "Joining clinical studies," later in this chapter), where you can get involved in research on such cutting-edge treatments as gene therapy and immune therapy (see Chapter 14). Your doctor may also suggest trying a combination of therapies, such as hormone therapy and radiation treatments.

Undergoing salvage therapy

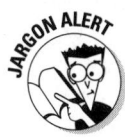

Salvage therapy is additional therapy that your doctor gives you when he knows for sure that the cancer is a problem for you again. If you already had radiation treatments, your doctor may recommend salvage therapy in the form of hormone treatments. If you already had a prostatectomy, your doctor may give you salvage therapy in the form of radiation or hormone treatments. Sometimes a combination of therapies is the best approach.

Salvage surgery is another option you may want to consider when initial radiation treatments don't work. The *salvage prostatectomy* (taking out the prostate after radiation has been given initially) is a very difficult surgery, even for experts, and can result in more complications. However, a salvage prostatectomy may be your best shot at eradicating the cancer or at least containing it. When the surgeon removes the prostate by salvage prostatectomy, pathologists may discover that cancer has spread beyond the prostate. Depending on how advanced the pathologist thinks the cancer is, the doctor may recommend watchful waiting or hormone therapy.

Exploring adjuvant treatments

Your doctor may suggest an *adjuvant therapy,* which is additional therapy given after the main procedure; for example, if you had radiation therapy, the doctor may recommend hormone therapy as an adjuvant therapy. If you had a prostatectomy, the doctor may recommend that you have hormone therapy or radiation (or both). Unlike salvage therapy, when the doctor knows that the cancer is definitely there, doctors recommend adjuvant therapy when indications suggest that the cancer is likely to still be there, but the doctor isn't absolutely sure about this.

Your doctor may also recommend that you have both radiation therapy and hormone therapy if the cancer is still present after surgery. However, if the cancer is advanced and your doctor doesn't feel that radiation therapy will be effective, he may recommend hormone therapy alone to slow the cancer down. Hormone therapy often effectively delays the growth of cancer cells for at least several years. However, hormone therapy doesn't work permanently, and can cause many side effects, such as mood swings and hot flashes.

Joining clinical studies

If your cancer recurs, you may be eligible to join a *clinical study* (also known as a clinical trial or research study), which is a formal research study for testing a hypothesis about a medication, new form of surgery, lifestyle changes, or other treatments. Clinical studies may also involve comparisons of already established therapies. When you participate in a clinical study, you may have the option to try new and experimental drugs and other treatments that otherwise wouldn't be available to you.

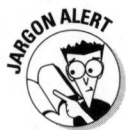

Researchers perform many different types of clinical studies. For example, *prevention trials* seek to identify ways to help avoid a medical problem from occurring in the first place, *screening trials* attempt to find better ways of identifying an illness, and *quality of life trials* seek to improve the living conditions for people diagnosed with the disease.

Coping with your emotions

When you find out that prostate cancer is a problem for you again (or may be a problem — your doctor will need to confirm it with testing), you may have a very hard time dealing with it emotionally. Maybe you thought that you were cured because of your surgery, radiation treatments, or another therapy. Maybe you've been fine for years, so you figured that you were safe. And now you have indications that your cancer may be present again, and you feel like you're right back where you started.

It may not sound like good news when your tests or symptoms indicate that you have prostate cancer again. Nobody can be happy to find out that they must cope with cancer again.

But having these warnings can actually be a good thing, because when you know that problem may be back, you can work with your doctor to resolve it. Your doctor may not be able to completely eradicate the cancer, but he can offer you many therapies and plans to help you live an extended life. Take advantage of the options your doctor offers you.

A recurrence of cancer can also be very hard on your partner, your children, and others who love you. They may have assumed you were cured. Now they have to deal with all the fears and worries all over again. (Read more about helping your family cope with your cancer in Chapter 23.)

A large part of the knowledge that doctors use when treating people comes from clinical trials. You may be thinking, "Helping advance medical science is wonderful, but this is my body. Is it safe to join a clinical study?" All reputable clinical trials require careful review by both government and local institution boards. The primary objective of these review groups is to ensure that the study is as safe as possible. These review groups also make sure that all possible risks and benefits are clearly understood by patients before they enter a study.

Subjects for clinical studies are carefully chosen. For example, for a prostate cancer study, you must fit the specific criteria that the researchers have set. The criteria may be based on age, race, previous treatments, or other factors.

The three types of clinical trials are Phase I, Phase II, and Phase III. Phase I is a study in which all patients are tested with new therapies to see if they are safe and to find out the proper method or dosage to administer. Phase II studies generally are trials where all the patients are tested with the therapy to determine whether or not it works. Phase III trials are performed when the treatment in the Phase II trial looks good but the researchers are still unsure whether the treatment is better than the older treatment or, in some cases, better than no treatment. In the Phase III trials, researchers compare one treatment with another.

The disadvantages of joining a clinical study include the following:

- ✔ You may not receive the treatment or medication being tested. When researchers perform Phase III trials, they use a control group and an experimental group, and the selection process (who gets picked for which group) is "randomized." Thus, although you have to volunteer to participate in the study, the choice of what treatment you receive is made for you by a process much like flipping a coin. The control group receives either the older therapy or a placebo (sugar pill) drug or treatment. In some randomized trials, subjects don't know whether they're getting the real drug or treatment or the placebo. Even the doctors treating the patients don't know who's getting the real drug or treatment — only the doctors overseeing the study know. This is called a double-blind randomized study. In these ways, therapies can be correctly assessed without interference from patient and/or doctor biases.

- ✔ The drug or treatment being tested may prove to be completely ineffective at treating prostate cancer.

- ✔ The drug or treatment being tested may cause minor or major side effects. After all, it's still in the testing stages. The side effects may be difficult to deal with, such as extreme nausea and diarrhea.

- ✔ It may be many years before clinical researchers have enough evidence to determine whether the drug or treatment being tested really works. In the meantime, your own personal time clock is ticking away, and you can only join so many clinical studies. (Probably only one or two, at most.)

In general, the advantages of joining a clinical trial far outweigh the disadvantages. (I very much encourage my own patients to participate when possible.) Here are some of the advantages of joining a clinical study:

- ✔ You may have the chance to try drugs or treatments that wouldn't otherwise be available to you. If the clinical trial is a study with a control group, the researchers may give the drug that's being tested to the control group subjects after a certain period of time. So you may eventually have the chance to try the new anti-cancer therapy. In that case, sometimes the new therapy becomes available early to everyone.

- ✔ Your clinical progress is monitored very carefully. In most cases, your progress is monitored much more carefully than with regular treatments from your doctor (outside a clinical study).

- ✔ You have access to expert medical care normally only available at large hospitals or university medical centers. Of course, you can also see your primary care doctor during the course of the study, as well as your urologist and oncologist. Thus, your therapy and subsequent medical management will be carefully monitored by a variety of specialists.

✔ The cost to you is no different than if you were receiving routine care. Sometimes the cost of the treatment in the trial is free.

Talk to your doctor to find out if you may qualify for a current clinical study. You can also check out the ClinicalTrials.gov Web site (www. clinicaltrials.gov), where you can search a database to find prostate cancer clinical trials that are actively recruiting new subjects. You may find a clinical study that's just right for you.

Part VI
Handling Work and Family

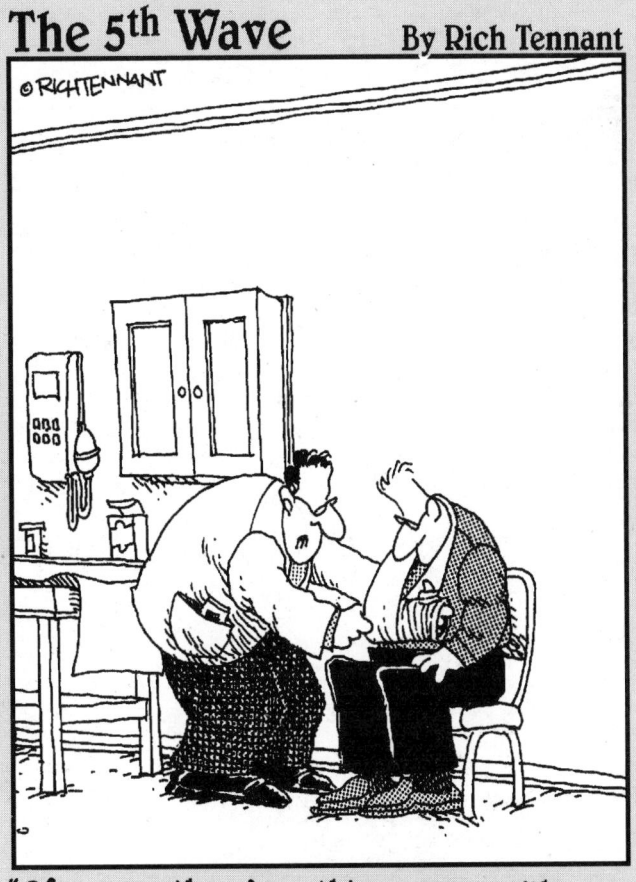

The 5th Wave
By Rich Tennant

©RICHTENNANT

"Of course there's nothing wrong with your arm, but it will keep people from focusing on your cancer treatment."

In this part . . .

*P*rostate cancer is undeniably a major player in your life, affecting you at both work and home. In Chapter 22, I talk about having prostate cancer on the job, and I tell you what to do if your symptoms or a treatment's side effects make it hard (or impossible) to work anymore. I also offer tactics on coping with your boss and co-workers. In Chapter 23, I talk about explaining prostate cancer to your family and friends, and I offer you advice on how to deal with aggravating comments, such as "You have a 'good' kind of cancer." Chapter 24 is devoted to your loved ones who don't have prostate cancer — they care about you, and they want to help. I also offer specific advice for your wife or significant other.

Chapter 22

Coping with Cancer on the Job

. . . .

In This Chapter

▶ Revealing your prostate cancer to people at work

▶ Understanding the laws that cover serious illness

▶ Considering short-term or long-term disability leave

▶ Thinking about Social Security disability

. . . .

Many women joke about the general reluctance men have when it comes to asking for help. Some men drive around for hours looking for their destination instead of just stopping and asking a convenience store clerk for directions. (Of course, this isn't true for all men.) Some men behave the same way with their prostate cancer. They don't tell anyone at work about it. They keep their cancer a deep, dark secret, and they only let a few trusted people at work in on it — if they tell anyone at all.

Instead, these men see their doctors and make their own treatment plans without ever letting anyone know about it. After waiting as long as they possibly can, they announce one day that they're going to be off for a few weeks because they have cancer. Or they may avoid discussing it with anyone by putting in for vacation time instead of sick leave. Most of these men have no idea that prostate cancer is a common medical problem, and that shared information can make their path to wellness much less rocky.

This chapter tells you how to explain the basics of the disease to your boss and co-workers. I also talk about federal laws, such as the Family and Medical Leave Act and the Americans with Disabilities Act, that protect you so that you can take time off for necessary treatment. In addition, I describe the short-term work disability option that's offered by most companies. If your company offers this option, you should consider applying for it. And finally, I cover Social Security disability benefits and tell you how to apply for them.

Explaining Prostate Cancer to Your Boss and Co-Workers

When explaining your prostate cancer to your boss and co-workers, keep one key issue in mind: You can greatly limit the scope of the information that you provide to others. Your prostate cancer is not a mandatory tell-all situation. Remember, though, that any information you share with one person in your company may well make the rounds of the entire company — even when that one person was sworn to secrecy. (It's very hard for most people to keep a secret.) So if, for example, you don't want everyone at work to know that you're having trouble with incontinence, refrain from telling people about it. Your problem with incontinence isn't really relevant to the workplace, anyway.

What to say

The main thing you can say about prostate cancer is that you have it, and you're working on obtaining treatment. You may also wish to say that you're planning on having surgery, radiation treatment, or hormone shots (or that you've already had one of these treatments). But you don't have to tell anyone about the treatment method you're considering or have already undergone.

If you need to take time off from work for treatment, tell your boss that you have a medical reason. (Unless you're going the super-secret route and using vacation days.) In some cases, you may need a note from your doctor. Doctor's notes can be aggravating (like you're back in grade school all over again, and the principal is checking up on you). Sadly, some people abuse medical leave, so your company may demand verification of your illness.

You may need more than a few weeks off, especially if you have a prostatectomy. The recovery period for surgery may be a month, but most men need at least six weeks before they're fully up to speed. If your job is very physical, you'll need at least two months off to recover. With radiation therapy, the amount of time needed to recover varies. With brachytherapy (see Chapter 12), patients are usually out of the hospital the same day, but taking off at least a week is a good idea. With external beam radiotherapy, you need to visit the x-ray facility several hours a day for a month to six weeks, so plan ahead.

What you don't have to say

If people ask you impertinent and embarrassing questions — particularly questions that relate to possible problems with impotence or incontinence — you don't have to answer them. Nor is it necessary for you to laugh at any jokes made by others about these problems. These jokes probably don't seem like knee-slappers to you, and they wouldn't be hilarious to others at the company if they were in the same situation.

Identifying Laws that Cover Serious Illness

Because people develop a broad array of serious illnesses (such as cancer, heart disease, and diabetes), Congress has passed several laws to protect workers when they're sick. These laws enable workers to take time off when they're sick or when they need to provide care for a very ill family member. The laws also provide protection against discrimination and require employers to offer reasonable work accommodations to their disabled workers.

Cancer moved up their retirement plans

Jack and Eva had their retirement all figured out — or so they thought. Jack was 55, and he was going to work in the Mega Corporation until he was 60, at which time he'd have plenty of money in his 401(k) retirement plan. Eva was a self-employed artist who was a year younger than Jack. She was planning on scaling back to part-time work when Jack retired.

Then Jack was diagnosed with prostate cancer, which shocked both him and Eva. Jack's cancer made them rethink all their hopes and dreams for the future. Jack had a prostatectomy, and the doctor said that it looked pretty good, although the pathology report indicated that some of the cancer escaped the prostate gland. The results of the pathology report could mean nothing, or they could mean that the cancer might spread in the future — months or even years later.

Eva told Jack that she wanted him to change his retirement plan. His work was extremely stressful. Eva often saw Jack take a few extra shots of bourbon to "calm his nerves." She also worried about the general effect of stress on Jack's

life; she wondered if it could lead to a resurgence of the cancer. (Some studies indicate that stress can raise the prostate specific antigen [PSA] level, although it's not known whether stress increases the risk of cancer.)

Jack was resistant to an early retirement at first, but after a while, he realized that working a 60-hour-plus week was not making either him or Eva happy. He also realized that his plan of delaying his happiness until he was 60 years old wasn't a good idea. So Jack took an early retirement at age 55 and became a part-time consultant with his old corporation.

Jack loved consulting. He found that consulting was much less stressful than being on the front lines of management. Eva also cut back on her workload. The two of them concentrated much more on each other and the "now" of life.

As Jack and Eva found out, sometimes you have to adjust your plans to accommodate what life throws at you (including prostate cancer). And when you do make new plans, sometimes you're happier than you were before.

Family and Medical Leave Act

The Family and Medical Leave Act (FMLA), which was passed in 1993, requires most employers to give workers time off for illnesses suffered by them or someone in their family. The FMLA provides for up to 12 weeks of *unpaid* leave each year. Because most people have trouble making ends meet without pay for three months, they either take only a few unpaid weeks off, or they take short-term paid disability from work.

The FMLA is good for men with prostate cancer because it enables them to take a few days (or a week or so) off work to recover from treatment. (If you have a prostatectomy, you'll need to take at least four to six weeks off. Most people take a short-term disability from their company after having a prostatectomy. I cover short-term disabilities later in this chapter.)

If you take an FMLA leave, your company is required by federal law to either hold your job open for you or give you a comparable job when you return. The time you take off under the provisions of the FMLA may be intermittent, meaning that you can take a day off here and there. You don't have to take off weeks or months at a time. Taking intermittent time off is especially beneficial if you need to receive radiation therapy, hormone therapy, or other treatments that may cause you to feel ill for a few days, and you don't want to use your sick time — or maybe you don't have any sick time left. However, if you want to use the FMLA provisions, you must tell your supervisor about your prostate cancer.

Be sure to ask your doctor for the best estimate of how much recuperation time you'll need before you can return to work. Ask her for both the average and the worst-case scenario. When you relay this information to your boss, be sure that you don't underestimate. If you overestimate, and then you come back sooner than planned, you'll be better off than if you underestimate but can't come back to work when the boss is expecting you.

For more information on the Family and Medical Leave Act, write to the Equal Employment Opportunity Commission (EEOC) at 1801 L St. NW, Washington, DC 20507. You can also contact the EEOC by phone at 202-663-4900. To read about the key provisions of the FMLA, take a look at the Employment Law Guide on the U.S. Department of Labor's Web site at www.dol.gov/asp/programs/handbook/fmla.htm. The Department of Labor enforces the provisions of the FMLA.

Americans with Disabilities Act

The Americans with Disabilities Act (ADA), which was passed in 1990, covers employers of 15 or more employees, and protects workers against employment discrimination. The law protects you if you have cancer; it also protects you if you've been cured of cancer, because people who have had cancer are sometimes discriminated against in the workplace. The ADA also requires employers to make work accommodations to workers who have temporary or permanent disabilities.

If your prostate cancer makes it difficult for you to work without accommodations, ask for what you need. For example, if your job requires you to sit for long hours, and your old chair is extremely uncomfortable — a problem that is further complicated by problems relating to your cancer (such as weak bones or a sore butt from radiation treatments) — don't suffer in silence. Ask for a new chair. Most employers will agree to this simple request.

If you think that you've been discriminated against because of your prostate cancer, contact your human resources office for further information. If that doesn't work, consider filing a formal complaint with the Justice Department.

For more information on the ADA, call the toll-free information line at 800-514-0301. You can also visit the ADA Home Page on the Department of Justice's Web site at www.usdoj.gov/crt/ada/adahom1.htm.

Other federal and state laws

Your state law may require employers to give more time off to workers with medical problems or disabilities than the federal law stipulates, or it may require disability time off to be paid rather than unpaid. Ask your doctor if your state has any specific laws regarding the time off that can be taken for a temporary or permanent disability.

If you're a military veteran who served in Vietnam during the Vietnam War and was subsequently diagnosed with prostate cancer, you can apply for the Agent Orange program. This program may provide you with monthly compensation and/or medical benefits if you are approved. You don't have to prove that your cancer was somehow caused by Agent Orange or your being in Vietnam — it's assumed that this was the cause. To find out more about the Agent Orange program, read Chapter 3 and contact your local Veterans Administration (VA) office.

Thinking about Applying for Short- or Long-term Disability

When you're undergoing cancer treatments, it may be difficult or impossible for you to work. If you're having a prostatectomy, you'll definitely need to take time off work. You may also need time off for radiation treatments and hormone therapy or other treatments. As a result, you may want to take a short- or long-term disability leave from your company.

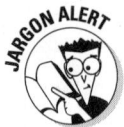

Short-term disability is time off due to a medical condition. (Not all companies offer short-term disability programs, but many do.) A short-term disability leave can, by most definitions, last anywhere from a few weeks to about six months. According to "A Quick Guide to Disability Insurance," a pamphlet published by the Health Insurance Association of America (a trade association of private insurance companies), some states require employers to provide short-term disability benefits, including California, Hawaii, New York, New Jersey, and Rhode Island. (You can read this pamphlet online at `www.hiaa.org/consumer/disability.cfm`. You can also call the Health Insurance Association of America toll-free at 866-872-3434 to request a free copy of a similar title for consumers: "A Disability Income Insurance Guide.")

The short and the long of disability plans

Several major categories of disability benefit programs exist. They vary in a variety of ways, such as how long they last, who administers them, and whether or not the federal or state government is involved. They also vary in whether your employer pays all or part of the premiums for your disability insurance. The different categories and their many rules and ramifications are far too complex for me to delve deeply into here, but I can offer you a brief overview of disability options.

You may have both short- and long-term disability options available where you work. Not all companies have such programs. (In general, medium and large corporations are more likely to offer them as part of your benefits package.) When you receive short-term disability benefits, you usually get all or part of your regular paycheck amount, but it's taxable (unless you paid for all the insurance premiums yourself). If you receive a long-term disability leave, however, you only get a percentage of your regular paycheck amount (often about 50 percent to 60

percent), but the amount is non-taxable. For more details on these tax issues, request IRS Publication 907, "Tax Highlights for Persons with Disabilities." (It's also available on the Web at `www.irs.gov/pub/irs-pdf/p907.pdf`).

The Social Security disability program, which is a lifelong disability program for those who can no longer work, and for whom the possibility of returning to work is very slender, is another program that you may be eligible for. You may qualify for a Social Security disability if you've worked long enough in the past (contact the Social Security Administration to find out if you're eligible, but most men older than age 50 have probably worked enough years to qualify) and you've paid into the Social Security system. In addition, other family members may also be eligible for benefits (based on your past earnings and current disability), such as your children under age 18 or your spouse who is caring for your child under age 16.

To find out about the insurance laws in your state, contact your state insurance office. You can find a listing of state insurance offices on the Internet at www.hiaa.org/consumer/state_insurance.cfm.

A *long-term disability,* which is also covered by some employers, is generally a medical problem that prevents you from working indefinitely. However, corporate definitions vary. As of this writing, no state or federal laws require companies to provide long-term disability coverage, but many companies do offer it as part of their benefits package.

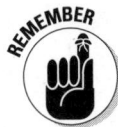

Ask your Human Resources department (formerly called the personnel department) for information on whether you're eligible for short- and long-term disability benefits. Many companies cover their employees with a short-term disability plan, but you usually have to sign up for a long-term disability plan. You can't suddenly sign up for a long-term disability benefits package when you're diagnosed with cancer. However, your company may have insured you for long-term disability long ago — you just may not be aware of it. Or maybe you signed up for it long ago and have completely forgotten about it. Double-check by asking questions.

Checking Out the Social Security Disability

If you're like many people who have prostate cancer, you can continue to stay on the job, only taking time off to recover from your treatments. If your illness has made it impossible for you to keep working, and your doctor has recommended that you stop working altogether, you should probably consider applying for a monthly Social Security disability payment.

Considering your eligibility

If you're under age 62, and you've been working and paying into the Social Security system for years, you may be eligible to apply for monthly Social Security disability benefits. (The eligibility rules and the application process are a little complicated, however, and individual circumstances vary, so contact your local Social Security office to find out whether you've been working long enough to qualify for disability benefits.) For more information on Social Security disability, go to the Social Security Administration Web site at www.ssa.gov/disability.

If you're eligible to receive monthly benefits, other members of your family, such as your children under age 18 or your spouse who's caring for your child under age 16, may also be eligible for benefits. The average monthly Social Security disability payment for a person with a spouse and one or more children was $1,360 as of June 2002 (according to the Chief Actuary of the Social Security Administration). To obtain a very rough estimate of how much you'd receive if you qualified for disability income (or retirement income) — based on your current age and income — check out the following Web site: www.ssa.gov/OACT/quickcalc/calculator.html.

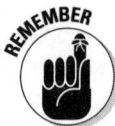

Your gross earnings determine whether you're eligible for Social Security disability benefits. For example, if your gross earnings were more than $780 a month in 2002, your income would have been considered too high for you to qualify for Social Security disability. The dollar amount changes slightly each year, so check with the Social Security Administration Web site (www.ssa.gov) to see what the current amount is.

The disqualifying gross earnings amount isn't a king's ransom. (Even the Social Security Administration doesn't think that.) It's just that, in contrast to Social Security retirement income, the Social Security disability program has income limitations.

When you receive Social Security disability, you're also eligible for Medicare benefits, which will cover your doctor visits, hospital care, and most medical treatments. (As of this writing, Medicare doesn't provide coverage for outpatient prescriptions.) If you're approved for disability benefits, you'll also receive Medicare benefits about 24 months later.

If you're age 62 or older, be sure to contact the Social Security Administration to find out if you're eligible to receive retirement benefits. Social Security retirement benefits don't have any upper financial limitations — you can be a millionaire and still be eligible for them, as long as you paid into the system for a long enough period of time.

Participating in the application process

According to the Social Security Administration, in order to apply for a monthly disability payment, you need to provide the government with the following information:

- ✔ A phone number where you can be reached, as well as contact information for a friend or relative.
- ✔ A list of all the illnesses, injuries, and conditions that make you unable to work, as well as the date when you became unable to work.

✔ The names, addresses, and phone numbers for all the physicians, hospitals, and clinics you went to, as well as the dates when you were seen. (Whether they were consulted for prostate cancer or not.)

✔ A list of all the prescription and nonprescription drugs you take.

✔ A list of all the jobs you've had for the last 15 years, with a description of the one job that you held for the longest period.

✔ A list of all the education and training you've received to date.

✔ Your complete medical records. (The Social Security Administration will request this information from your doctor, or you can provide it to them.)

✔ Your most recent W-2 form, or, if you're self-employed, your most recent tax return.

✔ Information about family members, such as minor children, who are also applying for benefits. (Social Security numbers and proof of birth dates are required.)

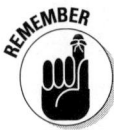

After you fill out and mail all the many forms that are involved in your application for Social Security disability, don't expect to hear about your claim by return mail. You're working with the government, after all! You may have to wait about three to six months or even longer before you hear anything, and even then, no matter how strongly documented your application is or how truly sick you are, you may still receive a denial to your claim. Don't give up. Appeal the decision.

Appealing a denial

If your claim is denied, don't take it personally and don't give up. Understand that the whole process has several layers of applications and appeals. Experts say that it's very important not to give up too early.

If you're denied when you first apply for Social Security disability, your next step should be to appeal to the *reconsideration level,* which is the next rung of the appeals process. Keep in mind that when your claim is being reconsidered at this level, you may *still* be denied. Again, don't take it personally. You should receive a decision about three to six months after you've filed your reconsideration appeal.

If you are denied at the reconsideration level, appeal again. On the next rung of the appeals ladder, your case will be heard by an administrative judge, and this hearing will be scheduled about four to six months after you request it.

Finding an attorney to help with your Social Security disability claim

Unless you're an experienced attorney yourself (and even if you are a lawyer, do you *really* want to take on this problem when you're so sick?), you may decide that your best course of action is to seek an attorney to help you with your Social Security disability claim.

Don't worry, hiring a lawyer isn't going to cost you big bucks. Some lawyers specialize in helping people with Social Security disability claims. They work on a *contingency basis,* which means that when your claim is approved, the lawyer will receive a preset percentage of your lump sum payment. Until you receive your payment, you don't have to pay the attorney anything. In addition, if you're approved for a disability and you receive a lump sum to cover past months (in addition to the amount you'll receive monthly from now on), federal law stipulates that the lawyer can't charge you more than either 25 percent of the past due award *or* $5,300, whichever is *less.*

You may want to hire an attorney who is a member of the *National Organization of Social Security Claimants Representatives* (NOSSCR), because this is the only organization that specializes in Social Security claims, and member attorneys are regularly updated with proposed and actual changes to the Social Security regulations. The NOSSCR also has an extensive referral network that can be accessed if the situation is unusual and requires a second legal opinion. You can write the NOSSCR at 6 Prospect St., Midland Park, NJ 07432. You can also contact the organization by phone at 800-431-2804, or visit its Web site at www.nosscr.org.

Before you agree to work with a particular attorney, ask her the following questions:

✔ How many people have you assisted with applications for Social Security disability claims? (It should be at least 20 to 30 people.)

✔ Of the people you've assisted, what percentage was approved by the Social Security Administration? (The percentage should be at least about 75 percent or more of the attorney's cases.)

✔ How many people with prostate cancer or other forms of cancer have you assisted with applications? (You need an attorney who is conversant in the technical terminology of cancer. She should also be very proficient in translating medical jargon into everyday layman's language.)

Experts report that this is the point where many claims prevail. So don't give up before then!

I can't promise that you'll ultimately be granted a disability payment, no matter how good you are at filling out the myriad of forms, or how many times you appeal denials. But if you're denied at the very first application point and you don't appeal, you'll just never know what would have happened if you had just kept going. So stay the course. Realize that the whole process (from the initial application and on through the appeals) often takes more than a year; sometimes it even takes as long as two years.

And keep in mind that if you're ultimately approved for disability payments, your approval date will be backdated roughly to when you originally applied, and you'll receive a large lump sum payment. Social Security rules are rather complicated, so the payment won't coincide with the month you applied. But the starting date for your payment will usually be sometime within the first year of when you first applied, and the lump sum will usually be thousands of dollars.

Chapter 23

Helping Friends and Family Understand Prostate Cancer

. . . .

In This Chapter

▶ Talking about prostate cancer with your family and friends

▶ Helping your partner deal with your cancer

▶ Describing cancer and its implications to your children

. . . .

*Y*ou know how painful it was for you to hear that you have prostate cancer. But you may not realize how hard it was for your partner and other family members to discover that someone they love has the big "C." They don't have cancer themselves, but they still experience a similar range of emotions, including fear and anger. It may also be difficult for people outside your family who care about you, such as your friends, to hear about your cancer. Some men don't ever tell their friends or family members about their cancer diagnosis, because they think that they can save others from the pain. Yet the people who care about you can tell something's wrong, whether you share the specifics with them or not.

As you struggle to cope with selecting the best treatment and dealing with the side effects you may experience, it's not easy to think about the difficulties others may be experiencing in response to your cancer. In fact, their emotional difficulties may not seem that important: After all, you're the one who's sick. You're the one who has to think about mortality, not them. Actually, they also have to think about life and death, both yours and theirs. You can't avoid thinking about death when someone you love is diagnosed with cancer, no matter how treatable the doctor says it is. The diagnosis is like an elephant in the room: Even if nobody's talking about it, everyone knows that it's there.

This chapter talks about how to help your partner, family members, and friends understand what you're going through. It also helps you understand that your diagnosis is devastating to the people who care about you. You shouldn't spare them from knowing that you have a problem. If you hide your problem from your family members, particularly your partner, they may feel betrayed or diminished in their importance to you. They want to help you. Tell them how.

Explaining Your Illness

Your partner, family members, and friends and may be very distressed, shocked, and dismayed when they discover that you have prostate cancer. What you tell them about your illness, and how you plan to cope with it, is really up to you and your doctor. In the following sections, I offer some helpful suggestions for you to consider when discussing prostate cancer with the people you care about.

Talk about the basics

When talking about your prostate cancer, the main point to convey is that the disease is treatable in most people, and you intend to work hard at getting the best treatments. Tell your friends and family that you didn't cause your illness with something you did (or failed to do), and that you don't know why you have the disease. Assure them that you're working on handling it as best you can.

Don't assume that they know what you know

Whether you know a lot or just a little bit about prostate cancer, don't assume that other people know as much as you know. Most men don't even know that they *have* a prostate gland; most women are unaware of the gland, as well.

When you're talking with others about prostate cancer, start with the basics. Tell them that the prostate gland is a male-only gland that's involved with urination and reproduction, and that sometimes it develops minor or major problems. Prostate cancer is a major problem, even when it's highly treatable. Tell people that the prostate can develop other problems, as well, such as infections or blockages. Be sure to tell them that prostate cancer isn't infectious, and let them know that the disease is nobody's fault. Tell your partner that nobody gets prostate cancer from sex. Some people are more at risk than others (Chapter 3), but you didn't cause yourself to have cancer, and nobody else did either. It just happens.

Give people time to think about and react to what you tell them about your diagnosis. The information can be hard to take in at first. When you say that you have prostate cancer, most people hear the word "cancer" as though it was booming from a loudspeaker — they don't hear much of anything else. Their brains need some time to process this scary information before they can really understand what prostate cancer is, how it affects you, what treatments you're considering, and so on.

Discuss myths and realities

Many different myths about prostate cancer exist, such as "It's only an old man's disease," "Nobody dies from it," or "Everybody dies from it." You can read more about the major myths and realities of prostate cancer in Chapter 25. Make sure that you're familiar with these myths and realities so that you can help your family and friends know the real deal.

Tell them how to help you

Your family and friends will appreciate your telling them how to make your life easier. You may want them to sit and listen to you, drive you to a treatment, or perform another task. Ask for what you need, and both sides will benefit.

In addition, tell them what you *don't* need. For example, if a friend is constantly collecting tabloid articles about the latest "cure" for cancer, she's not really being helpful to you. Tell your friend that your doctor has a good treatment plan for you to follow. Try to channel that friend's interest to information-gathering: Perhaps she can help you find a good specialist, if you need one.

Dealing with Your Partner's Reactions

Being sensitive, caring, and concerned about how your partner feels can be difficult when you feel like you've been emotionally hit over the head with a sledgehammer. But your partner is also terribly upset and maybe even devastated by your prostate cancer diagnosis. Follow these suggestions to help maintain the caring relationship you both need now more than ever.

Maintain good communication

If you're in a long-term serious relationship with another adult, your significant other will wonder what's going to happen to you when you're diagnosed with prostate cancer: She may wonder, "Will you get really sick? Will you get sick slowly? How does this generally work out?" She may worry about your imminent death, or she may fear that you may become severely disabled. She may want to know what effect your treatments will have on you and whether or not the treatments are worth the side effects you may experience. Tell your partner what you know, even if you don't know much. You need to share the information you have with your partner, because it can help alleviate fears and concerns. Whenever possible, enlist your partner's help in gathering information about prostate cancer treatments.

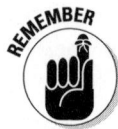

Experts report that maintaining good communication with your significant other is vital while you're undergoing treatment for prostate cancer (and afterwards). Yet some men try to pretend that they aren't having any problems. Or they deny that their cancer is causing any changes in the life they share with their partners.

One study on the quality and type of marital communication between men with prostate cancer and their wives revealed that several men didn't tell their spouses that they'd been diagnosed with prostate cancer, because they felt that this information would upset their wives too much. The motives of the men in the study may have been very positive — but they were quite misguided. After a man is diagnosed with prostate cancer, the most clueless wife on the planet will know that *something* is wrong.

If your partner is *not* told what the problem is, she may well jump to the erroneous conclusion that you're having an affair. Or she may imagine that you are dealing with another issue altogether. When you don't communicate the problem to your partner, you deprive yourself of the love and support that you may need very urgently. If you avoid the problem and pretend that it doesn't exist, you may create a festering sore in your relationship — something that's not really fair to you or your partner.

Ask for (and accept) your partner's help

After the initial shock of the diagnosis, you and your partner should talk about possible problems that may occur as a result of your cancer. Most of the problems will be yours to face directly, but, because of her love for you, your partner also will be affected by your disease. Whenever possible, involve your partner in your ongoing treatment.

For example, if you have your surgery at a major medical center far away from home, have your partner come along with you for moral support and maybe to hold your hand. Even if you receive your treatments locally, having someone who cares about you at your side — ready to cheer you up, tell you stupid jokes, or just be there — can be very helpful. And believe it or not, this involvement can help your partner, too: She gets the opportunity to be there and see what's going on. Sure, hospitals can be very scary places, but imagining and worrying about what's happening to you can be much worse than being by your side and having the chance to ask the doctor any questions that may arise.

Prepare for possible treatment side effects

You should also anticipate that some physical problems that affect both you and your partner, such as temporary impotence or loss of sex drive, may occur as a result of your treatments, so ask your doctor to tell you everything that may happen. If you both know about the possibility of decreased sex in the near future, you won't be so dismayed if it happens. Neither of you will *like* it, but you'll both be better prepared, and you won't rush into the "Oh no! What do we do now?" mindset. (See Chapter 19 for info on resolving erectile problems.) Have your partner come with you to the doctor's office, so the doctor can explain the risks of impotence and answer any questions your partner may have. Some partners plan ahead for possible problems with impotence, reading up on different medications and treatments. If you and your partner obtain this information upfront, you'll have it if you need it.

Tell your partner that there's a good chance that you may have a low sex drive for awhile, especially if you're receiving hormone therapy. You don't want your partner to think that she's no longer appealing to you.

Hot flashes and mood swings are other side effects of hormone therapy that can be difficult to live with. But if your partner realizes ahead of time that the side effects are the result of a treatment you need to extend your life, she may be better able to tolerate them. Of course, she may sometimes respond to your extreme crabbiness by yelling back at you. Understand that you're both human, and you both face a tough situation. (Ask your partner to read Chapter 24, which gives advice to partners for dealing with the side effects of your treatment.)

Cope with the need for more/less time alone

At times, you may feel like you need some time alone as you struggle with the side effects of your cancer treatments. If you experience this feeling, tell your partner that it's nothing personal, but you just need a little time to yourself.

On the other hand, you may feel that you need to spend *more* time with your partner. In this case, tell your partner you need some extra tender-loving care. Don't expect your partner to magically know that you need more or less alone time. Even if she normally reads you very well, her radar may currently be a little off because of her distress over your illness. So tell her what you need.

Keep in mind that your partner may have similar issues: She may want more time to herself, or she may want to spend more time with you. Openly discuss what you both need from each other.

Work through powerful emotions

You and your partner may have strong emotional reactions to your diagnosis. (See Chapter 16 for more about coping with stress.) Some of the common emotional reactions you may experience, which are also reactions that will directly affect you and your significant other, include:

- ✔ **Anger:** You may react to your diagnosis with extreme anger or rage. Your cancer is not your partner's fault, but she may have to cope with your outbursts. If you have a temper tantrum over nothing (as a result of your underlying anger about having cancer), apologize to your partner. Tell her that it's not her fault. Of course, she may also be unfair to you at times. If she gets angry with you for no apparent reason, allow her to apologize.

- ✔ **Depression:** You may experience depression as a result of feelings of helplessness and hopelessness. If you feel depressed, don't ignore the problem; talk about it with your partner and your doctor. (See Chapter 16 for more on depression and how to deal with it.) Understand that your partner may also suffer from depression and need to see a therapist. Because she loves you, she may have trouble dealing with your having such a serious illness. Imagine how upset you'd feel if the roles were reversed.

- ✔ **Jealousy:** Even if you've never had a passing acquaintance with the green-eyed jealousy monster, you may become very watchful of your partner after being diagnosed with prostate cancer. Jealousy can stem from insecurity and fear, as well as from the fact that your whole life may be in a turmoil as a result of your cancer diagnosis. Your partner bears the brunt of your jealousies. If your partner has always been faithful to you in the past, set aside your petty jealousies and fears. Coping with someone who not only has a serious illness but is also unfairly playing the blame game can be extremely difficult.

✔ **Withdrawal:** You may react to your prostate cancer diagnosis by pulling away from your partner and refusing to discuss how you feel. This behavior can drive your partner crazy. She may find it hard to understand why you won't talk about the problem. Facing your diagnosis head on and talking about it with your partner can help you both enormously, because you can then acknowledge the problem and brainstorm what to do about it.

✔ **Denial:** You may react to your diagnosis by ignoring the problem and doing nothing. Or you may think that you're ignoring it, when it's really rattling around inside your head. You don't do yourself or your partner any good when you deny that you have cancer. She may be at her wit's end trying to make you face the facts. Denial can be costly, so don't make the mistake of ignoring your illness.

✔ **Anxiety:** Before your cancer diagnosis, you may have felt that the world was generally an okay place. Now threats may seem to loom from every corner. If your whole life can be negatively affected by one afternoon at a doctor's office, you may wonder what other bad things may happen. Anything seems possible. Your partner may also experience extreme anxiety upon hearing your cancer diagnosis, wondering what's going to happen next and whether her normal, happy life will be destroyed forever. Tell your partner that you know the diagnosis is very hard to deal with. Your acknowledgement of her feelings can help a lot.

✔ **Guilt:** When you're diagnosed with prostate cancer, you may feel irrationally guilty about being sick. Your partner may also experience intense guilt about any negative feelings she may have toward you. After all, it isn't nice to think bad thoughts about or be mean to a sick person. And yet, everybody sometimes has angry thoughts about someone they're close to. Your partner doesn't have to feel guilty, because people with prostate cancer can still act annoying or aggravating at times. You can help your partner feel better by telling her that you don't expect her to turn into a perfect person because you're sick. Like it says in the old Billy Joel song, you love her just the way she is.

Explaining Cancer to Your Kids

It can be hard to talk to your children about cancer, no matter how old they are. They count on you to be around forever, and they don't want to think about the possibility that this assumption can be wrong. But the word "cancer" is a scary word that connotes disability and death, no matter how much you try to sugarcoat it. The following sections give advice on explaining cancer to children and young adults.

Understanding your children's fears

If you have prostate cancer, your children will experience the same fears felt by most children whose parents have been diagnosed with a serious illness. The biggest fear is the horrific loss that they'll feel if you die. The younger the child, the more difficult it may be to imagine a world without you in it.

Fear of loss and death

Your child's knowledge of cancer can sometimes generate nightmarish dreams of monsters bearing down on her or of others attacking her. You don't want your child to feel bad, of course, but some bad feelings come with this territory. You may be able to help your child deal with the problem by making sure that she understands that it isn't fair that you have cancer, and by telling her that other people feel the same way she feels about that nasty old cancer monster. Tell her that the cancer monster should be beat up and killed forever.

Unless you're severely ill and it's very unlikely that any treatment will help you (which only occurs in a small number of cases), tell your child that you expect to live for a very long time. Don't tell your child that you are going to live forever, because no one lives forever, but do tell her that you hope to live for many years. Let her know that you need to have some treatments in order to help you continue to live a good life. Assure the child that you love her and that you know she loves you.

You don't have to provide explicit details about your treatment, other than the fact that you've chosen to have surgery, radiation treatments, hormone therapy, or some other option. However, your children may be very curious about your treatment; if they are, sharing some details or showing them brochures may help them understand what you're going through. You may also be able to reassure them that prostate cancer really is treatable and often curable. But don't push it. Offer the information, and if your child wants more, she'll ask for it. Observe your child's body language. If she's cringing away, staring at the clock, or standing there with arms folded and feet akimbo, she's probably heard quite enough about this cancer thing.

Fear of catching cancer, like a cold

Another big fear for young children is that they may be able to catch your prostate cancer, as if it were a cold or virus. For most pre-adolescents, their primary experience is with illnesses that are contagious, like the flu or strep throat; few of them have had experience with chronic ailments. (Adults are more likely to have chronic ailments such as diabetes, arthritis, and so on.)

Telling (or not telling) people about your cancer

Don, who is 60 years old, has advanced prostate cancer. His cancer is being treated with hormone shots. He told his adult daughters about his medical problem, but he refuses to tell his granddaughters, who are 9 and 11 years old — he doesn't want his daughters to tell them either. He thinks that the children are too young to know about his cancer and that telling them would unnecessarily frighten them. Don's daughters believe that their children have a *right* to know about their grandfather's cancer.

Because of the dispute, a lot of friction has occurred at family gatherings. Don's wife Laura has stood by his refusal to tell their grandchildren about his cancer, but her daughters have been trying to get her to change Don's mind. She told the daughters to back off, but they just won't do it.

You may have a similar problem, only it may be that you don't want to tell your adult children, your parents, or someone else about your prostate cancer. When it comes to sharing information about your health, the choice is yours to make. Therefore, Don has the right to withhold information about his cancer from his grandchildren, and his daughters should rethink their rigid position that he *must* tell his grandchildren that he's sick. At the same time, Don should consider that he may be suffering from a little denial, pretending that he's just fine. If your family gets into a heated disagreement about your prostate cancer, you may want to ask a third party, such as a counselor or therapist, to act as a mediator, because handling such a conflict on your own can be very difficult with so much emotion swirling around. (See Chapter 16 for more info about how therapists can help you deal with stress and depression.)

To assuage this fear of catching prostate cancer, assure your children that cancer is not a contagious disease. Let them know that you can't get it by kissing someone with the disease, using the same towel, or drinking from the same cup. They may say, "We knew that, Dad!" but they may also be secretly relieved that you told them your cancer isn't contagious.

Fear of the true cause

The next question for most children may be, "If it's not contagious, then how *did* you get cancer?" This is an obvious question with a not-so-obvious answer, because in most cases, you don't know why it happened to you. And you may be quite angry that it did. Limit your answer to say that doctors really don't know how or why some people get cancer and others don't, except in a few cases. For example, doctors know that lung cancer is nearly always caused by smoking. But no one really knows for sure what the true causes of prostate cancer are.

Shocking news for your kids

When Ken was diagnosed with cancer, he was only 44 years old. He had three sons, who were 4, 7, and 10 years old. They were horrified when they heard the "C" word, and at first, they were terrified that their father would die any day. Six years have passed since the initial diagnosis, and now Ken is receiving hormone treatments for the cancer. His children no longer fear that when they come home from school, Dad may not be there. But they're still scared for their father. They also wonder if prostate cancer may happen to them when they're grown men.

Actually, they should be careful when they grow up. The sons of men with prostate cancer should have their prostate specific antigen (PSA) levels tested every year beginning at age 40, rather than at age 50 like most other men. The sons of men with prostate cancer are in no way doomed to develop prostate cancer; they just need to be cautious.

Dealing with "magical thinking"

Children who are adolescent or younger may sometimes experience *magical thinking,* which means that they may think or fear that they somehow made you sick by having bad thoughts about you.

For example, maybe you told your teenage son that he couldn't use the car because you needed it, and no matter how much he begged or pleaded with you for the keys, you just wouldn't relent. So he may have become really mad at you and thought to himself that he wished that you would die or go away, because you're such a mean and horrible father. And then days or weeks later you received the cancer diagnosis. The child may think that he actually *made* you get sick by wishing it on you. In his mind, your cancer is all his fault. Even if your child doesn't express such fears to you (and it's likely that he won't, because it may seem too awful to say out loud), he may still be experiencing them.

Magical thinking is most common among children, but adults may be suscep-tible to it, as well. For example, maybe your wife was angry with you for something that happened the day before you received your diagnosis of prostate cancer. Intellectually, she *knows* that she didn't make you sick. But she still may think or worry that she somehow wished you into getting sick.

Be generous with your children, partner, friends, and extended family mem-bers who may be harboring some magical thinking. Make a general statement such as "Some people actually think that they can make other people really sick with angry thoughts. Scientists have proven that this just isn't so." (The "scientists have proven" part is a little bit of an overkill, but it gives your statement the ring of authority that some people may need to hear to over-come their magical thinking. If anyone asks you how scientists have proven this — which is highly unlikely, because they'll be so relieved to hear from you that it wasn't their fault — tell them that you're not quite sure. Maybe you read it somewhere.)

Providing hope along with a needed dose of reality

When you're talking about prostate cancer to your children, concentrate on the hope angle, but don't exude a fake kind of hyper-happiness that would be hard for anyone but a small child to swallow. Let's face it: Cancer is cancer. Some people die from it; you can't get away from that fact. You don't believe that you'll be one of those people. You intend to do everything possible to stay alive for a long time.

Treating young men and women equally

Some studies indicate that men with prostate cancer are likely to talk to their adult sons about their cancer and fail to mention the problem to their adult daughters. Don't make this mistake. Although you don't need to provide your adult or teenage daughters with any embarrassing personal details of how prostate cancer is affecting you, you should at least tell them about the diagnosis. The information is important for them to know so that they can warn their current or future sons of the potential genetic risk.

Your daughters also need to know that you're sick, that you're not mad or disappointed in them in some way, and that you haven't lost interest in them. Your daughter may also be disappointed if she finds out that you told your son about the problem but not her. Old sibling rivalries can be needlessly stirred up, generating extra tension. You can avoid any rivalries by telling your daughters as well as your sons about the cancer diagnosis.

Chapter 24

Helping a Loved One Cope with Prostate Cancer

. . . .

. . . .

Maybe you don't have prostate cancer yourself, but you're the partner, family member, or friend of a man who's been diagnosed with the disease. You may feel devastated, concerned, and confused. Or maybe you're experiencing other emotions, and it seems like feelings are flooding over you like a tidal wave. At the same time you're awash with emotions, you also fervently want to help the person you love. But he may not be very receptive to TLC (tender loving care). He's coping with his own fears and anxieties. He may also be struggling to play the macho-man role that's dictated by society: the man as the strong one who solves problems and prevails over bad guys. Cancer is a bad guy that's tough to beat. Cancer can be beat, but it can be a tough fight (for him and you).

Struggling to figure out what you can do to help make your loved one's life easier and coping with your own emotions and fears can be tough acts to balance, especially when the man with cancer is your partner.

This chapter is for people who love men with prostate cancer. I offer advice on coping with your emotional reactions as you struggle to help your loved one. I also advise the partners of men with prostate cancer — the people on the front lines of support and help. Sometimes they forget that they shouldn't shut down their own feelings or needs, holding a sort of Scarlett O'Hara, "Tomorrow I'll think about what I need" point of view. You can take the self test at the end of this chapter to discover if you're trying too hard to ignore your own needs.

Dealing with Your Own Fears and Emotions

You're worried about your loved one after finding out that he has prostate cancer, and you can't help experiencing many other emotions. In the following sections, I talk about how to deal with the key emotions of anger, fear, and self-blame.

Being scared and angry is normal

The first emotion that hits you is probably the shocking and unthinkable fear that your loved one might die, followed by the fear of losing someone you care about deeply. Another common emotion is anger. You may wonder why this had to happen to him and to you, because you care about him so much. Fear and anger are normal reactions when you find out that a loved one is very ill. Some people lash out at others when they're angry, while others turn their anger inward, which can lead to depression. Others may even get angry at the person with cancer; when they finally realize who they're angry at, they feel very guilty.

Feeling this way is okay. After you have a chance to deal with the shock, try to maintain a positive attitude whenever possible. Remember, prostate cancer is treatable and often curable, so there's a good chance your loved one isn't going anywhere. Try to keep a level head and be there for your loved one, who is also struggling with his own powerful emotions of fear and anger.

If you're feeling overwhelmed, simply taking some deep, slow breaths can help calm down your racing pulse and pounding heart. You may also find that exercise can help you deal with your raging emotions. Even taking a walk can help calm you down. (You may also want to read my suggestions for dealing with stress in Chapter 16; the info focuses on men with prostate cancer, but it works for others, too!)

The fear can be pretty overwhelming at times. You may not be able to keep yourself from thinking of not only your loved one's possible death but your own, as well. You aren't the one who's been diagnosed with prostate cancer, but the disease may make you think about life in general, and how precious and short it really is. You may start thinking about your own life, as well as your own health. You may decide that now is a really good time to get that checkup you've been delaying for years. (And it is!) On the other hand, some people are so shocked and upset by their loved one's cancer diagnosis, that they start seriously neglecting their own health. Don't make this common mistake.

Avoid playing the blame game

When you find out that your loved one has prostate cancer, you may blame him, thinking that he should have gone to the doctor sooner. Or you may blame yourself, thinking that *you* should have made him go to the doctor sooner. You may also want to blame the doctor, because he didn't detect the problem earlier. Or you may want to blame the cancer on your partner's job: The high stress must have hurt his immune system somehow, allowing the cancer to sneak in. When you think about it, you can blame just about any person or circumstance. But ultimately, blaming is a fruitless and useless coping method; it loses its sheen pretty quickly.

When you realize that blaming only makes you feel worse and gets you nowhere, you can choose to accept the existence of the cancer. Accepting the cancer doesn't mean that you have to like the situation: You won't. And acceptance doesn't mean doing nothing. With acceptance, you can stop agonizing endlessly over why your loved one developed prostate cancer and start concentrating on helping him resolve the problem.

Deal with your frustration: No, prostate cancer isn't fair

It just doesn't seem fair that your loved one has been diagnosed with this illness. Why didn't it happen to someone who's a bad person? Or why didn't it happen to someone who's very old or otherwise very sick? Or why does anyone at all, ever, have to get cancer? These and other thoughts can make you more angry and fearful as you seek reasons and explanations. But remember, everything in life can't be figured out. The reason for why some people get prostate cancer and others don't is one of those things that medical science just can't explain yet. No matter how smart you are or how hard you strain your brain to try to make sense of it, you really can't. It doesn't fall into the realm of good common sense, and you need to accept that and focus on helping your loved one gather information and formulate a treatment plan.

Comforting Your Loved One

Your loved one — whether he's your partner, your brother, or someone else you really care about — needs your love, comfort, and reassurance more than ever. First, he needs your love and support as he decides on the best treatment option. Then he needs you during treatment. He may also suffer side effects from the treatments, such as impotence and incontinence, which can be really aggravating and temporarily threaten his personal identity. Even if he doesn't tell you how he's feeling or what side effects he's experiencing, your continued love and support mean a lot to him.

Talking about common fears

Many men hate talking about their fears and anxieties, but that doesn't mean that they don't have them. They do. Your loved one may experience many different emotions (see Chapter 23), including fear, anger, and anxiety. Sometimes detecting the underlying emotion is not so easy, especially when you're stressed out yourself. Talking about your emotions can help a lot.

If you have a hard time getting your loved one to open up, try thinking of activities that you can do together to help relax him, such as a picnic or some other type of casual outing. Participating in activities that he's enjoyed in the past can help provide a feeling of familiarity and bring some hope to his situation. Feeling more relaxed, he may be more open to talking about his feelings and fears. Be sure to read "Helping your loved one express his feelings," later in this chapter — this section can help everyone, not just the partner of the man with prostate cancer.

Understanding common reactions

Some men react to the diagnosis of prostate cancer by pretending that everything's just fine, while others become paralyzed with fear. These reactions don't represent good coping strategies. If your loved one displays one of these reactions for more than a few weeks, you need to jolt him back into the real world and tell him to take action.

If he reacts to his cancer diagnosis by basically pretending that it doesn't exist, at best, he'll go to the doctor, decide upon a plan of treatment, and then get treated. And at worst, he won't get treated at all. Either way, he may not discuss the treatment with you, or he may refuse to talk about his concerns. In fact, he may pretend that everything is just fine. Some men can get almost delusional when it comes to their denial of the need for treatment and their failure to see a doctor. Your loved one may need someone who loves him to insist that he go see a physician.

Like many men, he may struggle mightily to continue on with his regular life, acting as though nothing has happened. He may figure that if he talks about his cancer too much, it'll drive him crazy. He may also be afraid to talk to others about his cancer. Your loved one may think that others will treat him differently if they find out about his cancer (and sometimes they do; see the "Biting comments" sidebar in this chapter), or he may worry that his boss or co-workers will write him off or pity him. He may not be willing to risk taking the chance to prove himself wrong. Talk to him about the laws that protect his job (like the Family and Medical Leave Act and the Americans with Disabilities Act, which are both covered in Chapter 22). Tell him that taking care of his medical problem is more important than worrying about what the world at large thinks of him.

It hasn't been proven in any research study, but it seems that men are much more intimidated by health problems than women are. Men, to the disappointment of their loved ones, don't seem to cope that well when they're first diagnosed with prostate cancer. It isn't uncommon for the loved one to do all the talking and asking of questions at the doctor's office, while the man just sits there in apparent shock. Understand that this behavior is usually only temporary.

Your loved one may experience many different emotions as he struggles to deal with the idea of having cancer. He may also think that asking for help is unmanly and, as a result, be reluctant to ask you for any assistance. Offer to help him. Give your loved one suggestions for ways you can help him, such as driving him to treatments, picking up his medicine at the pharmacy, or any other ideas that come to your mind, and tell him that you really want and even need to help. If your loved one rejects all these ideas, ask him to think of something else you can do, and explain that helping him actually makes you feel much better. This explanation may help your loved one overcome the tendency avoid requesting assistance, and it may also help him address his situation and move forward with a plan for treating his cancer.

Trying too hard to hide her own feelings

Sometimes women play a sort of tough-guy protective role. When Amanda found out that her brother Eddie had prostate cancer, she hid her feelings from him as long she could. She didn't want to add to his already heavy burden. She cried many tears down the shower drain so that she wouldn't upset Eddie. But when she finally broke down sobbing in front of Eddie, to her surprise, he comforted her, and he didn't get upset. Eddie told Amanda that consoling her made him feel better. He may also have been secretly relieved, because he may have wondered why Amanda hadn't previously shown any emotion over his cancer.

You don't do any favors to the people you love by pretending that you're not feeling any emotions. I advise you to be positive when you can — but nobody can keep it up all the time, and you shouldn't try to.

Biting comments

Other people may make comments about cancer that can really set your teeth on edge. They may be well-meaning statements, but they can still cause considerable distress. The following table shows some comments that are frequently made to men with prostate cancer. The table shows how these comments are often interpreted by men with prostate cancer. It also provides a more appropriate statement that can be used instead of the aggravating comment.

Comment	What's Heard Instead	What Can Be Said
You're lucky that you have this kind of cancer.	You're lucky you have cancer.	I'm sorry you have cancer.
How much longer do you have?	When are you going to die?	I'm sorry you have cancer.
You can just have an operation.	You can just risk impotence and incontinence.	Have you decided what to do?
What does your partner think?	Is your partner going to leave you?	It must be hard on your partner, too.
Isn't that an old man's disease?	Because you have prostate cancer, you must be old.	It must have been hard to get the diagnosis.
Is your doctor any good?	Is your doctor at all competent?	Do you need help finding a doctor?
This disease makes you impotent, doesn't it?	You're going to be impotent, and your partner probably won't want you anymore.	The disease has side effects to keep in mind.
If you pray hard enough, maybe you'll get better.	You must not have prayed hard, because you're still sick.	I'll pray for you to recover.

Advice for Wives and Significant Others

Finding out that your significant other has been diagnosed with prostate cancer can deliver a shocking and devastating blow to your life. After all, who can plan for something like this? The answer: No one. The diagnosis of prostate cancer always hurts. Even though *your* body isn't being attacked by cancer cells that are growing out of control, the knowledge that someone you love has cancer can hurt a lot, too. You may find that your mind teems with questions, such as "What's going to happen?" "How do we get rid of this disease?" "*Can* we get rid of this disease?" or "What are the side effects of treatment?" You may also find that you have many more feelings and many more questions, but not enough answers.

Talking to others who are facing the same problem can sometimes help you cope with the situation. If you can't find any local prostate cancer support groups in your area, or you just can't find the time to attend the meetings, try joining an Internet support group (see Chapter 10 for more on support groups). Internet support groups provide both an opportunity and a place to exchange information and concerns. The Circle is a moderated *listserv,* where people can send and receive e-mails from the entire group of about 400 people. (The membership is growing.) For more information on The Circle, go to `www.prostatepointers.org/circle`.

Keep in mind, however, that support groups may sometimes include people who don't understand the disease or who may have especially bad problems (which is why they need support). When they talk about their plight, it may scare you silly. Remember, support groups are for support; they're *not* for medical insight or advice. If you need medical advice, see your doctor.

Tracking medical information

Gina has found that maintaining a folder at home with all her husband's test results and medical reports really helps her obtain some feeling of mastery over the prostate cancer problem. Many people feel helpless when their partner becomes very ill, and Gina was no exception. But she finds the record-keeping to be a useful and important task that she can handle; it's also something she can do to help her husband, Fred.

Gina also keeps copies of her husband's x-rays in the folder. The records proved to be useful when Fred and Gina were consulting a new doctor about his cancer. The x-rays didn't arrive in time for the appointment, so Gina just pulled out the copies from her folder. Gina thinks that men who are very upset and sometimes overwhelmed by their prostate cancer will appreciate it if their partner helps organize their medical information. Before you start creating a home medical folder for your significant other, ask him if it's okay. If you adopt Gina's idea, it may help ease your significant other's life and also make you feel (and be) an important part of the solution to the tough problem of prostate cancer.

Enveloped by her husband's cancer

When her husband Jack was diagnosed with prostate cancer, Debbie felt terribly afraid for a long time. She was afraid that her husband would die soon. She was afraid that she'd be left all alone. At times, she was overwhelmed with vague fears that she couldn't even identify. Debbie was even afraid that she'd always feel afraid, and that she'd never feel "normal" again. She felt like she was afraid of everything and nothing — her emotions were all kind of mixed up inside of her. For Debbie, life just didn't seem good anymore. Instead, everything seemed ominous and perilous.

Debbie's blood pressure, which had never been a problem before, started to go up dangerously high. In addition, her overall anxiety became so severe and so constant that she went to see a psychiatrist for help. Her doctor prescribed BuSpar (generic name: buspirone), an anti-anxiety drug. The medication helped her, and she was on it for several months.

After taking the drug, the coping mechanisms she developed (such as learning everything she could about prostate cancer) and a reclaiming of some of her old interests helped her feel like she had some semblance of control. Debbie started to feel like she was living her life again. She still wasn't happy about Jack's prostate cancer, but the constant panic and fears were no longer a problem for her.

Debbie discovered that when your loved one suffers from a severe health problem (and prostate cancer certainly qualifies!), your own health can sometimes suffer, as well. As a result, you may become overwhelmed with anxiety or depression. If you do become overwhelmed by your feelings, seek help. You may need medication, like Debbie did, or you may just need to speak to a trusted person, such as a clergyperson or a therapist. Think about what kind of help you may need, and then go get it.

Coping with your loved one's volatile emotions

Sometimes being aware of your partner's volatile emotions and their underlying causes can help you deal with them. You can point out the problem to your partner when he's calm. But if your partner's emotions are flying out of control and threatening your relationship, seek couples counseling. Find a counselor who understands how devastating a life-threatening disease can be to a family. Some of the emotions your partner may experience after being diagnosed with prostate cancer include

✔ **Anger:** When your partner is first diagnosed with prostate cancer, he may become very angry. He may explode, striking out at everyone around him. You may find that your significant other becomes intensely irritated at things that normally don't bother him. You may also find that you're often the focus of his anger. You're too helpful, or you're not helpful enough. You're too sad, or you're not sad enough. You're asking too many questions, or you're not asking enough questions. You can't do anything right. Little annoyances, such as leaving the cap off the toothpaste, can get mixed up with his rage over his diagnosis, and then suddenly you're the worst person in the world, and everything's all your fault.

If your partner is flying into rages, don't try to talk him out of his anger when he's in the middle of one. Instead, strike while the iron is cold. In other words, sit down and talk about the angry outbursts when your partner is calm. Tell him that when he flies into a rage, you're going to leave the house and come back when you think he's calm again. Make sure that you tell him this ahead of time, because some men may experience an intensity in their rage when the person they're screaming at walks out. If he knows about your plan ahead of time, he can be better prepared.

✔ **Depression:** Your partner may be depressed. When turned outward, depression can resemble anger. Depression is not a dark mood once in awhile, because everyone has their good days and bad days. Instead, a consistently negative outlook colors the person's entire life. Depression is highly treatable; most physicians treat depression with antidepressants. If your partner is resistant when it comes to seeing a psychiatrist, he can tell his primary care physician about the problem and often receive a prescription. Read more about depression in Chapter 16.

✔ **Fear of abandonment:** Your partner may be very shaken and disconnected as a result of this sudden and shocking change to his world. If he talks a lot about the next husband or boyfriend you're going to have after he's gone, don't just brush his concerns aside or think that he's being silly. Maybe he *is* being silly, but if he mentions your next lover more than few times, he may really be trying to tell you that he's worried you're going to abandon him. He may think to himself, "Who wants a sick guy, someone who might get sick again later on?" He may also find it difficult or impossible to express these fears aloud to you. Reassure him that you're going to stick around.

✔ **Insecurity:** Your loved one may talk a lot about how rich you'll be when he dies and you receive his life insurance money. These comments may be tremendously aggravating to you. He's probably not purposely trying to annoy you, but you shouldn't brush off such comments, either. He may need you to say that no amount of money can replace him. So say it. And tell him to lay off the comments about how you'll be a rich woman after he's gone, because they're hurtful.

✔ **Jealousy:** Your partner may also have some temporary but serious feelings of jealousy as a consequence of this sudden and shocking change to his world. Because it seems as though his world changed in one day when he was diagnosed with cancer, he may feel as though anything can change in one day. Your strong and steady love may not seem so certain to him anymore.

✔ **Anxiety:** Maybe your partner never worried much about his car before (unless something was obviously wrong with it), but now every little noise in the engine worries him. He may also be distraught if you or your children come home a little late, because he imagined that something terrible happened to you.

Helping your loved one express his feelings

When your partner is diagnosed with prostate cancer, you may expect him to become more open about sharing his feelings. Instead, he may pull back more and try to ignore the problem. He may also actively resist discussing it.

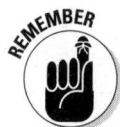

If you find yourself wondering why on earth your partner isn't more forth-coming about his feelings, keep this fact in mind: Many men just weren't brought up to openly express their feelings with others; instead, they were given the impression that feelings and emotions are for women, and that real men don't talk about the things that are bothering them.

So what can you do to get him to openly express his feelings? Try teaching him to think more like a woman, right? Wrong! Don't bother attempting this tactic. You probably couldn't overcome years of socialization if you wanted to, no matter how hard you tried. But you can encourage him to do action-oriented things that may help him express his feelings, such as looking up information, talking to other men with the same problem, or joining a prostate cancer sup-port group. And if he finally decides that he's ready to talk about how he feels, hold back any sarcastic comments, such as "well, finally!" and just sit there and listen. You may also want to hold his hand if you think it'll make him feel more comfortable. You know this guy, and you can usually tell what he needs by observing his behavior and listening to his words.

Dealing with the effects of treatment

If your partner is open to the idea, you can discuss treatment issues for prostate cancer and help him analyze which treatments may have the best results. Your partner's doctor may not offer any choices if his cancer is an advanced case. With advanced cases, patients really only have one best option, such as hormone therapy or maybe chemotherapy. If his cancer is not advanced, he'll have many treatment options available to him, such as surgery or radiation treatments. If your partner decides to have radiation treatments, he can choose between external and internal radiation. If your partner is considering surgery, he needs to decide if he wants to undergo nerve-sparing surgery. You can help your loved one make other choices, too, such as which doctor will perform his treatment.

Cancer isn't a punishment for bad behavior

When Carole's husband Sam was diagnosed with an advanced case of prostate cancer that required hormone shots and other treatments, he kept saying over and over again that it just wasn't fair. He led a clean honest life, and he worked very hard. And now, because of his sickness, he might not get to enjoy the retirement that he struggled so hard to earn.

Carole told Sam that he was right: He was a great husband and provider, and it wasn't fair that he now had prostate cancer. But she also pointed out that prostate cancer isn't a punishment handed down to men who cheat on their wives,

embezzle from their companies, or commit even worse infractions. These men may get prostate cancer, but nice guys may also get diagnosed with the illness. And no one knows why this is.

If your partner rages on about the unfairness of having cancer, tell him that he's right — cancer isn't fair. But also remind him that it isn't a punishment for bad behavior. Let him know that you're going to work with him and do everything you can to help him overcome this very unfair problem.

Before your partner receives treatment, you need to consider how cancer is going to affect your relationship. Temporary or long-term impotence can be a problem for some men with prostate cancer, but those who consider their options beforehand often report that they have more satisfaction later on. In other words, if you consider the possibility of impotence (even though many men with prostate cancer have no problems or only temporary problems with impotence) and think about how you can go about resolving it, you'll be prepared if it actually happens. (You can read more about impotence in Chapter 19.)

If your partner has a low (or no) sex drive during treatment, especially during hormone therapy, don't blame him, and don't let him blame himself. Telling your partner that sex is great but it's not everything, can help a lot. Remember (and remind your partner) that impotent men can still pleasure their partners sexually.

Keep your partner's privacy in mind when talking to others about how his treatment has affected him. Men are especially sensitive (understandably) about problems with impotence or incontinence. Your sister may swear that she'll never tell a soul that you and Johnny haven't had sex for three months, but secrets can be difficult to keep. Imagine how embarrassed and upset Johnny would be if someone made a comment about his impotence. If you need to talk to others about the consequences of your loved one's treatment, talk to someone who must uphold confidentiality, such as a medical doctor, a clergyperson, or a therapist. If people press you for details (and sometimes they will!), thank them for their interest and tell them that the matter is private.

Are you an obsessive caregiver?

The following test can help you determine whether you're overdosing on your caregiving role. (Being an obsessive caregiver is bad for you *and* your partner.) Answer true or false to the questions and then read the analysis that follows.

1. Every decision (or nearly every decision) is based on how it may affect my partner, including whether I get my hair cut, go to a movie with a friend, or even take my car in for repairs.

2. I can't remember the last time I went out with a friend or relative without my partner coming along, too. After all, he's sick! He really shouldn't be left alone.

3. I've gained or lost more than ten pounds since my partner was diagnosed with prostate cancer. I either can't eat, or I have to eat something all the time in order to relieve my stress.

4. I constantly think about *LBPC* (Life Before Prostate Cancer). Everything was perfect before my partner was diagnosed with prostate cancer. My life was idyllic, unlike it is now.

5. My partner's choices always take precedence over the choices of others.

6. When people make annoying remarks about cancer, such as "You're lucky you have this kind of cancer," I practically jump down their throats. How can they be so horribly insensitive? Why did I ever like these people, anyway?

If you answer "true" to many of these statements, or even to one or two of them, you may have a problem with caregiver obsession. You need to break away and get a new perspective.

In response to question 1: Sure, you love your partner, and maybe you think that the world revolves around him. But you also need some down time of your own, even if you don't realize it. Everyone needs to get away, even if only to visit a local museum or go for a walk in the park.

Question 2: If you can't remember the last time you went out with a friend or relative without your partner, now is the time to go! Being with others can lift your spirits and help remind you that the world isn't fixated on cancer.

Question 3: If you've recently lost or gained more than ten pounds without trying, you may be suffering from depression. If you can't get your weight under control, you may need to see a therapist or join a support group (or do both: see a therapist *and* join a support group).

Question 4: Idealizing your life before cancer is normal, but the fact is, everyone has their ups and downs. Life wasn't perfect before your partner was diagnosed with prostate cancer, although it may have been a whole lot better than you realized at the time. But don't beat yourself up over it. You didn't know. Enjoy the moments as best you can, and appreciate the time you do have with your partner, whether it's months, years, or whatever.

Question 5: Sick people often get first priority in their family. The family eats what the sick person wants to eat, and goes where the sick person wants to go. You need to consider yourself and other family members, too. If you have children, they need to know that they're still important and that they don't have to be sick to get attention. If you live only with your partner, give yourself a break — make what you want for dinner and go ahead and see the movies you want to see. You may be surprised to discover that your partner likes it when you please yourself as well as him.

Question 6: People sometimes say dumb things about cancer; it can be aggravating and grating. You have to realize that, in most cases, they don't mean to hurt you or your partner. If you're becoming too obsessed with cancer and caregiving, you need to give yourself a break. Think about it.

Taking time off from prostate cancer

When George was first diagnosed with prostate cancer, he and his wife Lena worked hard at obtaining information on prostate cancer all week long. But then they made sure to take the weekend off from talking or thinking about prostate cancer. Instead, they went to the movies, went out to dinner, went for walks, and enjoyed the kinds of activities they like doing together. They weren't going to let their whole lives be held hostage to prostate cancer. George got the treatment he needed, but whenever possible, they held to their pattern of taking weekends off from cancer.

Making time for yourself

Some issues can't be resolved by discussing them with your partner or creating a plan of action. In a situation like this, you can't help feeling alone and scared, and your partner can't promise to be around for your entire life anymore. If you're a very nurturing person who likes to fix situations for others, you may have a very tough time dealing with your feelings when faced with issues you can't resolve.

Be careful not to fall into the common trap of giving up your life and centering everything around your partner and his cancer. In this situation, you still eat and sleep, but now the focus of everything in your life is your sick partner and his needs and wants. To help illustrate this point, here's an example: When you're on an airplane, the flight attendants show you how the little oxygen masks pop out if they're needed in a dire emergency. The flight attendants also tell you to put on your mask before putting a mask on your child, which is the reverse of your natural reaction.

Why do the flight attendants tell you to put your mask on first? If you put the oxygen mask on yourself first, you'll be more likely to remain conscious so that you can take care of your child. Conversely, if you follow your natural inclinations and put a mask on your child first, you can pass out from lack of oxygen, leaving your child on her own. Your partner isn't a child, and he doesn't need an oxygen mask. But he does need your help. What he doesn't need is for you to totally neglect your physical and emotional health, drowning yourself in caregiving duties. He may need a lot more help than he ever needed before. But he doesn't need everything you have. Save some time for yourself, if only to keep something left for him. Remember, you're important, too.

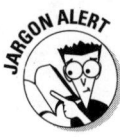

A *caregiver* is a person who provides physical or emotional assistance to another person with a serious problem. Your partner will probably be capable of handling all or most of his medical needs. But you may need to be an emotional caregiver, providing as much support and empathy as possible. Unfortunately, caregivers (especially women) can sometimes become a little (or a lot) obsessed with their caregiving role, making everyone and everything subordinate to the sick person. This behavior isn't healthy. Check out the "Are you an obsessive caregiver?" sidebar in this chapter to find out if you may be going overboard with your caregiving role.

To keep yourself from becoming an obsessive caregiver, follow these tips:

- ✔ **Stay healthy.** Make sure you get annual checkups (and go to your dentist at least once a year, too). Don't neglect your health, thinking, "Oh, it's not that important; it's not like his cancer." If you keep neglecting your own health, you can become ill — maybe very ill. You can't help your partner much, if at all, if you're extremely sick.

- ✔ **Pursue your own interests.** Go to a movie that you like (and your partner hates) or play tennis with friends. Don't give up your whole life. Don't let cancer win. If you devote everything you have to your partner and his illness, you may find yourself becoming angry and resentful.

- ✔ **See a therapist if you think that you may be depressed or anxious.** Talk to someone who understands what it's like to live with a person who has cancer or a severe illness. Your doctor may be able to recommend a therapist. You may also be able to get a good recommendation from members of a support group.

- ✔ **Get enough sleep.** Most people grossly underestimate the importance of a good night's sleep; they drag around during the day, half-asleep and miserable. Don't take cancer concerns to bed with you: Instead, lay your worries aside. Try thinking about floating away on a raft to a wonderful and beautiful safe place.

- ✔ **Don't neglect the rest of your family.** Continue to see your adult children and other family members. They may not be sick, but they are still important.

Part VII
The Part of Tens

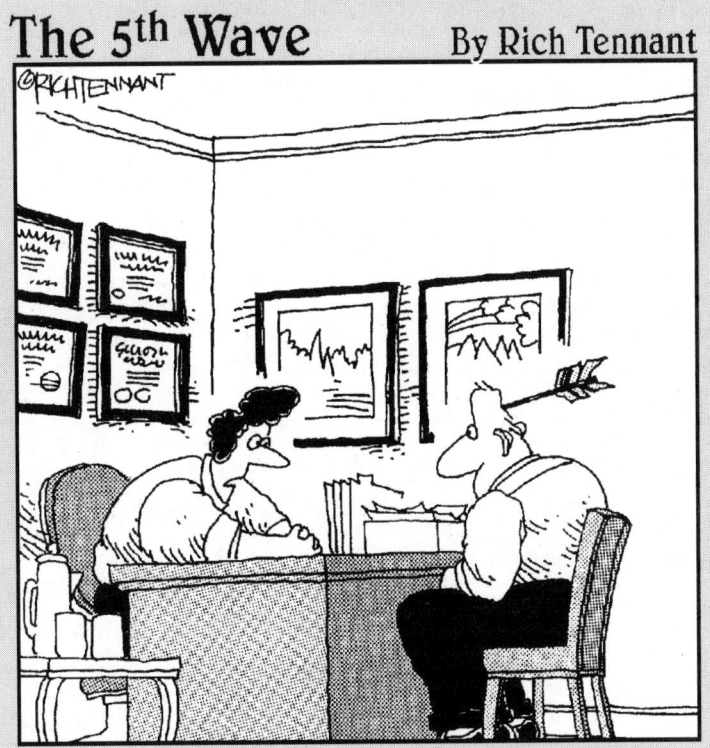

The 5th Wave   By Rich Tennant

"I don't mean to appear unenlightened, Mr. Grove, but I don't think this is the time to explore alternative forms of treatment."

In this part . . .

If you like quick and easy-to-read lists, you'll love this part. I offer you ten myths and realities about prostate cancer, ten must-do's when you have prostate cancer, and ten ways to beat the blues that can hit you hard when you're diagnosed with cancer.

Chapter 25

Ten Myths and Realities about Prostate Cancer

A lot of people think that they know at least the basics about prostate cancer, and some people believe that they really have the essentials of prostate cancer down — even though they're not doctors or cancer experts. But people's beliefs about prostate cancer, and cancer in general, are often flat out wrong. In this chapter, I describe the leading myths about prostate cancer and explain what the real deal is for each case.

Myth #1: Prostate Cancer Is Solely an Elderly Man's Disease

If you're diagnosed with prostate cancer in your late 40s or 50s, you may find that most people are amazed, because they think that only older men (age 65 years old or older) can get prostate cancer. The reality is that older men *do* have a greater risk for prostate cancer, but younger men can also develop the disease.

If a younger man believes that you have to be old to die from prostate cancer, and then he is diagnosed with the disease, he may think that he doesn't have to worry. He may then avoid or delay treatment for years, based on this erroneous assumption. Don't make the same mistake.

Myth #2: If You Have Cancer, You'll Know Because of the Symptoms

Some forms of early cancer have symptoms, but prostate cancer, especially in its early stages, usually has no symptoms at all. Only when men are in the advanced stages of prostate cancer do they often experience severe urinary or back problems. By then the illness is treatable but not often curable. Whether you have symptoms or not, make sure that you get your prostate specific antigen (PSA) blood level checked every year after age 50, and every year after age 40 if you're black and/or have a family history of prostate cancer — both groups are at higher risk than others to develop prostate cancer. So get those checkups!

Myth #3: When Diagnosed With Prostate Cancer, Death Is Inevitable

As myths about death go, this one has a long life. The reality is that everyone eventually dies. Many men with prostate cancer die of other illnesses. Although studies haven't provided any conclusive results, most doctors (including me) believe that early detection gives physicians a chance to provide effective treatments for many patients, including those patients whose prognosis would have been poor 20 or 30 years ago. I may sound like a broken record, but this point is important: Men ages 50 and older should have annual checkups, including a rectal exam and a prostate specific antigen (PSA) blood test (discussed in Chapter 5).

Myth #4: Nobody Dies of Prostate Cancer

Strangely, people may also believe the opposite of the "everyone must die" myth about prostate cancer — that no one ever dies of prostate cancer. Some people may actually tell men with prostate cancer that they have a "good kind" of cancer. One nurse told a man with prostate cancer that she learned in nursing school that nobody dies from prostate cancer. She was wrong. Sadly, some people do die of prostate cancer. In fact, it's the second leading cancer killer for men in the United States. Maybe the cancer was detected in a later stage, or maybe it was discovered early on, and everything "right" was done, and yet the patient died anyway. Doctors and patients regard death as a failure, and I'm no exception. I fight against it as much as I can. But it's just not right to say that this is a game that everyone wins, because it isn't. However, in most cases, when your doctor catches prostate cancer in the early stages, it's not only treatable, it's curable.

Myth #5: You Caused Your Cancer

You probably know that smoking causes lung cancer and oral cancer. Some preliminary studies suggest that smoking *may* sometimes also be involved in causing prostate cancer. However, it makes no sense to blame yourself for your illness. Experts don't know for sure what causes prostate cancer. I think that researchers will eventually find that the disease is caused by many different factors. Skip the guilt trips and focus on obtaining the best treatment possible. Adopt a healthy lifestyle, because it may help keep the cancer at bay. For example, if you smoke, stop now! I give you some other good suggestions for developing a healthy lifestyle in Chapter 17.

Myth #6: Surgery or Radiation Is Always Best

Understandably, most surgeons favor the prostatectomy as the best option for many cases of prostate cancer. Radiation oncologists often lean toward recommending radiation treatments for many men with prostate cancer. To determine which treatment is best, each individual situation needs to be considered, including the man's age, how advanced his cancer is, his attitude about side effects and quality of life issues, and other factors. For example, if a man is 70 years old and has diabetes, surgery may be a poor choice, because his life expectancy is less than 10 years. Conversely, if a man is 55 and otherwise healthy, and his cancer is *localized* (or confined to the prostate), a prostatectomy may be the best answer. Patients need to consider the choices they're offered and analyze what's best for them. (This is no easy task.) I cover the decision-making process in Chapter 9.

Myth #7: You'll Become Permanently Disabled

Many men continue to work after being treated for prostate cancer, while some take four to six weeks off (or longer) to recover from surgery or other treatments. Some men decide to retire — a decision they may have been delaying before the diagnosis of prostate cancer. If you have prostate cancer and you're a military veteran who served in Vietnam during the Vietnam War, you may be eligible for disability compensation from the Veterans Administration. (Check out Chapter 3.)

Myth #8: Impotence Always Follows Treatment

Unlike the other myths, there may actually be a bit of truth behind this one. Half of all men who receive treatment for prostate cancer will experience some impotence (or problems with potency), albeit temporarily. However, some men have few or no problems.

Specifically, treatment for prostate cancer *may* cause *erectile dysfunction* (impotence) in men because of the effects of surgery or radiation on the nerves and blood vessels that control erections. In addition, hormone shots can cause impotence by drastically lowering your sex drive. But if your doctor performs the nerve-sparing prostatectomy (that I describe in Chapter 11), or you have radiation therapy, you have good odds of retaining or getting your potency back in a year (or sooner).

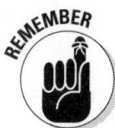

Even if you do have continual problems with erectile dysfunction, medications (such as Viagra) and treatments can help you. Even if all else fails, and erections are just not happening, you may still be able to have orgasms. (Read more about all of this in Chapter 19.)

Myth #9: Prostate Cancer Always Makes Men Incontinent

Incontinence, or problems with bladder control, may result from the prostatectomy or radiation treatments, but it's often only a temporary problem. Some remedies and treatments can help if the incontinence is severe. Only about 20 percent of all men with prostate cancer ever have any form of troublesome incontinence, and in most of these men, the problem is temporary. In those few men with persistent incontinence (2 percent to 10 percent), some good solutions are available, such as medications or, if necessary, surgery. Thus, all but a few men end up without incontinence problems and can sing about how dry they are. Check out Chapter 20 for more information on incontinence.

Myth #10: Your Partner Will Dump You

Some individuals think that if you have prostate cancer, your partner will get frustrated and walk out on you. Although very few studies on the subject have been performed, abandonment doesn't seem to be a problem for men with prostate cancer. Sure, some men who are diagnosed with prostate cancer are walked out on, and some even decide to leave their partners. But in most of these cases, the relationship was in trouble before the cancer diagnosis. The illness may have provided a little push over the edge for a relationship that was already hovering on the cliff of serious problems.

Support groups can often help with relationship problems that occur after diagnosis. I talk about support groups in Chapter 10. I also provide a chapter dedicated to helping the significant others of men with prostate cancer: Chapter 24. You can even find some online support groups for significant others that can be very helpful in alleviating a lot of the concerns, questions, and tension that living with someone with prostate cancer can generate. Help is out there.

Chapter 26

Ten Must-do's for Everyone Battling Prostate Cancer

In This Chapter

▶ Finding and working with a good doctor

▶ Carefully considering all your treatment options

▶ Asking questions

▶ Taking action

*W*hen you first discover that you have prostate cancer, you're often so rattled that you really can't think straight at all. I'm a surgeon who specializes in treating prostate cancer, and I was shocked to find out that I had the disease — so I know firsthand what it feels like to get that diagnosis. Later, when you start to recover from the initial shock of receiving a cancer diagnosis, you can begin working on a battle plan for dealing with this assault on your body and your life. I hope that my list of ten must-do's helps you win the war against prostate cancer.

Locate a Good Doctor You Can Trust

You can't beat or treat prostate cancer on your own. You need the expertise of a good physician. Maybe you already have a talented and capable doctor right now — a physician who you feel is straight up and honest with you, giving you the information that you need. If not, read Chapter 6 to discover how to find a good specialist. Listen to his or her recommendations. Ask questions. Be an active participant in your medical treatment.

Tell Your Loved Ones (At Least Your Partner) About Your Cancer

You may think that you're a strong, tough guy by keeping your prostate cancer to yourself, but most men need the support and love of their partners and their family members during this difficult time. Sure, they may be scared, and yes, they'll be hurt emotionally, but they'll be hurt even more if they have to wonder what's wrong with you. So tell them. Start with your partner. A benefit of starting with your partner is that she often will help you gently explain to other family members that you have prostate cancer and what your diagnosis means. Your partner can help you research a doctor or gather information on different forms of treatment. Your partner can also help you create a medical file or amass other information that's useful. But often, it's the love and caring that you benefit from the most. Don't deprive yourself by thinking that you don't need the support. You do.

Consider Bringing Someone to Your Doctor Visits

When your doctor says that she wants you to come in and discuss your treatment, it's a good idea to at least consider bringing your partner or a friend with you. Because you may still be suffering from disbelief over the diagnosis, you may have great difficulty understanding what your doctor is saying. You may have heard about the prostate cancer last week or several weeks ago, but the thought still flashes like a huge beacon in your brain, with neon lights showing "You have cancer!" over and over. You may not be able to hear or attend to anything else. Your partner, family member, or friend can pay attention to what your doctor says and make sure that you obtain the information you need. You may also want to ask your partner to bring a notebook or some paper to write down what the doctor recommends, so that the information can be reviewed later.

Ask Your Doctor Questions

If you don't understand something that your doctor says, now is not the time to hold back on your questions. Ask them. Your doctor may have been asked the same questions about a zillion times, but so what. If you're confused about your disease, your treatment, or anything else connected with prostate cancer, empower yourself by asking your doctor to explain the things you don't understand.

If your doctor's explanation still isn't clear, or if you need information and the doctor isn't available for some reason, you can find some helpful information online. I provide some Web addresses for you to check out in Appendix B.

Adopting a Healthy Lifestyle

Although it may be difficult to dump bad health habits like chronic excessive drinking and smoking, you'll feel much better when you end these addictions. Some studies indicate that drinking and smoking may be linked to the development of prostate cancer. But even if they have nothing to do with the disease, these habits take a toll on your entire body and rob you of the positive energy that you need to fight the cancer. Talk to your doctor about tips on ending smoking and drinking habits.

You may also wish to consider taking vitamins or supplements. Some preliminary studies indicate that supplements like selenium or vitamin E may help prevent prostate cancer in the first place or may prevent it from recurring. Ask your doctor if he recommends these supplements, which I cover in Chapter 18.

Consider Different Treatment Options

Some cases of prostate cancer don't have a lot of treatment options, especially if the cancer is an advanced case, but the fact is that many men *do* have options to choose from. Your doctor may have one treatment that he feels is best, and he may try to steer you toward that treatment, but it's a good idea to ask around and consider other forms of treatment, too. If you think about your options and then go back to what your doctor recommended in the first place, that's okay. If you decide that another form of treatment would be better, you've made a reasoned choice that way, too. Read more about choosing a good treatment plan in Chapter 9.

Get a Second Opinion on Treatment, but Don't Endlessly Search

Even if you have complete confidence in your physician, discussing treatment options with another doctor is still a good idea. You're not being disloyal to

Dr. Wonderful by going to see Dr. Smart, you're just exploring your options. You can still go back to Dr. Wonderful, whether Dr. Smart agrees with him or not. It's your choice.

Make sure you don't search endlessly for doctors' opinions on what you should do about your prostate cancer. Take your time and seek opinions, but don't get in a rut. Too many opinions and too much reading can actually increase your stress. Eventually, you have to make a decision. Find a competent and caring doctor you can trust, and then give up the search.

When You Decide on a Treatment, Don't Delay Needlessly

After you consider different treatment options and then decide on the best one for you, don't delay your treatment. Get it over with. Sure, you can find many reasons not to have treatment: your daughter's graduation, the big contract you're working on at the office, and on and on. Rethink your priorities. Your mental health and wellness, and occasionally even your survival, can depend on your taking action against the prostate cancer. Three months should provide adequate time to consider the options, obtain second opinions, and schedule your treatment, unless your doctor advises otherwise.

Research Prostate Cancer

If you know very little about prostate cancer, this book is a great place to start your research. But don't stop here. Read the pamphlets and books that your doctor recommends. If friends, family members, or others give you newspaper articles, read them. The Internet can also offer helpful information on prostate cancer and the various treatment options.

Do your homework, but retain a healthy skepticism. Realize that some authors take a strong stand for some treatments, and that sometimes these strong stands are more marketing than conviction. Be especially wary of anyone who claims that changing your diet or taking herbs and supplements is all you need to do to cure your cancer. No evidence supports the theory that diets or supplements will cure your cancer, so don't take any unnecessary risks.

Talk to Others Who Have Prostate Cancer

Find out if your friends or relatives know anybody who's had prostate cancer in the past few years. (Treatments have changed a lot, so it's best to talk to someone who's been treated recently.) Consider joining a support group for men with prostate cancer. (Read Chapter 10 for info on support groups, and check out Appendix B at the end of this book for a list of support groups.) You have to understand that what worked well for Bob, whose prostate cancer was treated with radiation, may not work for you, because your cancer may be more or less advanced. But talk to him anyway, because he can probably offer some good advice.

Chapter 27

Ten Ways to Beat the Blues

*F*eeling very upset and distressed when you find out that you have prostate cancer is normal. You may continue to feel this emotional anguish when you experience treatments that frighten and upset you — whether you admit it or not. You may find yourself slipping into despair or even depression, which is signaled by such symptoms as poor appetite, early-morning awakenings, low energy, and an inability to find pleasure in activities that you normally enjoy.

This chapter highlights ten ways to beat the severe sadness that can envelope you when you're confronted with prostate cancer. You may need help from a support group (see Chapter 10), or you may need to consult with a therapist or a religious counselor (perhaps with your partner at your side). If your depression becomes severe, seek treatment from your doctor. (You can read more about depression and stress in Chapter 16.) You don't deserve cancer (nobody does), but you have it. Empower yourself by increasing your emotional strength. You can also follow my ten ways to beat the blues.

Enjoying Activities with Your Family

Maybe you never really had the opportunity to spend some good quality time with your partner and/or children because of work constraints and worries. And now that you have cancer, you may not feel like going off on family picnics or taking long walks in the park. But hanging out with your kids (even your grownup kids!) in the backyard and immersing yourself in the love of your family members can serve as a good pick-me-up tonic.

If you're like some men, you may think that the best thing to do is to conceal your cancer from the people you care about. But such a tactic can lead to feelings of isolation, anxiety, and depression. It can also confuse the people who care about you, because they'll know that something is wrong, even if you don't tell them what it is. Cherishing the people you care about and thinking how fortunate you are to have such people in your life is one good way to beat the blues. Availing yourself of their love and comfort is another key part of the entire self-affirming process.

Realizing that Prostate Cancer Is Highly Treatable

Many good treatments for prostate cancer are available. You need to take advantage of your options and discover what works best for you, whether it's surgery, radiation treatments, hormone therapy, or a combination of treatments. Reading this book can help you gain some good information, and talking to your physician can solidify your knowledge base even further. Tell yourself, "I will do my best to beat this," and then, with the help of your physician, go do it.

Praying Helps

Many people find solace from regular prayer. Praying can help you give the control over your fears and anxieties to a higher power. You don't have to go to a specific place of worship on a regular basis in order to pray. Tapping into your religious faith and the power of prayer can be very consoling. Don't worry about whether you're praying "the right way." Just speak from your heart when you pray to your higher power, and then give up your emotional pain to that entity. Also, talking to a religious counselor, such as a priest, pastor, or rabbi, may be just what you need.

During Treatment, Imagine Cancer Cells Dying

Some treatments can be tough, especially when you're worried about having them. The prospect of having surgery or *brachytherapy* (where the doctor sews irradiated seeds into your prostate to kill the cancer cells), or of taking hormone medications, can be frightening.

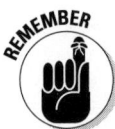

You may worry, "What if this treatment doesn't work?" But remember, treatments often *do* work. And if the treatment you receive doesn't work, you and your doctor can try something else. But no matter what treatment you try, before you have the treatment (and during, if you're conscious), imagine those nasty cancer cells being destroyed by the treatment. Just killed dead, end of story. That oughta make you feel better.

Getting Out of the House Can Lift Your Spirits

When you're in the midst of the blues, you may have a hard time motivating yourself to do much of anything. But you eventually have to get off that couch or out of bed, even if it's only to go to the bathroom or get something to eat. After you perform these essential functions, keep moving! Get out of the house. Go for a walk or take a ride in the car. Sign up for yoga classes or judo lessons, or learn meditation. Activity is the enemy of depression. When you get yourself in motion, you often build up the momentum to pull yourself out of a depressed mood.

Exercising Can Infuse You with Energy

If you have prostate cancer, you're probably not worried about getting in great shape or losing weight. But vigorous exercising has an emotional benefit, as well: It leads to the production of brain chemicals called *endorphins*, which act as natural mood elevators. (The natural highs produced by endorphins are actually one of the upsides of being an athlete.) You don't have to be a jock to get those endorphins going. Even a brisk walk can be effective.

Accept that Having Cancer Is Undeniably Tough

Accepting that having prostate cancer is awful and unfair, and that nobody deserves to have it (certainly not you!), may sound like a strange way to deal with your condition. And yet, some men report that when they stop raging over why they have cancer, and accept that they have it and are going to deal with it, they feel better. Of course, they're not walking around with big gaping smiles like the ones on those old yellow smiley-face buttons. But accepting that you have cancer, and that it must be dealt with, can help you concentrate on working with your doctor to kill those nasty cancer cells.

Reuniting with an Old Friend or Family Member

Calling a friend you haven't talked to for a long time, maybe years, can help beat the blues. If you can, try to meet with an old friend, even if it means some major juggling with your schedule. Of course, don't forego having treatment for cancer, because that's something that shouldn't be delayed, especially if your doctor is pressing you to act. But do try to find time to make contact with someone you care about and haven't connected with for awhile.

Maybe you'll tell this person about the cancer, and maybe you won't. But wouldn't it be great to see him or her again? Just the thought of seeing an old friend may cheer you up. Seize the day.

Participating in Activities You Enjoy

Another good way to beat the blues is to engage in activities that you enjoy but haven't experienced in a long time, such as playing chess with your pals or fishing in the local river. If you're feeling unmotivated, tell a friend that you're feeling down and you need him to drag you off to go skating, swimming, or whatever. After you start engaging in these activities again, you may have a hard time staying in a deep funk.

Considering Therapy When Depression Overwhelms You

If nothing you try helps you beat the blues, and you feel yourself sinking into a mire of depression and distress, you need to get professional help. Some therapists specialize in treating people with life-threatening and life-changing problems such as cancer. Ask your doctor if he can recommend a therapist, and talk to others who have dealt with therapists. Then consult with the therapist and discover how to empower yourself to deal with your prostate cancer without giving up. If you're having suicidal thoughts, you need to see a therapist as soon as possible. Depression is highly treatable, even when you have a very serious problem such as cancer.

Appendix A

Glossary

n this glossary, I provide brief definitions for important terms used in this book. The terms are important for people with prostate cancer (as well as others interested in knowing more about prostate cancer) to understand.

advanced cancer: Cancer that has spread to the lymph nodes, the bones, or other organs of the body.

alternative remedies: Nontraditional treatments for preventing and treating prostate cancer (such as taking herbs or vitamins).

androgens (also called anabolic steroids): Hormones produced predominantly by males. The presence of male hormones such as testosterone may make prostate cancer grow faster.

anti-androgens: Medications that are given to block the action of androgens and thus delay the spread of prostate cancer.

antioxidants: Cancer-fighting substances. Scientists are studying whether antioxidants in selenium and vitamin E can prevent prostate cancer. Many vegetables contain antioxidants, especially tomatoes.

benign prostatic hyperplasia (BPH): An enlargement of the prostate caused by an overgrowth of noncancerous cells. BPH can be a very painful condition.

biopsy: A tissue sample that is analyzed to determine if a person has a disease. A *prostate biopsy* refers to one or more tissue samples taken from the prostate gland for the purpose of determining whether a man has prostate cancer.

blood urea nitrogen (BUN) test: A blood test that measures the level of urea nitrogen (a toxin) in the blood. Urea nitrogen levels may be abnormally high in the presence of prostate cancer.

bone scan: An imaging test used to determine if prostate cancer has spread to the bones.

brachytherapy: A prostate cancer treatment in which radioactive seeds are implanted in the prostate to destroy the cancer cells.

catheter: A tube that is temporarily inserted into the bladder to remove urine when it is difficult or impossible for the man to urinate on his own, such as after a prostatectomy or when a blockage is present, or when the urethra needs time to heal after surgery.

chemotherapy: The treatment of advanced cancer with cancer-killing drugs. This treatment usually is used when hormone therapy is no longer working.

clinical study (also called a clinical trial): A formal medical investigation of a therapy or treatment. Joining a clinical study often gives men with prostate cancer an opportunity to use therapies or treatments that are otherwise not available.

cryosurgery: A procedure that uses very cold temperatures to freeze, and therefore destroy, cancer cells in the prostate.

cystitis: Inflammation of the bladder, usually caused by a bladder infection.

cystoscope: An instrument that is used to see inside the bladder.

cystoscopy: Procedure in which the doctor inspects the inside of the bladder with a cystoscope.

digital rectal examination (DRE): A manual examination of the prostate that is performed by inserting a lubricated finger into the rectum. With the exam, doctors can check for abnormalities that may indicate prostate cancer or other diseases.

endocrine therapy: See *hormone therapy.*

endorectal coil: A device that's inserted in the rectum and monitored with magnetic resonance imaging (MRI). This device shows the prostate gland in more detail than is possible with an ultrasound. Some doctors use endorectal coils when performing brachytherapy. Endorectal coils are also sometimes used to help doctors stage cancer.

erectile dysfunction (ED — also known as impotence): Difficulty starting or keeping erections.

external beam radiotherapy (EBRT): Radiation therapy provided by machines that aim special radiation beams at the prostate to destroy cancer cells. Patients usually receive individual treatments five days a week for at least four weeks.

free prostate specific antigen (free PSA): An inactive form of the prostate specific antigen in the blood. Some doctors use the free PSA test in conjunction with the regular PSA test (usually expressed as the percent free PSA) to help evaluate the likelihood that the prostate contains cancer.

Gleason score: A measurement used to evaluate the appearance of prostate cancer cells in terms of how aggressive they are. The further from normal cells they look, the more advanced the cancer.

hormone therapy: Treatment using drugs or surgery to stop or block natural male hormones for the purpose of halting or delaying the spread of cancer.

impotence (also known as erectile dysfunction)**:** The inability to have or maintain an erection. Impotence sometimes results from treatments for prostate cancer.

intensity modulated radiotherapy (IMRT): A relatively new method of external beam radiotherapy (EBRT) in which each radiation beam is "shaped" to produce a pattern of radiation intensities that work together to destroy cancer cells without destroying the surrounding healthy tissue. This approach allows radiation oncologists to focus more radiation on the prostate cancer without increasing side effects.

interstitial cystitis: A painful bladder condition that causes frequent urination and pain. Interstitial cystitis is more common among women, but men may also experience this condition.

Kegel exercises: Special exercises, performed by the bladder *sphincter* (the muscle that contracts to control the release of urine), that can help you retain urine better and longer.

laparoscopic radical prostatectomy: Total removal of the prostate gland using long instruments and TV cameras that are inserted through very small incisions in the abdomen. These incisions are smaller than the incisions made in the standard radical retropubic prostatectomy, so they may be less stressful for the patient. This procedure is relatively new, but it's likely to become more common in the future.

localized prostate cancer: Cancer that is confined to the prostate itself and that hasn't spread.

luteinizing hormone-releasing hormone (LH-RH) agonists: Drugs used in hormone therapy to block the production of testosterone. (Testosterone accelerates the growth of prostate cancer.)

lymphadenectomy: The surgical removal of the lymph nodes. With a radical prostatectomy, the lymph nodes in the pelvic area are often removed along with the prostate.

lymph nodes: Tiny organs that work to rid the body of toxins and dangerous substances. Cancer sometimes spreads from the prostate to the lymph nodes.

metastasis: The spread of cancer from the prostate to the bones, the lymph nodes, or other parts of the body.

nerve-sparing radical prostatectomy: Procedure that removes the entire prostate and seminal vesicles, and attempts to spare the nerve bundles that control erections. If successful, the man will be able to have a normal sex life.

oncologist: A doctor who specializes in treating patients with cancer. Types of oncologists include specialists in radiation therapy (radiation oncologists), chemotherapy (medical oncologists), and surgery (in this case, urological oncologists).

orchiectomy: A form of hormone therapy that involves the surgical removal of the testes.

pathologist: A medical doctor who analyzes tissue samples, such as biopsies, to determine if disease is present.

penile implant (also called a prosthesis): Cylinders that are permanently installed in the two natural "sausage-shaped" chambers of spongy tissue (corpus cavernosa) inside the penis. The cylinders can be malleable but rigid, or hollow and inflatable. Penile implants enable a man to have an erect penis so that he can have sexual intercourse.

peripheral zone: The outer part of the prostate gland.

prostate specific antigen (PSA) test: A test that measures levels of prostate specific antigen in the blood. High and/or rising levels of PSA may indicate the presence of prostate cancer. The PSA test is used to help diagnose prostate cancer, as well as to determine if treatment for prostate cancer has been effective.

prostatic intraepithelial neoplasia (PIN): Precancerous cells that may indicate that cancer is present or developing. Only high-grade PIN (PIN 3) is considered a risk for prostate cancer.

prostatitis: An inflammation of the prostate that is often caused by infection.

PSA density: A ratio between the prostate specific antigen (PSA) blood levels and the size of the prostate gland (measured in cubic centimeters). The comparison is made to help the doctor determine how likely it is that prostate cancer is present in the prostate. Generally, the higher the PSA density, the higher the likelihood of prostate cancer.

PSA velocity: A measure of how fast PSA levels are going up. If PSA levels are rising quickly, it may be an indication that treatment isn't working. If PSA levels are going down, it may be an indication that treatment is working. PSA velocity is often expressed as PSA doubling time.

radiation therapy (also known as radiotherapy): Treatments, such as brachytherapy or external beam radiotherapy (EBRT), that use radiation to treat prostate cancer. Radiation therapy may be successful at curing early forms of prostate cancer. Radiation may also be used to alleviate bone pain in patients with advanced cancer.

radical prostatectomy: The surgical removal of the prostate and the seminal vesicles through an incision between the scrotum and anus (perineal), an incision in the lower abdomen (retropubic), or several very small incisions in the abdomen using special instruments (laparoscopy).

seminal vesicles: Organs that supply nutritive fluid to sperm. (The seminal vesicles are attached to the prostate and are routinely removed with the prostate during a radical prostatectomy.)

staging: The process of determining how extensive the tumor is within the prostate, whether it has extended outside the prostate, and whether it has spread to the lymph nodes, bones, or other organs. The Tumor Node Metastasis (TNM) system is a commonly used staging system.

sural nerve graft: A procedure where nerves are taken from a man's leg and ankle and grafted in place of the erection-controlling nerve bundles removed during a radical prostatectomy. If the procedure is successful, the nerves will grow and replace the old nerves, restoring sexual potency.

testosterone: A male hormone, produced by the testicles, that may hasten the growth of prostate cancer.

three-dimensional conformal therapy: An external beam radiation therapy (EBRT) approach in which computers help aim extremely targeted beams of radiation from different directions, all at the same time, at the prostate in order to destroy cancer cells without damaging the surrounding normal tissue. This procedure allows radiation oncologists to give more radiation to the cancer in the prostate without increasing side effects.

transitional zone: The area located toward the middle of the prostate gland. The transitional zone is the area where benign prostatic hyperplasia (BPH) develops and grows. In most cases, prostate cancer starts in the peripheral zone, but it may also start in the transitional zone (although this is rare). Transitional zone cancers can be hard to detect, and they are also often slower-growing than cancers in the peripheral zone.

transrectal ultrasonography: A procedure in which a special probe (inserted rectally) uses sound waves to show pictures of the prostate and the surrounding organs. A special biopsy needle can be passed through the probe to sample pieces of tissue from specific areas of the prostate.

transurethral resection of the prostate (TURP): A common surgical procedure that's used to treat serious cases of BPH. When doctors perform this procedure, they remove the excess tissue from the prostate (which blocks urination) with an instrument that is inserted through the urethra.

Tumor Node Metastasis (TNM) system: A cancer classification system that is used (in all forms of cancer) to stage how advanced the cancer is.

urethra: The canal that carries urine from the bladder through the penis to the outside.

urinary incontinence: Loss of control over the release of urine.

urologists: Surgical doctors who specialize in the urogenital or urinary system and its diseases. Urologists can diagnose and treat cancers of the kidneys, bladder, prostate gland, penis, and testicles.

watchful waiting (also called expectant management or surveillance)**:** The decision to *not* treat localized prostate cancer with surgery, radiation, hormone therapy, or any other treatment options. Instead, the physician monitors the patient's prostate cancer by checking PSA levels and looking for signs and symptoms of cancer growth. If the PSA levels start to go up or the signs and symptoms of cancer growth become more apparent, treatment may be started.

Appendix B

Resources

· ·

*I*n this appendix, I provide useful resources that may be valuable to you, your family, and your friends. I hope that you find these resources helpful.

Note: I don't personally endorse any of the resources listed here (and neither does the publisher), nor am I responsible for their content.

Finding Support in Organizations and Support Groups

You can find national and regional support groups and organizations that provide a wealth of information, education, and encouragement.

✔ Canadian Prostate Cancer Network, P.O. Box 1253, Lakefield, Ontario K0L 2H0, Canada; phone 705-652-9200; Web site: www.cpcn.org/. (This organization offers a support group.)

✔ CaP Cure (Association for the Cure of Cancer of the Prostate), 1250 4th Street, Suite 360, Santa Monica, CA 90401; phone 800-757-2873 or 310-458-2873; Web site: www.capcure.org.

✔ Man to Man, American Cancer Society, 1599 Clifton Road NE, Atlanta, GA 30329; phone 800-227-2345; Web site www.cancer.org/docroot/SHR/content/SHR_2.1_x_Man_to_Man.asp?sitearea=SHR. (This organization offers a support group.)

✔ National Prostate Cancer Coalition, 1158 15th Street NW, Washington, DC 20005; phone 888-245-9455 or 202-463-9455; Web site: www.pcacoalition.org.

✔ Prostate Cancer Exchange, 304 N Broadway, Suite 304, Jericho, NY 11753; phone 516-942-5000. (This organization offers a support group.)

✔ US TOO! International, Inc., 5003 Fairview Ave., Downers Grove, IL 60515; phone 630-795-1002 (prostate cancer toll-free support hotline: 800-808-7866); Web site: www.ustoo.org. (This organization offers a support group.)

Utilizing the Web

The Internet offers a variety of Web sites, e-mail lists, newsgroups, and online newsletters that provide opportunities to obtain information, meet others who have prostate cancer, and share what you know about prostate cancer.

Web sites

You can find many informative Web sites that have an interest in prostate cancer. Some popular sites (in addition to those listed earlier in this chapter) include

- American Cancer Society, Learn About Cancer page: `www.cancer.org/docroot/CRI/CRI_2x.asp?sitearea=LRN&dt=36`
- American Urological Associaton: `www.auanet.org`
- Cancer.gov (National Cancer Institute): `www.cancer.gov/cancerinfo/types/prostate`
- CancerLinks, Prostate Cancer page: `www.cancerlinks.com/prostate.html`
- ClinicalTrials.gov (National Institutes of Health): `www.clinicaltrials.gov`
- National Comprehensive Cancer Network (NCCN), Prostate Cancer Treatment Guidelines for Patients: `www.nccn.org/patient_gls/_english/_prostate_cancer/index.htm`

E-mail lists

An *e-mail list* (also called a *listserv*) is an arrangement whereby members automatically receive all e-mails that are sent by other members. (If you don't want to receive a large number of e-mails, some e-mail lists usually provide the option for you to go to a special Web site to read all messages.)

With e-mail lists, you may discover information that you need, and you may be empowered by an opportunity to talk to others who are also dealing with prostate cancer — or with others who are trying to help someone they love deal with prostate cancer. The large number of responses that you have to wade through is the primary disadvantage of some e-mail lists. Also, some people who post messages may seem to know what they're talking about, when, in reality, they offer information that's wrong, inadequate, or not helpful.

Some examples of prostate cancer e-mail lists are:

- ✔ The Circle: www.prostatepointers.org/circle
- ✔ Patient to Physician (P2P): www.prostatepointers.org/mlist/mlist.html
- ✔ The PROSTATE list: www.acor.org/prostate.html
- ✔ Prostate Problems mailing list: www.acor.org/diseases/prostate

Newsgroups

Newsgroups (also called *usenet groups*) are online special interest groups that generally discuss one specific topic. You can find newsgroups that discuss medical problems, famous authors, political issues, or many other topics. Several newsgroups focus on prostate cancer.

When you join a newsgroup, you can read all the messages that have been left by others, and you can leave your own messages for other members to read. You don't have to compose any messages to the group unless you want to.

Newsgroups often offer good, or at least interesting, information (as long as you read everything skeptically). Newsgroups can also provide strong moral support. In addition, many newsgroup *posters* (people who leave messages) offer direct Web links to useful journal articles. The primary disadvantage of newsgroups is that they're open to anyone who logs on: Some people may write aggravating or insulting messages, while others may try to sell products, either overtly or covertly. It's not always easy to spot frauds and scams, so be careful.

Contact your Internet service provider to find out how you can access newsgroups. You can find links to many disability, health, and medical newsgroups, including alt.support.cancer.prostate and sci.med.prostate.cancer, at www.makoa.org/usenet.htm.

Online newsletters

Some online newsletters are dedicated to prostate cancer. These newsletters often provide new information on treatments and medications for prostate cancer patients and their families, and refer to the results of clinical studies. When you subscribe, you receive the newsletter by e-mail. You may want to check out the following publications:

- *Aware:* This free online publication is published by the National Prostate Cancer Coalition. You can subscribe at www.pcacoalition.org/Aware/ Aware_Intro/aware_intro.html.

- *Prostate Forum:* This monthly publication, which is available by e-mail ($36) or snail mail ($46), is produced by a physician. It includes easy-to-understand synopses of the latest information on prostate cancer. You can subscribe by visiting the publication's Web site at www.prostateforum. com, writing to Rivanna Health Publications (P.O. Box 6696, Charlottesville, VA 22906), or calling 800-305-2432. You can also request a print version to be sent via regular mail.

Index

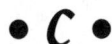

• C •

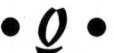

• *Q* •

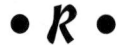

• *R* •

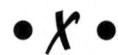

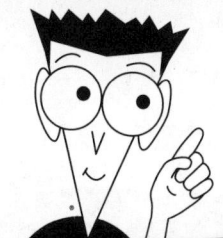
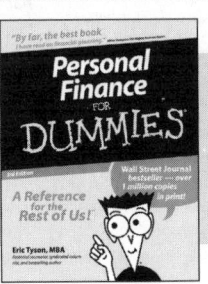
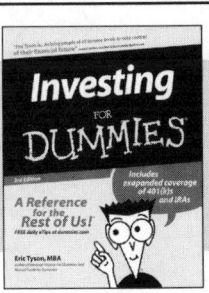
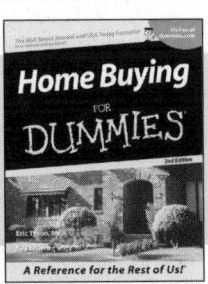
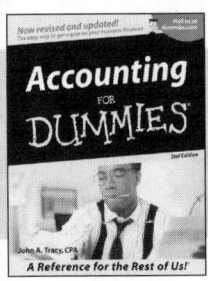
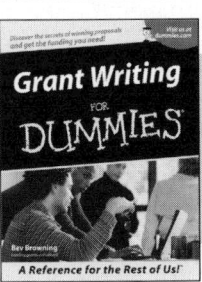
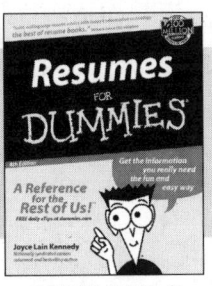
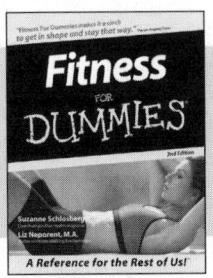
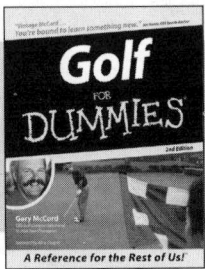
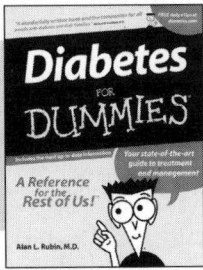
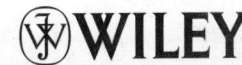

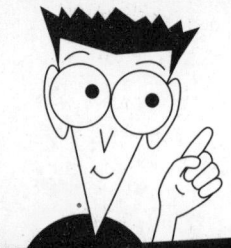

FOR DUMMIES®

A world of resources to help you grow

HOME, GARDEN & HOBBIES

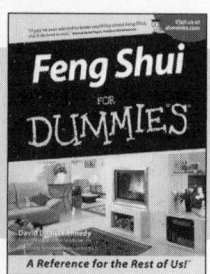

Feng Shui FOR DUMMIES
A Reference for the Rest of Us!
0-7645-5295-3

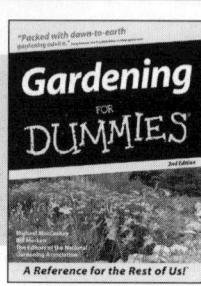

Gardening FOR DUMMIES
2nd Edition
A Reference for the Rest of Us!
0-7645-5130-2

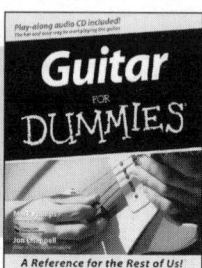

Guitar FOR DUMMIES
A Reference for the Rest of Us!
0-7645-5106-X

Also available:

Auto Repair For Dummies
(0-7645-5089-6)

Chess For Dummies
(0-7645-5003-9)

Home Maintenance For
Dummies
(0-7645-5215-5)

Organizing For Dummies
(0-7645-5300-3)

Piano For Dummies
(0-7645-5105-1)

Poker For Dummies
(0-7645-5232-5)

Quilting For Dummies
(0-7645-5118-3)

Rock Guitar For Dummies
(0-7645-5356-9)

Roses For Dummies
(0-7645-5202-3)

Sewing For Dummies
(0-7645-5137-X)

FOOD & WINE

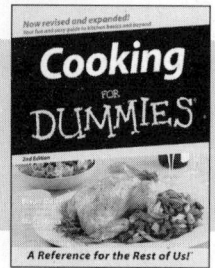

Cooking FOR DUMMIES
2nd Edition
A Reference for the Rest of Us!
0-7645-5250-3

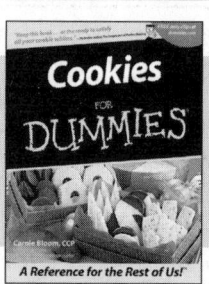

Cookies FOR DUMMIES
A Reference for the Rest of Us!
0-7645-5390-9

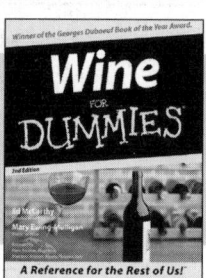

Wine FOR DUMMIES
2nd Edition
A Reference for the Rest of Us!
0-7645-5114-0

Also available:

Bartending For Dummies
(0-7645-5051-9)

Chinese Cooking For
Dummies
(0-7645-5247-3)

Christmas Cooking For
Dummies
(0-7645-5407-7)

Diabetes Cookbook For
Dummies
(0-7645-5230-9)

Grilling For Dummies
(0-7645-5076-4)

Low-Fat Cooking For
Dummies
(0-7645-5035-7)

Slow Cookers For Dummies
(0-7645-5240-6)

TRAVEL

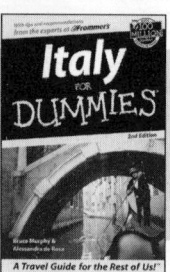

Italy FOR DUMMIES
2nd Edition
A Travel Guide for the Rest of Us!
0-7645-5453-0

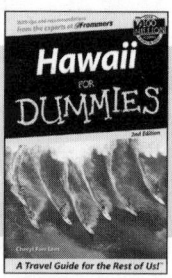

Hawaii FOR DUMMIES
2nd Edition
A Travel Guide for the Rest of Us!
0-7645-5438-7

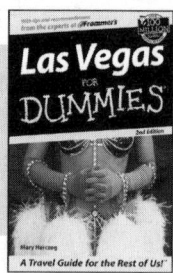

Las Vegas FOR DUMMIES
2nd Edition
A Travel Guide for the Rest of Us!
0-7645-5448-4

Also available:

America's National Parks For
Dummies
(0-7645-6204-5)

Caribbean For Dummies
(0-7645-5445-X)

Cruise Vacations For
Dummies 2003
(0-7645-5459-X)

Europe For Dummies
(0-7645-5456-5)

Ireland For Dummies
(0-7645-6199-5)

France For Dummies
(0-7645-6292-4)

London For Dummies
(0-7645-5416-6)

Mexico's Beach Resorts For
Dummies
(0-7645-6262-2)

Paris For Dummies
(0-7645-5494-8)

RV Vacations For Dummies
(0-7645-5443-3)

Walt Disney World & Orlando
For Dummies
(0-7645-5444-1)

FOR DUMMIES®

Plain-English solutions for everyday challenges

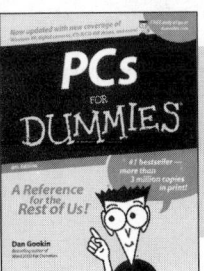
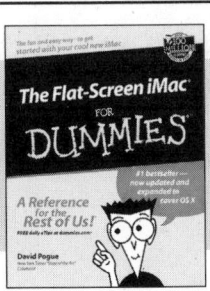
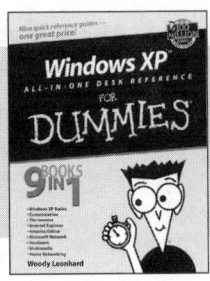
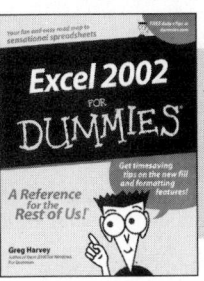
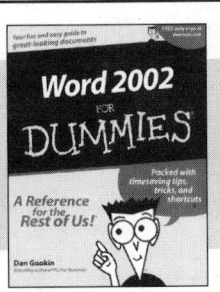
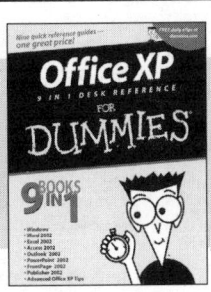
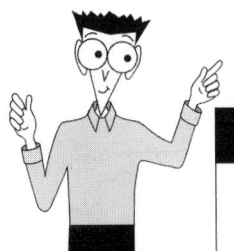

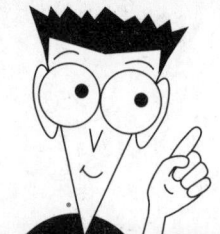

FOR DUMMIES

INTERNET

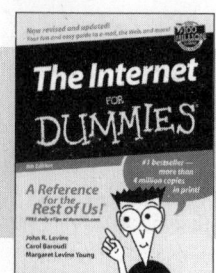

0-7645-0894-6

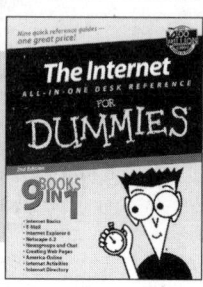

0-7645-1659-0

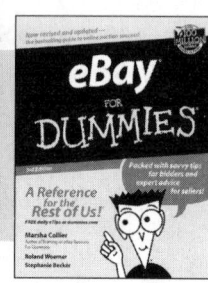

0-7645-1642-6

Also available:

America Online 7.0 For Dummies
(0-7645-1624-8)

Genealogy Online For Dummies
(0-7645-0807-5)

The Internet All-in-One Desk Reference For Dummies
(0-7645-1659-0)

Internet Explorer 6 For Dummies
(0-7645-1344-3)

The Internet For Dummies Quick Reference
(0-7645-1645-0)

Internet Privacy For Dummies
(0-7645-0846-6)

Researching Online For Dummies
(0-7645-0546-7)

Starting an Online Business For Dummies
(0-7645-1655-8)

DIGITAL MEDIA

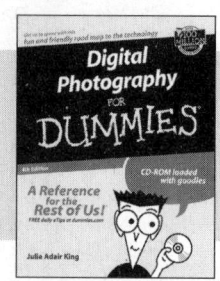

0-7645-1664-7

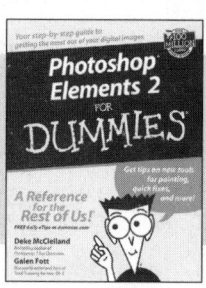

0-7645-1675-2

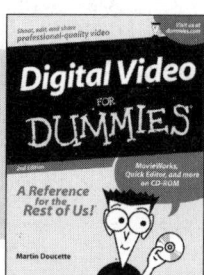

0-7645-0806-7

Also available:

CD and DVD Recording For Dummies
(0-7645-1627-2)

Digital Photography All-in-One Desk Reference For Dummies
(0-7645-1800-3)

Digital Photography For Dummies Quick Reference
(0-7645-0750-8)

Home Recording for Musicians For Dummies
(0-7645-1634-5)

MP3 For Dummies
(0-7645-0858-X)

Paint Shop Pro "X" For Dummies
(0-7645-2440-2)

Photo Retouching & Restoration For Dummies
(0-7645-1662-0)

Scanners For Dummies
(0-7645-0783-4)

GRAPHICS

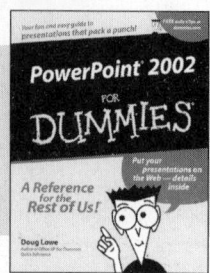

0-7645-0817-2

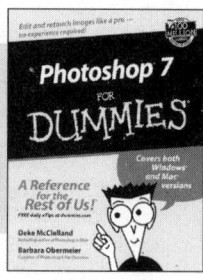

0-7645-1651-5

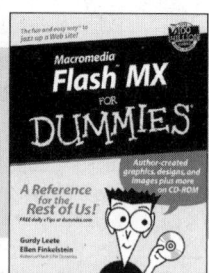

0-7645-0895-4

Also available:

Adobe Acrobat 5 PDF For Dummies
(0-7645-1652-3)

Fireworks 4 For Dummies
(0-7645-0804-0)

Illustrator 10 For Dummies
(0-7645-3636-2)

QuarkXPress 5 For Dummies
(0-7645-0643-9)

Visio 2000 For Dummies
(0-7645-0635-8)

FOR DUMMIES®

The advice and explanations you need to succeed

SELF-HELP, SPIRITUALITY & RELIGION

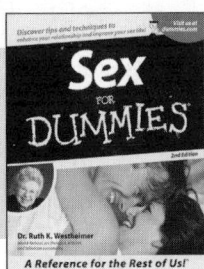

Sex FOR DUMMIES
2nd Edition
Dr. Ruth K. Westheimer
A Reference for the Rest of Us!
0-7645-5302-X

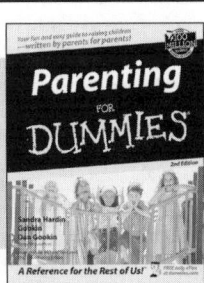

Parenting FOR DUMMIES
2nd Edition
Sandra Hardin Gookin
Dan Gookin
A Reference for the Rest of Us!
0-7645-5418-2

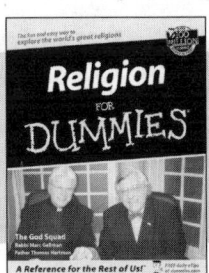

Religion FOR DUMMIES
The God Squad
Rabbi Marc Gellman
Father Thomas Hartman
A Reference for the Rest of Us!
0-7645-5264-3

Also available:

The Bible For Dummies
(0-7645-5296-1)

Buddhism For Dummies
(0-7645-5359-3)

Christian Prayer For Dummies
(0-7645-5500-6)

Dating For Dummies
(0-7645-5072-1)

Judaism For Dummies
(0-7645-5299-6)

Potty Training For Dummies
(0-7645-5417-4)

Pregnancy For Dummies
(0-7645-5074-8)

Rekindling Romance For Dummies
(0-7645-5303-8)

Spirituality For Dummies
(0-7645-5298-8)

Weddings For Dummies
(0-7645-5055-1)

PETS

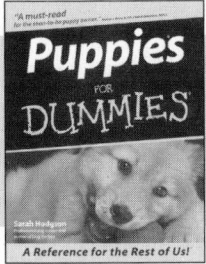

Puppies FOR DUMMIES
Sarah Hodgson
A Reference for the Rest of Us!
0-7645-5255-4

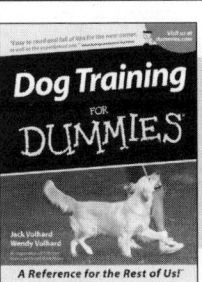

Dog Training FOR DUMMIES
Jack Volhard
Wendy Volhard
A Reference for the Rest of Us!
0-7645-5286-4

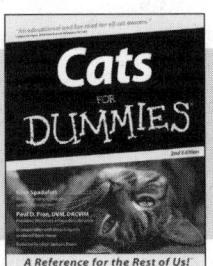

Cats FOR DUMMIES
2nd Edition
Paul D. Pion, DVM, DACVIM
A Reference for the Rest of Us!
0-7645-5275-9

Also available:

Labrador Retrievers For Dummies
(0-7645-5281-3)

Aquariums For Dummies
(0-7645-5156-6)

Birds For Dummies
(0-7645-5139-6)

Dogs For Dummies
(0-7645-5274-0)

Ferrets For Dummies
(0-7645-5259-7)

German Shepherds For Dummies
(0-7645-5280-5)

Golden Retrievers For Dummies
(0-7645-5267-8)

Horses For Dummies
(0-7645-5138-8)

Jack Russell Terriers For Dummies
(0-7645-5268-6)

Puppies Raising & Training Diary For Dummies
(0-7645-0876-8)

EDUCATION & TEST PREPARATION

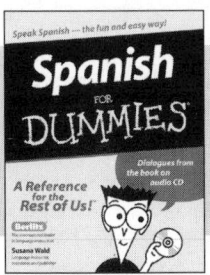

Spanish FOR DUMMIES
A Reference for the Rest of Us!
Susana Wald
0-7645-5194-9

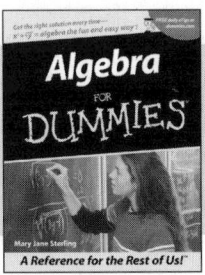

Algebra FOR DUMMIES
2nd Edition
Mary Jane Sterling
A Reference for the Rest of Us!
0-7645-5325-9

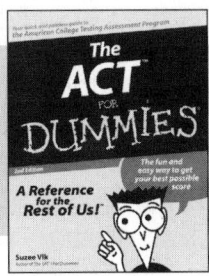

The ACT FOR DUMMIES
A Reference for the Rest of Us!
Suzee Vlk
0-7645-5210-4

Also available:

Chemistry For Dummies
(0-7645-5430-1)

English Grammar For Dummies
(0-7645-5322-4)

French For Dummies
(0-7645-5193-0)

The GMAT For Dummies
(0-7645-5251-1)

Inglés Para Dummies
(0-7645-5427-1)

Italian For Dummies
(0-7645-5196-5)

Research Papers For Dummies
(0-7645-5426-3)

The SAT I For Dummies
(0-7645-5472-7)

U.S. History For Dummies
(0-7645-5249-X)

World History For Dummies
(0-7645-5242-2)

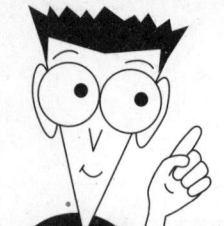
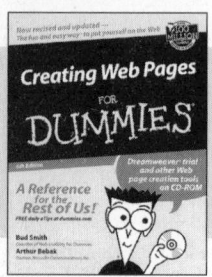
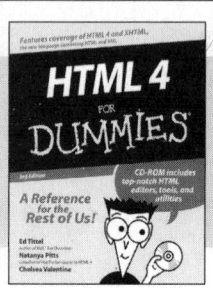
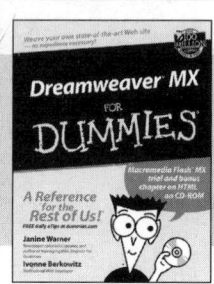
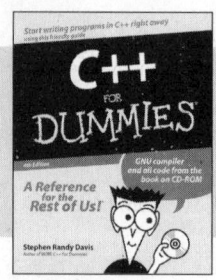
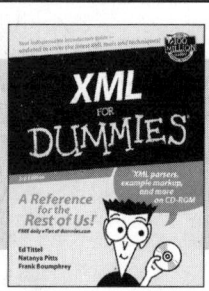
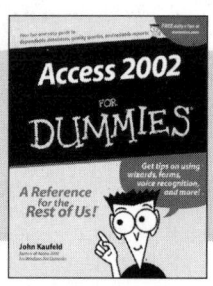
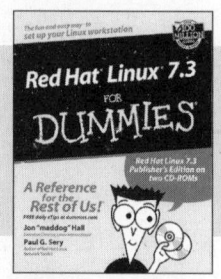
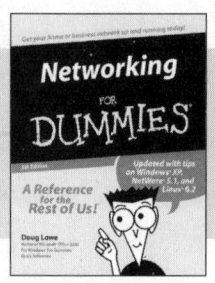
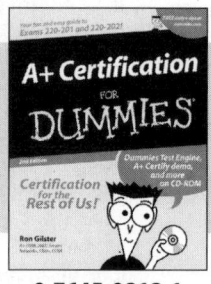
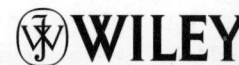